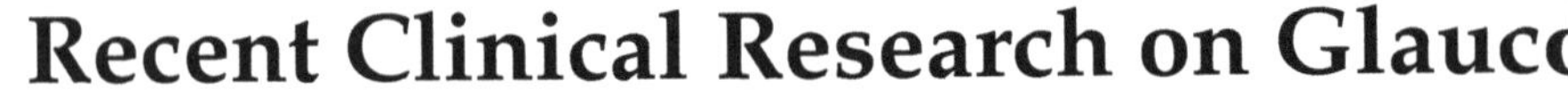

Recent Clinical Research on Glaucc

Recent Clinical Research on Glaucoma

Editors

Jose Javier Garcia-Medina
Maria Dolores Pinazo-Duran

MDPI • Basel • Beijing • Wuhan • Barcelona • Belgrade • Manchester • Tokyo • Cluj • Tianjin

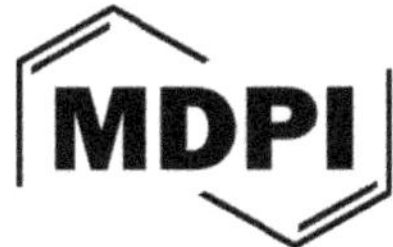

Editors
Jose Javier Garcia-Medina
University of Murcia
Spain

Maria Dolores Pinazo-Duran
University of Valencia
Spain

Editorial Office
MDPI
St. Alban-Anlage 66
4052 Basel, Switzerland

This is a reprint of articles from the Special Issue published online in the open access journal *Journal of Clinical Medicine* (ISSN 2077-0383) (available at: https://www.mdpi.com/journal/jcm/special_issues/recent_clinical_research_on_glaucoma).

For citation purposes, cite each article independently as indicated on the article page online and as indicated below:

LastName, A.A.; LastName, B.B.; LastName, C.C. Article Title. *Journal Name* **Year**, *Volume Number*, Page Range.

ISBN 978-3-0365-3835-8 (Hbk)
ISBN 978-3-0365-3836-5 (PDF)

Cover image courtesy of Jose Javier Garcia-Medina
Macular structure-function relationships of all retinal layers in primary open-angle glaucoma assessed by microperimetry and 8 × 8 posterior pole analysis of OCT

Contents

Journal of
Clinical Medicine

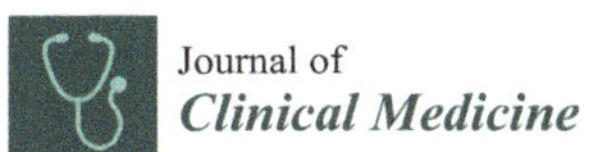

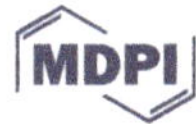

Editorial

Updates in Clinical and Translational Glaucoma Research

José Javier García-Medina [1,2,3,*,†] and Maria Dolores Pinazo-Durán [3,4,5,6,*,†]

1   Department of Ophthalmology, General University Hospital Morales Meseguer, 30007 Murcia, Spain
2   Department of Ophthalmology and Optometry, University of Murcia, 30120 Murcia, Spain
3   Spanish Net of Ophthalmic Research "OFTARED" RD16/0008/0022, Institute of Health Carlos III, 28029 Madrid, Spain
4   Ophthalmic Research Unit "Santiago Grisolia"/FISABIO, 46017 Valencia, Spain
5   Cellular and Molecular Ophthalmobiology Group, University of Valencia, 46010 Valencia, Spain
6   Department of Surgery, Faculty of Medicine and Odontology, University of Valencia, 46010 Valencia, Spain
*   Correspondence: jj.garciamedina@um.es (J.J.G.-M.); dolores.pinazo@uv.es (M.D.P.-D.)
†   These authors contributed equally to this work and shared the first authorship.

Citation: García-Medina, J.J.;
Pinazo-Durán, M.D. Updates in
Clinical and Translational Glaucoma
Research. *J. Clin. Med.* **2022**, *11*, 221.
https://doi.org/10.3390/
jcm11010221

Received: 15 December 2021
Accepted: 28 December 2021
Published: 31 December 2021

Publisher's Note: MDPI stays neutral
with regard to jurisdictional claims in
published maps and institutional affiliations.

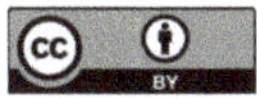

Glaucoma is a sight-threatening disease and the primum mobile of irreversible blindness worldwide [1]. Throughout the last decade, the interest in glaucoma diagnosis and therapy has been encouraged through outstanding biotechnological advances and the emergence of artificial intelligence to make the decision-making processes of glaucoma management easier [2,3]. Clinicians, biomedical engineers, and scientific researchers have been involved in improving knowledge of glaucoma risk factors and pathogenic mechanisms as well as refining innovative tools for glaucoma diagnostic performance, such as those wielded for corneal biomechanical properties, intraocular pressure (IOP) measurement, structural and functional glaucoma probes [4–9], and those regarding the discovery of IOP-lowering medical, laser, and surgical approaches [10,11].

The rising prevalence of diabetes mellitus, hypertensive blood pressure, cardiovascular diseases, respiratory illnesses, neurodegenerative disorders, etc., has had a great impact on global health, and can especially affect the course of glaucoma [12]. The COVID-19 pandemic, causing the severe acute respiratory syndrome coronavirus-2 (SARS-CoV-2), the government/volunteer lockdown, and subjective fear-related restrictions have had a great impact on glaucoma patients [13]. Nevertheless, glaucoma patients may also suffer from ocular disorders that can interfere with vision, quality-of-life, and well-being, such as dry eye disorders, cataracts, uveitis, and/or retinopathies, all of these influencing visual outcomes [14,15].

The primary goal of the Special Issue: "Recent Clinical Research on Glaucoma" is to show readers to review the interdisciplinary background that favors exploration and understand the outstanding preclinical translational research that is taking place in the glaucoma field. The authors of this Special Issue have addressed a series of relevant topics regarding glaucoma risk factors, clinical facts, diagnostic tools, glaucoma comorbidities, treatment, and follow-up, as well as the newest research. A total of 16 works were compiled in this Special Issue, including 1 review, 14 clinical articles and preclinical-translational research studies, and this editorial, which have been collected on this occasion to precisely illustrate the multidisciplinary characteristics of this Special Issue, with the articles synthesized below and ordered by their respective publication dates.

Sato and Kawaky [16] take a close look at the "Effects of ripasudil on open-angle glaucoma after circumferential incision of Schlemm's canal". Ripasudil hydrochloride hydrate (a Rho-associated coiled-coil containing protein kinase (ROCK) inhibitor), a new type of ocular hypotensive drug, was administered to open-angle glaucoma (OAG) patients who received an operation including a circumferential incision of the Schlemm's canal and phacoemulsification. The main conclusion was that Ripasudil probably influenced the distal outflow tract by resulting in significant IOP reductions [14].

Atanasovska Velovska et al. [17] provided an overview of the "Association of genetic polymorphisms in oxidative stress and inflammation pathways with glaucoma risk and phenotype". This work fully demonstrated that variability in the interleukin (IL)-1B and -6 gene polymorphisms encode significant risk for glaucoma, while the glutathion peroxidase and tumor necrosis factor gene polymorphism appear to be associated with the glaucoma phenotype.

Peris Martinez et al. [18] built upon the current knowledge of the diagnosis and management of glaucoma and keratoconus by using Corvis ST and Pentacam HD devices, through the "Evaluation of intraocular pressure and other biomechanical parameters to distinguish between subclinical keratoconus and healthy corneas". Therefore, this work demonstrated that the use of normalized biomechanical parameters provided by noncontact tonometry, combined with a discriminant function theory, is a useful tool for detecting subclinical keratoconus in the course of glaucoma.

Raga-Cervera et al. [19] analyzed the differential expression profile of miRNAs in the aqueous humor of OHT individuals and glaucoma patients in the analytical, observational, case–control study entitled "miRNAs and genes involved in the interplay between ocular hypertension and primary open-angle glaucoma. Oxidative stress, inflammation and apoptosis networks." In this work, the authors showed, for the first time, that eight miRNAs expressed differently in tears by comparing OHT and POAG patients. Therefore, Raga-Cervera et al. proposed that specific miRNAs and their target genes and corresponding signaling pathways can be useful to identify HTO individuals at risk of glaucoma neurodegeneration.

Jeon et al. [20] showed clinical research results on "Vessel Density Loss of the Deep Peripapillary Area in Glaucoma Suspects and Its Association with Features of the Lamina Cribrosa". These authors found that glaucoma suspects, with eyes having vessel density defects in the peripapillary area also displayed structural differences in the lamina cribrosa.

Additionally, dealing with the vascular densities of the optic disc areas, **Baek et al.** [21] observed normal-tension glaucoma (NTG) in their work "Optic Disc Vascular Density in Normal-Tension Glaucoma Eyes with or without Branch Retinal Vessel Occlusion". In conclusion, significant changes in the distribution of vascular densities for the optic disc (in the larger, medium, and small vessels) were observed in both eyes of NTG patients with branch retinal vessel occlusion compared to NTG patients without this condition.

Del Buey Sayas et al. [22] analyzed the "Corneal Biomechanical Parameters and Central Corneal Thickness in Glaucoma Patients, Glaucoma Suspects and a Healthy Population" by using an Ocular Response Analyzer (ORA). This work demonstrated that the biomechanical corneal parameters noticeably changed between the above study groups, suggesting that these variables play important roles in glaucoma diagnosis.

González-Hernández et al. [23] addressed artificial intelligence tools by means of their innovative article entitled "Fully automated colorimetric analysis of the optic nerve aided by Deep Learning and its association with perimetry for the study of glaucoma". These authors designed the Laguna-ONhE, an application for the colorimetric analysis of optic nerve images, which is capable of topographically assessing the cup and the presence of hemoglobin. Currently, this tool has been fully improved and automated with five deep-learning models. The authors evaluated glaucoma patients and glaucoma suspects by means of the latest Laguna-OHnE version in combination with perimetry or cirrus-optic coherence tomography, and the results were compared to those from normal eyes. In conclusion, the morphology, perfusion, and function of glaucoma and glaucoma-suspect eyes can be enhanced by using the procedures described herein to provide early sensitivity for better management of glaucoma.

Chen et al. [24] performed a nationwide-population-based study on glaucoma risk factors, precisely dealing with "Is Obesity a Risk or Protective Factor for Open-Angle Glaucoma in adults? A Two-Database, Asian, Matched-Cohort Study". This study aimed to analyze the risk of OAG among obese adults in Taiwan. Data processing of this matched-cohort study at the 13-year follow-up revealed that the obese adults had a higher incidence of OAG and that obese young adults displayed an increased chance of suffering OAG.

A systematic review and meta-analysis were performed by **Liu et al.** [25] on the "Multifocal visual evoked potentials for the detection of visual field defects in glaucoma". These authors evaluated the diagnostic precision of the mfVEP in glaucoma to find its best diagnostic indicator through the review of quantitative studies published up to 1 April 2021, including a total of 241 patients. The amplitude of mfVEP showed a good diagnostic precision in the prediction of visual field defects. Therefore, Liu et al. suggested that the analysis of the interocular mfVEP amplitude stands as a good indicator for glaucoma diagnosis.

Gené-Morales et al. [26] investigated the influence of exercise in IOP by their work entitled "Do age and sex play a role in the intraocular pressure changes after acrobatic gymnastics?" The authors described that the IOP was significantly reduced, and the central corneal thickness remained stable for five minutes after finishing a 90 min acrobatic gymnastics training session. Sex and baseline IOP levels appeared as predictors of IOP variations related to exercise. In summary, acrobatic gymnastics induced IOP reduction, with potentially predicting factors influencing the described changes.

Fernandez-Albarral et al. [27] investigated the role of inflammation and immune response and new therapeutic strategies for glaucoma in an animal model. This work was entitled "Is Saffron Able to Prevent the Dysregulation of Retinal Cytokines Induced by Ocular Hypertension in Mice?" The authors utilized a mouse model of unilateral laser-induced OHT, with the main goal of evaluating the production of inflammatory cytokine/chemokine and the changes following saffron treatment. The authors showed that safron extracts had the ability to regulate the expression of pro-inflammatory cytokines, VEGF, and fractalkine, thus protecting the retina from inflammation in the context of OHT.

Garcia-Medina et al. [28] carried out the work "Macular structure-function relationships of all retinal layers in primary open-angle glaucoma assessed by microperimetry and 8 × 8 posterior pole analysis of OCT". The authors fully demonstrated that glaucoma eyes displayed more structure–function relationships than healthy eyes. In addition, it was shown that the associations were positive for the innermost retinal layers but negative for the inner/outer retinal layers in glaucoma eyes. In summary, these data strongly suggest that the inner and outer retinal layers at the macula differ in structure–function relationships.

Lever et al. [29] described circulatory changes in early-to-moderate glaucoma in their work entitled "Microvascular and structural alterations of the macula in early to moderate glaucoma: an optical coherence tomography-angiography study". In this article, the authors reported that glaucoma severity reinforces the relationship between the thickness of the macular segment and the density of vessels. In conclusion, glaucoma individually influences the parameters of the OCT and OCTA.

Ko et al. [30], in their observational, cross-sectional study including 1228 eyes from 661 participants (POAG in early, moderate, and later stages, pre-perimetric glaucoma and normal), entitled "Vessel density in the macular and peripapillary areas in preperimetric glaucoma to various stages of primary open-angle glaucoma in Taiwan", focused on the comparison of the above groups in terms of the changes in peripapillary and macular vessel densities. With this work, the authors stated that the measurements of the peripapillary vessel density could help to distinguish glaucoma stages.

To summarize this collection of papers covering different glaucoma topics, as described above, being the Guest Editors of the Special Issue of the *Journal of Clinical Medicine* **Recent Clinical Research on Glaucoma**, we believe that all of these works can be useful for ophthalmologists, medical specialists, and interdisciplinary researchers to improve our understanding of the pathogenic mechanisms, clinical characteristics, diagnosis, and therapy underlying glaucoma for stimulating innovative "theranostic" glaucoma strategies for better eye and vision care. We sincerely hope that our readers can appreciate the substantial contribution of these works that may contribute to moving this important topic forward.

Author Contributions: J.J.G.-M. and M.D.P.-D. contributed equally to this Editorial. All authors have read and agreed to the published version of the manuscript.

Funding: This research received no external funding.

Conflicts of Interest: The authors declare no conflict of interest.

References

1. Flaxman, S.R.; Bourne, R.R.A.; Resnikoff, S.; Ackland, P.; Braithwaite, T.; Cicinelli, M.V.; Das, A.; Jonas, J.B.; Keeffe, J.; Kempen, J.H.; et al. Vision Loss Expert Group of the Global Burden of Disease Study. Global causes of blindness and distance vision impairment 1990-2020: A systematic review and meta-analysis. *Lancet Glob Health* **2017**, *5*, e1221–e1234. [CrossRef]
2. Okamoto, Y.; Akagi, T.; Kameda, T.; Suda, K.; Miyake, M.; Ikeda, H.O.; Numa, S.; Kadomoto, S.; Uji, A.; Tsujikawa, A. Prediction of trabecular meshwork-targeted micro-invasive glaucoma surgery outcomes using anterior segment OCT angiography. *Sci. Rep.* **2021**, *11*, 1–10. [CrossRef] [PubMed]
3. Ng, W.Y.; Zhang, S.; Wang, Z.; Ong, C.J.T.; Gunasekeran, D.V.; Lim, G.Y.S.; Zheng, F.; Tan, S.C.Y.; Tan, G.S.W.; Rim, T.H.; et al. Updates in deep learning research in ophthal-mology. *Clin. Sci.* **2021**, *135*, 2357–2376. [CrossRef]
4. Wu, Y.; Szymanska, M.; Hu, Y.; Fazal, M.I.; Jiang, N.; Yetisen, A.K.; Cordeiro, M.F. Measures of disease activity in glaucoma. *Biosens. Bioelectron.* **2022**, *196*, 113700. [CrossRef] [PubMed]
5. Tezel, G. Molecular regulation of neuroinflammation in glaucoma: Current knowledge and the ongoing search for new treatment targets. *Prog. Retin. Eye Res.* **2021**, *2021*, 100998. [CrossRef]
6. Bak, E.; Kim, Y.W.; Ha, A.; Kim, Y.K.; Park, K.H.; Jeoung, J.W. Pre-perimetric Open Angle Glaucoma with Young Age of Onset: Natural Clinical Course and Risk Factors for Progression. *Am. J. Ophthalmol.* **2020**, *216*, 121–131. [CrossRef]
7. Kazemi, A.; Zhou, B.; Zhang, X.; Sit, A.J. Comparison of Corneal Wave Speed and Ocular Rigidity in Normal and Glaucomatous Eyes. *J. Glaucoma* **2021**, *30*, 932–940. [CrossRef]
8. Berenguer-Vidal, R.; Verdú-Monedero, R.; Morales-Sánchez, J.; Sellés-Navarro, I.; del Amor, R.; García, G.; Naranjo, V. Automatic Segmentation of the Retinal Nerve Fiber Layer by Means of Mathematical Morphology and Deformable Models in 2D Optical Coherence Tomography Imaging. *Sensors* **2021**, *21*, 8027. [CrossRef]
9. Meier-Gibbons, F.; Töteberg-Harms, M. Structure/function/treatment in glaucoma: Progress over the last 10 years. *Ophthalmologe* **2021**, *118*, 1216–1221. [CrossRef]
10. Stacy, R.; Huttner, K.; Watts, J.; Peace, J.; Wirta, D.; Walters, T.; Sall, K.; Seaman, J.; Ni, X.; Prasanna, G.; et al. A Randomized, Controlled Phase I/II Study to Evaluate the Safety and Efficacy of MGV354 for Ocular Hypertension or Glaucoma. *Am. J. Ophthalmol.* **2018**, *192*, 113–123. [CrossRef]
11. Pereira, I.C.F.; van de Wijdeven, R.; Wyss, H.M.; Beckers, H.J.M.; Toonder, J.M.J.D. Conventional glaucoma implants and the new MIGS devices: A comprehensive review of current options and future directions. *Eye* **2021**, *35*, 3202–3221. [CrossRef]
12. Pinazo-Duran, M.D.; Zanon-Moreno, V.; García-Medina, J.J.; Arévalo, J.F.; Gallego-Pinazo, R.; Nucci, C. Eclectic Ocular Comor-bidities and Systemic Diseases with Eye Involvement: A Review. *BioMed Res. Int.* **2016**, *2016*, 1–10. [CrossRef]
13. Tejwani, S.; Angmo, D.; Nayak, B.K.; Sharma, N.; Sachdev, M.S.; Dada, T. Rajesh Composition of the All India Ophthalmological Society (AIOS) and Glaucoma Society of India (GSI) Expert Group includes the Writing Committee (as listed) and the following members: Devindra Sood, Arup Chakrabarti, Chandrima Paul, Chitra Ramamurthy, Harsh K Preferred practice guidelines for glaucoma management during COVID-19 pandemic. *Indian J. Ophthalmol.* **2020**, *68*, 1277–1280. [CrossRef]
14. Benitez-Del-Castillo, J.; Cantu-Dibildox, J.; Sanz-González, S.M.; Zanón-Moreno, V.; Pinazo-Duran, M.D. Cytokine expression in tears of patients with glaucoma or dry eye disease: A prospective, observational cohort study. *Eur. J. Ophthalmol.* **2018**, *29*, 437–443. [CrossRef] [PubMed]
15. Mokhles, P.; van Gorcom, L.; Schouten, J.S.A.G.; Berendschot, T.T.J.M.; Beckers, H.J.M.; Webers, C.A.B. Contributing ocular comorbidity to end-of-life visual acuity in medically treated glaucoma pa-tients, ocular hypertension and glaucoma suspect patients. *Eye* **2021**, *35*, 883–891. [CrossRef] [PubMed]
16. Sato, T.; Kawaji, T. Effects of Ripasudil on Open-Angle Glaucoma after Circumferential Suture Trabeculotomy Ab Interno. *J. Clin. Med.* **2021**, *10*, 401. [CrossRef] [PubMed]
17. Velkovska, M.A.; Goričar, K.; Blagus, T.; Dolžan, V.; Cvenkel, B. Association of Genetic Polymorphisms in Oxidative Stress and Inflammation Pathways with Glaucoma Risk and Phenotype. *J. Clin. Med.* **2021**, *10*, 1148. [CrossRef]
18. Peris-Martínez, C.; Díez-Ajenjo, M.A.; García-Domene, M.C.; Pinazo-Durán, M.D.; Luque-Cobija, M.J.; Del Buey-Sayas, M.Á.; Ortí-Navarro, S. Evaluation of Intraocular Pressure and Other Biomechanical Parameters to Distinguish between Subclinical Keratoconus and Healthy Corneas. *J. Clin. Med.* **2021**, *10*, 1905. [CrossRef]
19. Raga-Cervera, J.; Bolarin, J.; Millan, J.; Garcia-Medina, J.; Pedrola, L.; Abellán-Abenza, J.; Valero-Vello, M.; Sanz-González, S.; O'Connor, J.; Galarreta-Mira, D.; et al. miRNAs and Genes Involved in the Interplay between Ocular Hypertension and Primary Open-Angle Glaucoma. Oxidative Stress, Inflammation, and Apoptosis Networks. *J. Clin. Med.* **2021**, *10*, 2227. [CrossRef]
20. Jeon, S.-J.; Park, H.-Y.; Park, C.-K. Vessel Density Loss of the Deep Peripapillary Area in Glaucoma Suspects and Its Association with Features of the Lamina Cribrosa. *J. Clin. Med.* **2021**, *10*, 2373. [CrossRef]
21. Baek, J.; Jeon, S.-J.; Kim, J.-H.; Park, C.-K.; Park, H.-Y. Optic Disc Vascular Density in Normal-Tension Glaucoma Eyes with or without Branch Retinal Vessel Occlusion. *J. Clin. Med.* **2021**, *10*, 2574. [CrossRef]

22. Del Buey-Sayas, M.A.; Lanchares-Sancho, E.; Campins-Falcó, P.; Pinazo-Durán, M.D.; Peris-Martínez, C. Corneal Biomechanical Parameters and Central Corneal Thickness in Glaucoma Patients, Glaucoma Suspects, and a Healthy Population. *J. Clin. Med.* **2021**, *10*, 2637. [CrossRef]

23. Gonzalez-Hernandez, M.; Gonzalez-Hernandez, D.; Perez-Barbudo, D.; Rodriguez-Esteve, P.; Betancor-Caro, N.; de la Rosa, M.G. Fully Automated Colorimetric Analysis of the Optic Nerve Aided by Deep Learning and Its Association with Perimetry and OCT for the Study of Glaucoma. *J. Clin. Med.* **2021**, *10*, 3231. [CrossRef]

24. Chen, W.-D.; Lai, L.-J.; Lee, K.-L.; Chen, T.-J.; Liu, C.-Y.; Yang, Y.-H. Is Obesity a Risk or Protective Factor for Open-Angle Glaucoma in Adults? A Two-Database, Asian, Matched-Cohort Study. *J. Clin. Med.* **2021**, *10*, 4021. [CrossRef]

25. Liu, H.; Liao, F.; Blanco, R.; de la Villa, P. Multifocal Visual Evoked Potentials (mfVEP) for the Detection of Visual Field Defects in Glaucoma: Systematic Review and Meta-Analysis. *J. Clin. Med.* **2021**, *10*, 4165. [CrossRef] [PubMed]

26. Gene-Morales, J.; Gené-Sampedro, A.; Martín-Portugués, A.; Bueno-Gimeno, I. Do Age and Sex Play a Role in the Intraocular Pressure Changes after Acrobatic Gymnastics? *J. Clin. Med.* **2021**, *10*, 4700. [CrossRef] [PubMed]

27. Fernández-Albarral, J.A.; Martínez-López, M.A.; Marco, E.M.; de Hoz, R.; Martín-Sánchez, B.; San Felipe, D.; Salobrar-García, E.; López-Cuenca, I.; Pinazo-Durán, M.D.; Salazar, J.J.; et al. Is Saffron Able to Prevent the Dysregulation of Retinal Cy-tokines Induced by Ocular Hypertension in Mice? *J. Clin. Med.* **2021**, *10*, 4801. [CrossRef] [PubMed]

28. Garcia-Medina, J.J.; Rotolo, M.; Rubio-Velazquez, E.; Pinazo-Duran, M.D.; Del-Rio-Vellosillo, M. Macular Structure–Function Relationships of All Retinal Layers in Primary Open-Angle Glaucoma Assessed by Microperimetry and 8 × 8 Posterior Pole Analysis of OCT. *J. Clin. Med.* **2021**, *10*, 5009. [CrossRef] [PubMed]

29. Lever, M.; Glaser, M.; Chen, Y.; Halfwassen, C.; Unterlauft, J.D.; Bechrakis, N.E.; Böhm, M.R.R. Mi-crovascular and Structural Alterations of the Macula in Early to Moderate Glaucoma: An Optical Coherence Tomography-Angiography Study. *J. Clin. Med.* **2021**, *10*, 5017. [CrossRef]

30. Ko, C.-K.; Huang, K.-I.; Su, F.-Y.; Ko, M.-L. Vessel Density in the Macular and Peripapillary Areas in Preperimetric Glaucoma to Various Stages of Primary Open-Angle Glaucoma in Taiwan. *J. Clin. Med.* **2021**, *10*, 5490. [CrossRef] [PubMed]

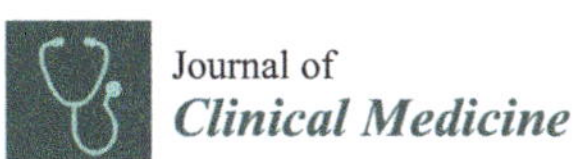

Journal of
Clinical Medicine

MDPI

Article

Vessel Density in the Macular and Peripapillary Areas in Preperimetric Glaucoma to Various Stages of Primary Open-Angle Glaucoma in Taiwan

Chung-Kuang Ko [1], Kuan-I Huang [2], Fang-Ying Su [3] and Mei-Lan Ko [4,5,*]

[1] Department of Neurology, China Medical University Hospital, Taichung 404, Taiwan; ko.chung.kuang@gmail.com
[2] Department of Ophthalmology, Shin-Kong Wu Ho-Su Memorial Hospital, Taipei 111, Taiwan; huangkuani@icloud.com
[3] Institute of Statistics, National Chiao Tung University, Hsinchu 300, Taiwan; fysu@hch.gov.tw
[4] Department of Ophthalmology, National Taiwan University Hospital, Hsinchu 300, Taiwan
[5] Biomedical Engineering and Environmental Sciences, National Tsing Hua University, Hsinchu 300, Taiwan
* Correspondence: aaddch@gmail.com; Tel.: +886-965-580-725

Abstract: Peripapillary and macular vessel density (VD) are reduced in myopic non-glaucomatous eyes, the dynamic range of VD may be decreased by myopia, and whether VD measurement has the potential in differentiating stages of glaucoma severity in patients with myopic glaucoma remains questionable. This observational, cross-sectional study aimed to clarify the changes in peripapillary and macular VDs in preperimetric glaucoma (PPG) and primary open-angle glaucoma in the early, moderate, and late stages. A total of 1228 eyes from 661 participants (540 normal, 67 PPG, and 521 glaucomatous) were included. Participants underwent free blood tests at the internal medicine clinic to retrieve systemic data. Patients with glaucoma were grouped by disease severity, defined by glaucomatous visual field mean defect, including early-(224 eyes), moderate-(103 eyes), and late-stage glaucoma (194 eyes), and further divided into advanced (158 eyes) and terminal glaucoma (36 eyes). Macular VD, peripapillary VD, circumpapillary retinal nerve fiber layer (cpRNFL) thickness, and ganglion cell complex (GCC) thickness were evaluated and divided into superior and inferior parts. One-way analysis of variance was performed, followed by Tukey's post-hoc test. The peripapillary VD was significantly different between the healthy and PPG groups and the early-, moderate-, and late-stage glaucoma subgroups (all $p < 0.001$). Peripapillary VD measurements are helpful in differentiating the various stages of glaucoma even in patients with myopic glaucoma.

Keywords: glaucoma; macula; peripapillary; optical coherence tomography-angiography; vessel density; myopia

Citation: Ko, C.-K.; Huang, K.-I.; Su, F.-Y.; Ko, M.-L. Vessel Density in the Macular and Peripapillary Areas in Preperimetric Glaucoma to Various Stages of Primary Open-Angle Glaucoma in Taiwan. *J. Clin. Med.* **2021**, *10*, 5490. https://doi.org/10.3390/jcm10235490

Academic Editors: Jose Javier Garcia-Medina and Maria Dolores Pinazo-Duran

Received: 26 October 2021
Accepted: 22 November 2021
Published: 23 November 2021

Publisher's Note: MDPI stays neutral with regard to jurisdictional claims in published maps and institutional affiliations.

1. Introduction

Glaucoma, which is the global leading cause of irreversible blindness in individuals aged 50 years and older, accounts for 11% of all blindness cases in 2020 [1]. In previous studies, Asians and Africans are disproportionately affected by glaucoma, and the number of patients with glaucoma worldwide is expected to increase to 111.8 million in 2040 [2]. Having a subtle chronic disease course, the pathogenesis of glaucoma has been theorized to correlate with microcirculatory defects in the retina. With regard to the prevention of glaucoma-related vision impairment, once detected, therapy for glaucoma can significantly preserve the visual field (VF) and slow its deterioration [3]. Early detection and treatment of glaucoma are very important in preserving vision, reducing morbidity, and diminishing the burden on healthcare systems. Optical coherence tomography angiography (OCTA) is a noninvasive, rapid, and high-resolution technique that provides three-dimensional images to illustrate blood supply status, different segmentations, and parameters to indicate the blood flow and microvasculature in the eyes.

The mean defect (MD) in the VF is an important categorical severity classification system for glaucoma. OCTA parameters such as vessel density (VD) have been shown to be moderately or highly correlated with VF parameters [4]. For visual function decline in glaucomatous eyes, OCTA parameters are better biomarkers than OCT parameters since vascular loss has a stronger correlation with VF MD than with structural changes [5–10]. Some researchers suggest that OCTA may provide useful additional information for monitoring progression in later disease stages [4].

It has been reported that peripapillary and macular VDs are reduced in myopic nonglaucomatous eyes [11–21], and the simultaneous presence of myopia and open-angle glaucoma results in a greater level of microvascular attenuation than that with either pathology alone [22]. In myopic eyes, reduced VD may increase the susceptibility to vascular and age-related eye diseases [23,24]. The dynamic range of VD may be decreased by myopia, and whether VD measurement has the potential in differentiating stages of glaucoma severity in patients with myopic glaucoma remains questionable.

The current study aimed to evaluate the changes in peripapillary and macular VDs in preperimetric glaucoma (PPG) and primary open-angle glaucoma (POAG) in various (early, moderate, advanced, and terminal) stages and to compare the potential of OCT and OCTA parameters in differentiating the stages of glaucoma severity, particularly in the myopic population.

2. Materials and Methods

2.1. Study Participants

Patients aged 20 to 80 years who visited the ophthalmologic outpatient department of our hospital between June 2019 and February 2020 were included. This cross-sectional, observational study was conducted and approved by the institutional review board ((IRB) number: NTUHHCB 108-025-E) of the National Taiwan University Hospital Hsin-Chu Branch, Taiwan, and in accordance with the tenets of the Declaration of Helsinki (1964). Informed consent was obtained from all the participants in the study.

All of the participants underwent a series of full ophthalmic examinations, including refractive error measurement by ARK-510A (Nidek Co., Gamagori, Japan), slit-lamp examination, gonioscopy, intraocular pressure (IOP) measurement by non-contact tonometer NT-530P (Nidek Co., Gamagori, Japan), open anterior chamber angle by gonioscopy, fundoscopy, visual field (VF) test by Humphrey Field Analyzer-840 (HFA-840; Carl Zeiss Meditec, Inc. Dublin, CA, USA), and axial length (AL) by AL-SCAN (Nidek Co., Gamagori, Japan). The bilateral eyes of every participant were evaluated and imaged. Then, they underwent a free blood test at the internal medicine clinic to retrieve systemic data, including mean arterial pressure (MAP), heart rate, serum triglyceride, high-density lipoprotein (HDL), low-density lipoprotein (LDL), serum sugar, HbA1C, alanine aminotransferase (ALT), creatinine, and uric acid.

All controls had best-corrected visual acuity (BCVA) better than 12/20. To avoid poor image quality, the study excluded participants older than 60 years without previous cataract surgery. Further exclusion criteria were as follows: history of ocular surgery aside from uncomplicated cataract surgery; uveitis; ocular trauma; vitreoretinal diseases; non-glaucomatous optic neuropathy; and retinopathy, such as diabetic retinopathy, hypertensive retinopathy, maculopathy; any other known disease that may cause optic neuropathy, retinopathy or VF loss, unreliable VF (false-positive and false-negative rate > 15%, fixation losses > 20%), and unreliable OCTA image quality, such as a signal strength index less than 40.

Control participants must show no evidence of retinal pathology or glaucoma in either eye, intraocular pressure of 21 mm Hg or less, no chronic ocular or systemic corticosteroid use, normal-appearing optic discs, and a normal result of VF examination. A normal VF was defined as a pattern standard deviation (PSD) within the 95% confidence limit and a normal glaucoma hemifield test result using a reliable VF test.

In this study, preperimetric glaucoma (PPG) was defined on the basis of lesions in decreasing circumpapillary retinal nerve fiber layer (cpRNFL) thickness or ganglion cell complex (GCC) thickness by OCTA without glaucomatous VF abnormalities. Glaucomatous VF abnormalities were defined as follows: (1) PSD beyond 95% normal limits ($p < 0.05$) and glaucoma hemifield test beyond normal limits; (2) various glaucoma stages were defined with 24–2 models as early (-2.0 dB $>$ MD ≥ -6 dB), moderate ($-6 >$ MD ≥ -12 dB), and late stage further divided into advanced (-12 dB $>$ MD ≥ -30 dB) and terminal stage (MD < -30 dB).

2.2. OCTA Measurements

All participants underwent OCTA (AngioVue, Optovue Inc., Fremont, CA, USA) examinations, which were reviewed manually to ensure correct segmentation and applicable quality. VD in the peripapillary area with a 4.5×4.5 mm^2 scan size was divided into superior and inferior hemifields. VD in the macular area was centered on the fovea with a scan size of 3×3 mm^2 with two concentric circles and diameters of 1 mm and 3 mm. It was further divided into center, superior, and inferior parts. The scan base was between the inner border of the internal limiting membrane and 10 μm above the outer border of the inner plexiform layer. The cpRNFL thickness was measured in an annulus centered on the optic disc with an outer and inner diameter of 4 mm and 2 mm, respectively. The GCC scan, including the nerve fiber, ganglion cell, and inner plexiform layers, covered a 7 mm $\times$ 7 mm area that is centered 1 mm temporal to the fovea. All images and data containing an optic nerve head analysis, including cup/disc ratio, rim area, and disc area, were automatically acquired using a built-in software.

2.3. Statistical Analysis

Categorical variables were expressed as percentages, while continuous variables as mean values and standard deviation (SD). Categorical variables were compared using the chi-square test and a two-sample independent *t*-test for other continuous variables.

The propensity score (PS) was derived using logistic regression to model the probability of receipt in the control or glaucoma groups (PPG + glaucoma (G)) as a function of all the potential confounders listed in Table 1. Matching analysis based on the PS was used for different groups of glaucomatous and control participants to reduce selection biases between each pair of groups. Glaucoma groups (PPG + G) were matched to control groups (using the greedy matching algorithm) at a 1:1 ratio, 1:9 PS-matching for PPG groups and control groups, 1:1 PS-matching for glaucoma eye (excluding PPG) and control groups, and 1:5 PS-matching for glaucoma eye (excluding PPG) and PPG groups. Sex and age were used as covariates.

The balance in baseline characteristics for different groups of glaucomatous and control participants among the PS-matched population was assessed using the Mantel–Haenszel test for sex and paired *t*-test for age.

To compare OCTA and OCT parameters within glaucoma severity groups, one-way analysis of variance was performed, followed by the Tukey's post-hoc test. Two paired sample *t*-tests were used to compare the percentage loss of the superior and inferior regions of the macular and peripapillary VDs and cpRNFL and GCC thicknesses within the control, PPG (mean control $-$ PPG)/mean control), and glaucoma groups (mean control $-$ glaucoma)/mean control).

Pearson's correlation coefficient was used to evaluate the relationship between structural thickness and VD. Multivariable linear regression models using a generalized estimating equation (GEE) model were utilized for correlations between outcome and predictive variables, while adjusting for within-patient and inter-eye dependence. After adjusting for age, sex, and AL, the working correlation matrix was defined as exchangeable (compound symmetry); that is, the two eye measurements were assumed to be equally correlated and independent of the sequence. Statistical analysis was performed using the SAS (version 9.4;

SAS Inc., Cary, NC, USA) and R (version 3.6.2) software. All tests were two-sided, and *p*-values < 0.05 were considered significant.

3. Results

Of the 1275 eyes of 690 participants aged 20–80 years that were initially enrolled in the study, 540 eyes from 290 control participants and 588 eyes from 371 glaucoma participants were eligible for the study. A flowchart for selecting the eligibility criteria is shown in Figure 1.

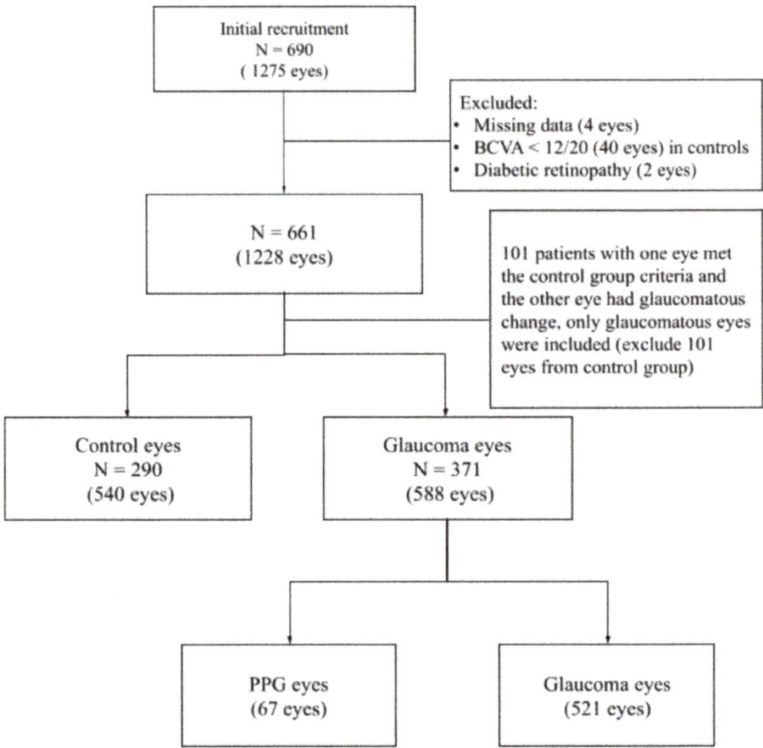

Figure 1. Flow chart of eligible eyes selection. After manual evaluation of the raw data to exclude ineligible eyes, we grouped the eyes into control eyes (540 eyes), PPG eyes (67 eyes), and glaucoma eyes (521 eyes) for the analysis. BCVA, best corrected visual acuity; PPG, pre-perimetric glaucoma.

All raw data were manually evaluated, and four eyes with missing data, 40 eyes in controls with best-corrected visual acuity <0.6, and two eyes whose fundus photography showed diabetic retinopathy were excluded. Furthermore, 101 patients who had one eye that met the control group criteria, while the other eye with glaucomatous change, were excluded; hence, only glaucomatous eyes were included. A total of 1128 eyes were included in the database with SVD, cpRNFL thickness, and GCC thickness. For further multivariable linear regression models with GEE analysis, 58 eyes that were selected from those who only had a single eye that met the inclusion criteria were excluded.

The demographics and characteristics of the control and glaucoma participants are summarized in Table 1 (Supplementary Table S1). No significant difference was found among the groups in terms of the prevalence of nephropathy, self-reported diabetes, self-reported hypertension, asthma, and CVA history (*p* > 0.05). The groups differed by age, sex, blood pressure, MAP, heart rate, HDL, Ante Cibum (AC) sugar, ALT, and eGFR (all *p* < 0.05). After matching for sex and age (Table 2, *N* = 200/200 in each group)

(Supplementary Table S2), significant differences were not observed in the factors mentioned above in both groups.

Table 1. Demographics and Characteristics of the Control and Glaucoma groups.

	Control (*N* = 290)	Glaucoma (*N* = 371)	*p*-Value
Age (years)	45.19 ± 14.23	51.95 ± 14.12	<0.001
<40	109 (37.6%)	76 (20.5%)	
40–60	142 (49.0%)	190 (51.2%)	
≥60	39 (13.5%)	105 (28.3%)	
Gender			<0.001
Male	91 (31.4%)	231 (62.3%)	
Female	199 (68.6%)	140 (37.7%)	
SBP (mmHg)	123.81 ± 17.91	128.77 ± 18.61	<0.001
DBP (mmHg)	73.26 ± 12.35	76.07 ± 12.1	0.004
MAP (mmHg)	90.11 ± 13.31	93.63 ± 13.07	<0.001
HR (/min)	79.34 ± 12.46	75.31 ± 12.03	<0.0001
TG (mg/dL)	106.84 ± 70.33	117.08 ± 55.63	0.192
HDL (mg/dL)	56.04 ± 13.75	51.86 ± 15.29	0.024
LDL (mg/dL)	113.89 ± 33.05	108.98 ± 30.45	0.292
AC sugar (mg/dL)	94.86 ± 14.73	104.39 ± 23.19	<0.001
HbA1c (%)	5.98 ± 0.65	6.01 ± 0.88	0.798
ALT (U/L)	21.54 ± 18.05	27.21 ± 19.37	0.007
Creatinine (mg/dL)	0.9 ± 1.22	0.95 ± 0.77	0.641
eGFR (mL/min/1.73 m^2)	99.83 ± 22.24	91.92 ± 21.34	0.001
Uric Acid (mg/dL)	5.24 ± 1.51	5.94 ± 1.36	<0.001

Note. SBP, systolic blood pressure; DBP, diastolic blood pressure; MAP, mean arterial pressure; HR, heart rate; TG, triglyceride; HDL, high-density lipoprotein (cholesterol); LDL, low-density lipoprotein (cholesterol); ALT, aspartate aminotransferase; eGFR, estimated glomerular filtration rate.

Table 2. Demographics and Characteristics of the Control and Glaucoma groups after Gender and Age Matching.

	Control (*N* = 200)	Glaucoma (*N* = 200)	*p*-Value
Age (years)	47.4 ± 15.2	49.3 ± 14.7	0.08
<40	62 (31.0%)	51 (25.5%)	
40–60	101 (50.5%)	107 (53.5%)	
≥60	37 (18.5%)	42 (21.0%)	
Gender			0.19
Male	88 (44.0%)	75 (37.5%)	
Female	112 (56.0%)	125 (62.5%)	
SBP (mmHg)	124.7 ± 17.9	126.9 ± 19.4	0.23
DBP (mmHg)	74.2 ± 11.8	73.3 ± 11.5	0.45
MAP (mmHg)	91.0 ± 12.9	91.2 ± 13.1	0.91
HR (/min)	78.4 ± 13.1	76.3 ± 12.4	0.10
TG (mg/dL)	114.7 ± 84.5	102.9 ± 52.2	0.29
HDL (mg/dL)	56.1 ± 15.0	54.7 ± 15.2	0.56
LDL (mg/dL)	107.2 ± 31.0	104.9 ± 31.2	0.70
AC sugar (mg/dL)	96.5 ± 16.1	101.9 ± 24.2	0.10
HbA1c (%)	6.0 ± 0.7	5.8 ± 0.7	0.25
ALT (U/L)	23.6 ± 20.9	25.8 ± 21.1	0.47
Creatinine (mg/dL)	1.0 ± 1.3	0.9 ± 0.4	0.45
eGFR (mL/min/1.73 m^2)	97.1 ± 21.4	95.6 ± 22.4	0.63
Uric Acid (mg/dL)	5.5 ± 1.8	5.6 ± 1.5	0.93

Note. SBP, systolic blood pressure; DBP, diastolic blood pressure; MAP, mean arterial pressure; HR, heart rate; TG, triglyceride; HDL, high-density lipoprotein (cholesterol); LDL, low-density lipoprotein (cholesterol); ALT, aspartate aminotransferase; eGFR, estimated glomerular filtration rate.

Table 3 (Supplementary Table S2) summarizes the ophthalmic characteristics of the control and glaucoma groups after matching for sex and age. Significant differences were not found in eye laterality between the groups. The glaucoma group had significantly longer AL and thinner central corneal thickness (CCT) as expected, higher CD ratio, lower rim area, and worse VA, VF, VD, cpRNFL thickness, and GCC thickness (all $p < 0.001$) than those in the healthy group. A significant difference ($p = 0.51$) was not observed in the IOP between the two groups because of ethical and medical concerns. Moreover, the patients in the current study did not stop using antiglaucoma eye drops; therefore, patients with glaucoma in the present study should be more precisely described as those with medically treated glaucoma.

Table 3. Ocular Data of the Control and Glaucoma groups after Gender and Age Matching.

	Control Eyes ($N = 343$)	Glaucoma Eyes ($N = 343$)	p-Value
OD/OS			0.76
OD	173 (50.4%)	177 (51.6%)	
OS	170 (49.6%)	166 (48.4%)	
VA (logMAR)	0.1 ± 0.2	0.3 ± 0.6	<0.001
AL (mm)	25.1 ± 1.7	25.7 ± 2.1	<0.001
<24	100 (29.2%)	75 (22.0%)	<0.001
24–25.9	145 (42.3%)	101 (29.6%)	
≥26	98 (28.6%)	165 (48.4%)	
IOP (mmHg)	14.9 ± 3.6	14.7 ± 4.1	0.509
CCT (μm)	547.1 ± 33.2	535.4 ± 37.9	<0.001
VF: Mean Defect	-1.2 ± 1.8	-8.2 ± 8.3	<0.001
Macular VD (%)			
Superior	50.1 ± 4.7	43.8 ± 7.4	<0.001
Center	18.7 ± 6.4	16.4 ± 7.0	<0.001
Inferior	49.6 ± 4.7	41.4 ± 8.1	<0.001
Peripapillary VD (%)			
Superior	51.6 ± 5.0	40.5 ± 10.7	<0.001
Inferior	52.7 ± 5.0	37.9 ± 10.5	<0.001
cpRNFL Thickness (μm)			
Superior	100.0 ± 9.6	78.2 ± 15.5	<0.001
Inferior	96.1 ± 9.1	72.0 ± 15.1	<0.001
GCC Thickness (μm)			
Superior	95.6 ± 5.5	78.4 ± 12.5	<0.001
Inferior	95.0 ± 5.5	72.3 ± 13.2	<0.001
Cup/Disc Ratio (%)	51.2 ± 18.6	79.2 ± 16.0	<0.001
Rim Area (0.01 mm^2)	131.1 ± 36.9	75.9 ± 39.8	<0.001
Disc Area (0.01 mm^2)	203.5 ± 49.4	212.1 ± 61.5	0.046

Note. OD, right eye; OS, left eye; VA, visual acuity; AL, axial length; CCT, central corneal thickness; VF, visual field; VD, vessel density; cpRNFL, circumpapillary retinal nerve fiber layer; GCC, ganglion cell complex.

Tables 4 and 5 (Supplementary Table S3) show the demographic and ophthalmic characteristics and ocular data, respectively, of the control, PPG, and glaucoma (G) groups after sex and age matching. The heart rate was significantly higher in the control group, whereas the AC sugar and HbA1C levels were significantly lower in the PPG group than those in the G group. The G group had significantly worse VA, thinner CCT, and longer AL than those in the control group. VF in the G group was significantly lower than that in the control and PPG groups. Significant differences in the hemifield macular VD, peripapillary VD, and cpRNFL and GCC thicknesses were noted among the three groups when compared in pairs (all $p < 0.05$) except for the center macular VD, which was only significantly lower in the G group than that in the control group.

Table 4. Demographics and Clinical Characteristics after Gender and Age Matching for Groups of Glaucomatous Subjects and Control Subjects.

	A vs. B N = 288:32		A vs. C N = 314:314		B vs. C N = 62:310		*p*-Value a	b	c
Age	44.7 ± 13.9	48.6 ± 15.7	47.7 ± 14.4	48.2 ± 12.9	46.9 ± 12.2	50.6 ± 14.1	0.12	0.52	0.33
<40	112 (38.9%)	9 (28.1%)	81 (25.8%)	95 (30.2%)	15 (24.2%)	75 (24.2%)	0.24	0.95	0.20
40–60	142 (49.3%)	18 (56.3%)	177 (56.4%)	150 (47.8%)	40 (64.5%)	163 (52.6%)			
≥60	34 (11.8%)	5 (15.6%)	56 (17.8%)	69 (22.0%)	7 (11.3%)	72 (23.2%)			
Gender							1.00	1.00	0.23
Male	72 (25.0%)	8 (25.0%)	156 (49.7%)	156 (49.7%)	43 (69.3%)	190 (61.3%)			
Female	216 (75.0%)	24 (75.0%)	158 (50.3%)	158 (50.3%)	19 (30.7%)	120 (38.7%)			
SBP	122.5 ± 17.7	130.3 ± 18.4	126.2 ± 18.4	125.9 ± 17.5	129.5 ± 16.0	129.0 ± 18.6	0.03	0.85	0.82
DBP	72.0 ± 12.0	76.8 ± 13.0	75.4 ± 12.0	74.5 ± 11.7	78.6 ± 12.5	76.0 ± 12.3	0.03	0.35	0.13
MAP	88.9 ± 13.0	94.7 ± 13.5	92.4 ± 13.2	91.7 ± 12.5	95.6 ± 12.7	93.6 ± 13.1	0.02	0.51	0.28
HR	79.4 ± 12.4	75.5 ± 9.8	78.8 ± 12.3	74.7 ± 11.5	74.9 ± 10.1	75.5 ± 12.3	0.08	<0.001	0.71
TG	105.7 ± 69.9	102.3 ± 45.6	122.7 ± 87.1	113.1 ± 49.7	108.6 ± 45.0	116.9 ± 57.2	0.64	0.27	0.52
HDL	55.9 ± 13.5	55.2 ± 12.4	52.4 ± 14.1	52.5 ± 14.8	52.0 ± 11.7	50.4 ± 15.5	0.77	0.96	0.63
LDL	113.7 ± 32.8	115.2 ± 35.1	113.6 ± 34.1	109.1 ± 29.1	119.2 ± 27.4	113.4 ± 31.7	0.89	0.35	0.47
AC sugar	94.1 ± 14.3	93.4 ± 8.1	96.9 ± 14.1	100.3 ± 19.8	95.4 ± 8.1	104.2 ± 22.5	0.70	0.12	0.001
HbA1c	6.0 ± 0.7	5.1 ± 0.3	6.0 ± 0.5	6.1 ± 1.1	5.4 ± 0.6	6.1 ± 0.9	0.02	0.33	0.01
ALT	20.2 ± 17.1	32.0 ± 21.9	22.2 ± 11.9	23.8 ± 16.2	31.1 ± 21.7	25.7 ± 18.3	0.03	0.38	0.18
Creatinine	0.9 ± 1.2	0.8 ± 0.2	1.0 ± 1.5	0.9 ± 0.8	0.9 ± 0.2	0.9 ± 0.8	0.49	0.47	0.27
eGFR	100.9 ± 21.3	99.2 ± 16.6	95.0 ± 21.4	95.9 ± 21.2	97.9 ± 17.7	93.0 ± 21.2	0.37	0.71	0.26
Uric Acid	5.1 ± 1.3	5.3 ± 1.3	5.7 ± 1.6	5.9 ± 1.3	5.9 ± 1.3	6.0 ± 1.4	0.51	0.46	0.85

Group A, control eyes; Group B, pre-perimetric glaucoma eyes; Group C, glaucoma eyes; a *p*-value, A vs. B; b *p*-value, A vs. C; c *p*-value, B vs. C; Unit. Age (years); SBP (mmHg); DBP (mmHg); MAP (mmHg); HR (/min); TG (mg/dL); HDL (mg/dL); LDL (mg/dL); AC sugar (mg/dL); HbA1c (%); ALT (U/L); Creatinine (mg/dL); eGFR (mL/min/1.73 m^2); Uric Acid (mg/dL); Abbreviations. SBP, systolic blood pressure; DBP, diastolic blood pressure; MAP, mean arterial pressure; HR, heart rate; TG, triglyceride; HDL, high-density lipoprotein (cholesterol); LDL, low-density lipoprotein (cholesterol); ALT, aspartate aminotransferase; eGFR, estimated glomerular filtration rate.

Table 5. Ocular Data after Gender and Age Matching for Groups of Glaucomatous subjects and Control subjects.

	A vs. B N = 288:32		A vs. C N = 314:314		B vs. C N = 62:310		*p*-Value a	b	c
OD/OS							0.68	0.58	0.68
OD	151 (52.4%)	18 (56.3%)	160 (51.0%)	153 (48.7%)	30 (48.4%)	159 (51.3%)			
OS	137 (47.6%)	14 (43.7%)	154 (49.0%)	161 (51.3%)	32 (51.6%)	151 (48.7%)			
VA (logMAR)	0.1 ± 0.2	0.2 ± 0.6	0.1 ± 0.2	0.3 ± 0.5	0.3 ± 0.6	0.4 ± 0.7	0.37	<0.001	0.20
AL (mm)	25.2 ± 1.8	25.6 ± 1.8	25.1 ± 1.8	25.7 ± 2.1	25.9 ± 1.9	25.6 ± 2.4	0.22	<0.001	0.37
<24	78 (27.1%)	7 (21.9%)	97 (30.9%)	71 (22.8%)	13 (21.0%)	86 (27.8%)			
24–25.9	121 (42.0%)	8 (25.0%)	118 (37.6%)	100 (32.0%)	16 (25.8%)	87 (28.2%)			
26	89 (30.9%)	17 (53.1%)	99 (31.5%)	141 (45.2%)	33 (53.2%)	136 (44.0%)			
IOP (mmHg)	14.6 ± 3.4	14.9 ± 3.3	14.8 ± 3.6	14.8 ± 4.0	15.1 ± 4.0	14.7 ± 3.8	0.66	0.84	0.45
CCT (μm)	543.9 ± 35.9	542.2 ± 31.0	544.0 ± 35.4	536.4 ± 34.1	530.7 ± 44.7	536.5 ± 36.0	0.80	0.007	0.34
VF	−1.4 ± 1.8	−1.4 ± 1.5	−1.2 ± 1.9	−9.0 ± 8.6	−1.0 ± 1.3	−10.3 ± 9.0	0.98	<0.001	<0.001
Macular VD (%)									
Superior	50.1 ± 4.8	47.3 ± 5.1	49.9 ± 5.3	43.5 ± 7.1	46.4 ± 6.7	42.9 ± 7.5	0.002	<0.001	<0.001
Center	18.4 ± 6.8	18.0 ± 6.4	18.6 ± 6.3	16.1 ± 7.0	17.8 ± 6.2	16.0 ± 6.9	0.72	<0.001	0.06
Inferior	49.5 ± 5.1	46.1 ± 4.8	49.4 ± 5.4	41.0 ± 7.7	45.7 ± 6.1	40.2 ± 8.0	0.001	<0.001	<0.001
Peripapil-lary VD (%)									
Superior	51.7 ± 5.2	47.1 ± 6.4	51.3 ± 5.3	39.1 ± 10.6	47.3 ± 5.9	37.9 ± 10.6	<0.001	<0.001	<0.001
Inferior	52.7 ± 5.4	48.5 ± 5.2	52.4 ± 5.4	36.6 ± 10.2	47.4 ± 5.1	35.4 ± 10.3	<0.001	<0.001	<0.001

Table 5. *Cont.*

| | A vs. B | | A vs. C | | B vs. C | | *p*-Value | | |
	N = 288:32		N = 314:314		N = 62:310		a	b	c
cpRNFL Thickness (μm)									
Superior	101.0 ± 10.1	85.6 ± 10.2	100.8 ± 10.0	76.0 ± 16.0	86.6 ± 10.3	75.1 ± 15.4	<0.001	<0.001	<0.001
Inferior	96.9 ± 9.4	85.1 ± 9.8	96.3 ± 8.9	69.3 ± 15.0	81.5 ± 10.7	67.8 ± 13.4	<0.001	<0.001	<0.001
GCC Thickness (μm)									
Superior	96.0 ± 5.9	86.3 ± 7.4	95.8 ± 5.4	76.6 ± 12.2	85.9 ± 8.0	76.3 ± 13.0	<0.001	<0.001	<0.001
Inferior	95.4 ± 5.9	83.5 ± 7.3	95.1 ± 5.6	70.5 ± 12.5	81.3 ± 8.1	70.0 ± 12.8	<0.001	<0.001	<0.001
C/D Ratio	49.8 ± 19.5	66.5 ± 18.6	51.5 ± 19.4	80.7 ± 15.6	70.5 ± 14.8	82.5 ± 13.4	<0.001	<0.001	<0.001
Rim Area	133.3 ± 37.2	109.3 ± 63.7	130.8 ± 37.1	72.0 ± 39.1	98.1 ± 50.8	69.8 ± 37.9	0.04	<0.001	<0.001
Disc Area	203.5 ± 48.4	218.9 ± 56.2	204.2 ± 49.4	212.6 ± 60.1	212.8 ± 48.8	216.4 ± 59.5	0.09	0.06	0.66

Group A, control eyes; Group B, pre-perimetric glaucoma eyes; Group C, glaucoma eyes; a *p*-value, A vs. B; b *p*-value, A vs. C; c *p*-value, B vs. C; Unit. VA (logMAR); VF (mean deviation); VD (%); thickness (μm); C/D ratio (%); Rim area (0.01 mm^2); Disc area (0.01 mm^2); Abbreviation. OD, right eye; OS, left eye; VA, visual acuity; AL, axial length; CCT, central corneal thickness; VF, visual field; VD, vessel density; cpRNFL, circumpapillary retinal nerve fiber layer; GCC, ganglion cell complex; C/D Ratio, cup to disc ratio.

Table 6 (Supplementary Table S4) summarizes the characteristics of the glaucomatous subgroups, which were divided according to the VF (MD) values, including the control (group 0), PPG (group 1), and early-(group 2), moderate-(group 3), and late-stage (group 4) glaucoma subgroups. Significant differences among the groups were not observed in terms of sex. Participants in the late-stage group were significantly older than those in the other groups, and their AL was significantly shorter. The peripapillary VD values were highest in the control eyes, followed by the PPG and early-, moderate-, and late-stage glaucoma eyes; all pairwise comparisons were statistically significant ($p < 0.05$, Tukey's honestly significant difference). Superior and inferior macular VDs showed significant differences between the control, early, moderate, and late glaucoma groups but could not be differentiated between the PPG and early glaucoma groups.

Table 6. One Way Analysis of OCTA parameters and OCT measurement among the glaucoma severity groups.

	Group 0 N = 540	Group 1 N = 67	Group 2 N = 224	Group 3 N = 103	Group 4 N = 194	*p*-Value	Tukey Test
Age (years)	44.4 ± 13.8	45.7 ± 12.7	48.3 ± 12.2	51.3 ± 12.8	56.1 ± 14.5	<0.001	4 > 0, 1, 2, 3
Axial Length (mm)	25.2 ± 1.7	25.9 ± 1.8	25.9 ± 1.8	26.3 ± 2.8	25.1 ± 2.2	<0.001	1, 2, 3 > 0, 4
Gender						0.463	
Male	169 (31.3%)	43 (64.2%)	137 (61.2%)	69 (67.7%)	132 (68.0%)		
Female	371 (68.7%)	24 (35.8%)	87 (38.8%)	33 (32.4%)	62 (32.0%)		
Macular VD (%)							
Superior	50.3 ± 4.8	46.6 ± 6.5	46.1 ± 6.0	41.2 ± 6.6	38.1 ± 7.5	<0.001	0 > 1, 2 > 3 > 4
Center	18.4 ± 6.4	18.1 ± 6.1	17.0 ± 6.6	14.7 ± 6.1	14.5 ± 7.0	<0.001	0 > 2; 0, 1, 2 > 3, 4
Inferior	49.7 ± 5.0	46.0 ± 5.9	43.7 ± 6.8	38.0 ± 7.2	35.2 ± 7.7	<0.001	0 > 1, 2 > 3 > 4
Peripapillary VD (%)							
Superior	51.8 ± 4.9	47.4 ± 5.8	43.6 ± 8.4	37.1 ± 10.2	29.5 ± 9.2	<0.001	0 > 1 > 2 > 3 > 4
Inferior	52.9 ± 5.2	47.6 ± 5.0	41.5 ± 8.1	33.2 ± 9.2	26.9 ± 7.8	<0.001	0 > 1 > 2 > 3 > 4
cpRNFL Thickness (μm)							
Superior	100.8 ± 9.7	86.8 ± 10.4	81.2 ± 13.5	74.0 ± 14.6	67.1 ± 14.9	<0.001	0 > 1 > 2 > 3 > 4
Inferior	96.8 ± 9.0	82.0 ± 10.7	74.6 ± 12.8	65.2 ± 14.0	61.1 ± 13.4	<0.001	0 > 1 > 2 > 3 > 4
GCC Thickness (μm)							
Superior	95.9 ± 5.8	86.0 ± 7.8	81.1 ± 10.2	73.9 ± 12.6	69.4 ± 12.4	<0.001	0 > 1 > 2 > 3 > 4
Inferior	95.3 ± 5.7	81.5 ± 8.0	75.0 ± 12.1	65.9 ± 10.4	64.2 ± 11.1	<0.001	0 > 1 > 2 > 3 > 4

Table 6. *Cont.*

	Group 0 *N* = 540	Group 1 *N* = 67	Group 2 *N* = 224	Group 3 *N* = 103	Group 4 *N* = 194	*p*-Value	Tukey Test
Cup/Disc Ratio (%)	49.7 ± 19.5	69.5 ± 16.0	77.5 ± 14.0	83.4 ± 13.7	89.5 ± 11.0	<0.001	$0 < 1 < 2 < 3 < 4$
Rim Area (0.01 mm^2)	133.3 ± 36.7	100.1 ± 50.2	78.5 ± 33.9	69.8 ± 38.2	51.6 ± 30.3	<0.001	$0 > 1 > 2, 3 > 4$
Disc Area (0.01 mm^2)	203.4 ± 48.6	213.9 ± 49.8	209.5 ± 51.8	221.0 ± 81.9	216.7 ± 60.6	0.006	

Group 0, control eyes; Group 1, pre-perimetric glaucoma eyes; Group 2, early glaucoma eyes with -2 dB $>$ VF(MD) ≥ -6 dB; Group 3, moderate glaucoma eyes with -6 dB $>$ VF(MD) ≥ -12 dB; Group 4, late glaucoma eyes with VF(MD) < -12 dB; OD, right eye; OS, left eye; VA, visual acuity; AL, axial length; CCT, central corneal thickness; VF, visual field; VD, vessel density; cpRNFL, circumpapillary retinal nerve fiber layer; GCC, ganglion cell complex; MD, mean deviation. The OCTA-based VD and OCT-based structural thickness of the two groups (advanced, terminal stage) are shown in Table 7. No significant difference was noted between the two groups in terms of peripapillary and macular VDs, cpRNFL and GCC thickness, or CD ratio.

Table 7. Comparison of advanced or terminal glaucoma with OCTA parameters and OCT measurement.

	Advanced Glaucoma (*N* = 158)	Terminal Glaucoma (*N* = 36)	*p*-Value
Age (years)	56.06 ± 14.44	56.47 ± 14.91	0.879
Male subjects	110(69.62)	22(61.11)	0.323
Macular VD (%)			
Superior	38.13 ± 7.44	37.84 ± 7.93	0.845
Center	13.98 ± 6.48	17.19 ± 8.88	0.064
Inferior	35.15 ± 7.56	35.64 ± 8.36	0.759
Peripapillary VD (%)			
Superior	29.68 ± 8.84	28.70 ± 11.02	0.635
Inferior	26.86 ± 7.33	27.16 ± 9.92	0.876
cpRNFL Thickness (μm)			
Superior	66.99 ± 13.61	67.75 ± 19.56	0.827
Inferior	60.94 ± 13.20	61.72 ± 14.21	0.753
GCC Thickness (μm)			
Superior	69.58 ± 11.95	68.56 ± 14.44	0.667
Inferior	63.96 ± 10.89	65.26 ± 11.81	0.536
Cup/Disc Ratio (%)	90.04 ± 9.79	87.11 ± 15.17	0.274
Rim Area (0.01 mm^2)	49.92 ± 25.06	59.03 ± 46.49	0.262
Disc Area (0.01 mm^2)	217.80 ± 59.97	211.69 ± 63.65	0.587
AL (mm)	25.07 ± 2.19	24.98 ± 2.24	0.818
VF (mean defect)	-20.24 ± 5.49	-31.71 ± 0.87	<0.001
VA (logMAR)	0.55 ± 0.79	0.91 ± 1.20	0.148

Note. Advanced glaucoma, -12 dB $>$ VF(MD) ≥ -30 dB; Terminal glaucoma, VF(MD) < -30 dB; Abbreviation. VD, vessel density; cpRNFL, circumpapillary retinal nerve fiber layer; GCC, ganglion cell complex; VA, visual acuity; AL, axial length.

The OCTA-based VD and OCT-based structural thickness of the two groups (advanced, terminal stage) are shown in Table 7 (Supplementary Table S5). No significant difference was noted between the two groups in terms of peripapillary and macular VDs, cpRNFL and GCC thickness, or CD ratio.

Multivariable linear regression models with the GEE for correlations between MD VF with OCTA parameters and OCT measurements are shown in Table 8. Positive correlations were found between MD VF with VD in the macula and peripapillary areas and cpRNFL and GCC thicknesses (all $p < 0.001$) except for the central macular VD. According to the β-value, the rates of increase were highest in macular VD (0.55%, 0.54% every dB), followed by peripapillary VD (0.47%, 0.53% every dB), GCC thickness (0.38 μm, 0.35 μm every dB), and cpRNFL thickness (0.24 μm, 0.25 μm every dB).

The superior and inferior hemifield asymmetries of the percentage loss of peripapillary and macular VDs and cpRNFL and GCC thickness were compared in the PPG and G groups (Table 9). In the PPG group, the GCC thickness showed significant intra-eye asymmetry, whereas the other factors did not. However, all factors were significantly more affected severely in the inferior hemifield of the glaucoma group ($p < 0.001$).

Table 8. Multivariable linear regression models with generalized estimating equation (GEE) model *
for correlations between visual field in mean defect with OCTA parameters and OCT measurement.

	β	SE	*p*-Value
Macular VD (%)			
Superior	0.55	0.05	<0.001
Center	0.16	0.10	0.123
Inferior	0.54	0.05	<0.001
Peripapillary VD (%)			
Superior	0.47	0.04	<0.001
Inferior	0.53	0.03	<0.001
cpRNFL Thickness (μm)			
Superior	0.24	0.03	<0.001
Inferior	0.25	0.03	<0.001
GCC Thickness (μm)			
Superior	0.38	0.03	<0.001
Inferior	0.35	0.03	<0.001
Cup/Disc Ratio (%)	−0.23	0.04	<0.001
Rim Area (0.01 mm^2)	0.07	0.01	<0.001
Disc Area (0.01 mm^2)	0.00	0.01	0.936

OCTA, optical coherence tomography angiography; VD, vessel density; cpRNFL, circumpapillary retinal nerve fiber layer; GCC, ganglion cell complex. * Adjusted for age, gender, axial length.

Table 9. Comparison of percentage loss hemifield asymmetry of corresponding regions of OCTA parameters between pre-perimetric glaucoma eyes and glaucoma eyes.

	PPG [†] N = 67	*p*-Value *	Glaucoma [‡] N = 521	*p*-Value *
Macular VD				
Superior	0.07 ± 0.13	0.94	0.16 ± 0.15	<0.001
Inferior	0.08 ± 0.12		0.20 ± 0.16	
Peripapillary VD				
Superior	0.09 ± 0.11	0.34	0.28 ± 0.21	<0.001
Inferior	0.10 ± 0.10		0.35 ± 0.20	
cpRNFL Thickness				
Superior	0.14 ± 0.10	0.36	0.26 ± 0.15	<0.001
Inferior	0.15 ± 0.11		0.30 ± 0.15	
GCC Thickness				
Superior	0.10 ± 0.08	<0.001	0.21 ± 0.13	<0.001
Inferior	0.14 ± 0.08		0.27 ± 0.13	

PPG, pre-perimetric glaucoma; VD, vessel density; cpRNFL, circumpapillary retinal nerve fiber layer; GCC, ganglion cell complex; * Two sample pair *t*-test; [†] PPG group = (Mean Control –PPG)/Mean Control; [‡] G group = (Mean Control – G)/Mean Control.

In Table 10, the r values of Pearson's correlation coefficient between the cpRNFL and GCC thicknesses and VD were 0.636 to 0.674, and higher positive linear associations were noted in the peripapillary area than that in the macular area. The associations were slightly higher in the superior region than that in the inferior region.

Table 10. Pearson correlation coefficient between OCTA parameters with OCT measurement in same region.

		r	*p*-Value
Superior	GCC Thickness Macular VD	0.658	<0.001
Inferior	GCC Thickness Macular VD	0.636	<0.001
Superior	cpRNFL Thickness Peripapillary VD	0.674	<0.001

Table 10. *Cont.*

		r	*p*-Value
Inferior	cpRNFL Thickness Peripapillary VD	0.666	<0.001

OCTA, optical coherence tomography angiography; VD, vessel density; cpRNFL, circumpapillary retinal nerve fiber layer; GCC, ganglion cell complex.

In Table 11, positive linear correlations were found between superior and inferior GCC thicknesses with macular VD (all $p < 0.001$) and between superior and inferior cpRNFL thicknesses with peripapillary VD ($p < 0.001$). According to the β-value, the GCC and cpRNFL thicknesses of the superior macular, inferior macula, and superior peripapillary areas increased at a rate of 1.04 µm, 0.94 µm, 0.90 µm, and 0.91 µm for every percent of VD, respectively. The macular area has a higher β-value than that in the peripapillary area.

Table 11. Multivariable linear regression models with generalized estimating equation (GEE) model * for correlations between OCTA parameters with OCT measurement in same region: change in structural thickness related with VD.

		β	SE	*p*-Value
Superior	GCC Thickness Macular VD	1.04	0.05	<0.001
Inferior	GCC Thickness Macular VD	0.94	0.05	<0.001
Superior	cpRNFL Thickness Peripapillary VD	0.90	0.06	<0.001
Inferior	cpRNFL Thickness Peripapillary VD	0.91	0.05	<0.001

OCTA, optical coherence tomography angiography; VD, vessel density; cpRNFL, circumpapillary retinal nerve fiber layer; GCC, ganglion cell complex; * Adjusted for age, sex, axial length.

Although myopia is a risk factor for glaucoma, the glaucoma group showed a longer AL than the control group. However, we found that approximately half of the patients had more VF defects in eyes with higher myopia than in the inter-eye asymmetry of the same individual (Table 12).

Table 12. Proportion of higher myopia with more VF defect in all patients with glaucoma.

Glaucoma Subjects, *N* = 318	*N*	%
Higher myopia with more VF defect [a]	161	50.6
Others [b]	157	49.4

VF, visual field; [a] In bilateral eyes: AL differences (mm) > 0 and VF differences (dB) < 0 or AL differences (mm) < 0 and VF differences (dB) > 0; [b] In bilateral eyes: AL differences (mm) $\leq$ 0 and VF differences (dB) $\leq$ 0 or AL differences (mm) $\geq$ 0 and VF differences (dB) $\geq$ 0.

4. Discussion

In the present investigation,

1. Significant differences in the hemifield macular VD and peripapillary VD were noted among the control, PPG, and glaucoma groups when compared in pairs (all $p < 0.05$) except for the center macular VD.
2. Peripapillary VD showed better potential in differentiating the various stages of glaucoma severity than macular VD even in the myopic population.
3. All parameters showed no significant differences between advanced and terminal glaucoma.
4. Positive correlations between VF defect with VD and thickness were noted, and rates of increase were highest in macular VD, followed by peripapillary VD, GCC thickness, and cpRNFL thickness.

5. The GCC thickness in the PPG group showed significant intra-eye asymmetry of percentage loss ($p < 0.001$), whereas peripapillary and macular VDs and cpRNFL thickness did not.
6. Only 50.6% of the patients had more VF defects in both eyes than that in the inter-eye asymmetry of the same individual.

Peripapillary VD measurement showed better potential in differentiating the stages (PPG, early, moderate, late) of glaucoma severity, whereas macular VD did not show a significant difference between the PPG and early-stage glaucoma groups in our study. However, the percent reduction in macular VD was significantly greater in the early glaucoma group than in the PPG group (all $p < 0.05$), as reported by Wang et al. [25]. The inconsistency may be attributed to our scan sizes being smaller than those of Wang's study, and the most vulnerable macular area was found to be outside the central 3×3 mm^2 area but inside the 6×6 mm^2 area [26].

There was no significant difference between the parameters of advanced- (-30 dB $<$ MD ≤ -12 dB) and terminal-stage (MD ≤ -30 dB) glaucoma. In the early stage of disease, both structural and functional data could help making judgements about the rate of progression. In the advanced stage, functional data, such as mean defect of VF, is more useful for follow-up in these cases. Severity in the advanced group (VF MD -20.2 ± 5.5 dB) may have reached the measurement floor of cpRNFL and GCC thickness, as supported by Moghimi et al. [27] and Phillips et al. [28]. Measurement floors of cpRNFL thickness and macular VD in our population may be higher than that in Americans [27]. Measuring the floor of peripapillary and macular VDs and cpRNFL and GCC thicknesses in the Asian population should be performed in the future.

Mikelberg et al. found that 70% of glaucomatous eyes had initial damage limited to a single hemifield, and 57% still had a single hemifield defect at the completion of follow-up [29]. Therefore, the asymmetry of the percentage loss of VD and structural thickness in the PPG and G groups was compared. All parameters were significantly more affected severely in the inferior hemifield of the G group. In the PPG group, GCC thickness and hemifield asymmetry could be seen in the PPG stage but not in peripapillary and macular VDs, which was supported by previous studies. Chen et al. reported that macular ganglion cell–inner plexiform layer (GCIPL) thickness asymmetry measurements have diagnostic ability comparable to that of cpRNFL, GCIPL, and optic nerve head analysis for PPG [30]. Chang et al. also found that macular perfusion density asymmetry was not significantly different between the healthy and PPG groups [31].

The peripapillary and macular VDs and GCC and RNFL thicknesses were significantly more affected severely in the inferior hemifield than that in the superior hemifield of the glaucoma group ($p < 0.001$). The literature shows that the inferior region of the macula is particularly susceptible to glaucomatous damage [32]. Other studies have shown that VD superior/inferior asymmetry may permit a more reproducible, objective diagnosis in detecting early stages of glaucomatous changes [33,34]. As POAG progresses, the damage becomes multifocal and diffuse, and asymmetry becomes smaller in the severe stages of the disease [34]. Intra-eye VD asymmetry may have the potential to detect early glaucoma with less influence of interindividual variation in factors, such as age, sex, race, AL, hypertension, diabetes, and other systemic drug-related factors. In the future, it may be interesting to see if the VF hemifield test matches upper and lower VD, cpRNFL, and GCC differences in various stages of glaucoma.

A recent meta-analysis showed that individuals with myopia have a higher risk of developing open-angle glaucoma than those without myopia. The overall odds ratio (OR) was 1.95 for any myopia compared with emmetropia. The pooled ORs were 2.92 for moderate/high myopia and 1.59 for low myopia, with a cutoff value of -3 D [23]. In our study, the glaucoma group had longer AL than the control group, whereas in comparing the inter-eye asymmetry of the same individual, only 50.6% of the patients with glaucoma had more VF defects in eyes with higher myopia. In contrast, Lee et al. reported that in inter-eye comparisons, more myopic eyes in myopic normal-tension glaucoma demonstrate more severe VF [35]. However, the literature showed that the rates of VF progression in the myopic group (0.356 and 0.361 dB/y for 10° to 24°, respectively, and glaucoma hemifield test maps) were not significantly different from those in the non-myopic group (0.349 and –0.364 dB/y; $p = 0.951$ and 0.973, respectively) [36]. Other studies have reported that myopia may be a protective factor against optic disc/RNFL or VF progression in those with open-angle glaucoma [37–39]. Whether inter-eye asymmetrically higher myopia is associated with inter-eye asymmetrically progressive open-angle glaucoma remains questionable. Further studies are needed to clarify the association between the inter-eye asymmetry of myopia and open-angle glaucoma progression.

Our study population included more myopia patients and had a longer mean AL than those of other studies in healthy [27,40,41], PPG [40], and glaucoma groups [27,40]. The mean macular and peripapillary VD values of the glaucoma group in our study were lower than those in other studies [27,40]. However, for the healthy and PPG groups, no significant difference in the mean VD values was noted between our populations and other studies [27,40,41]. It has been reported that peripapillary and macular VD may be reduced in high myopia non-glaucoma patients [11–21]. While comparing the non-glaucoma population with that of Korean studies, our control group had shorter AL, lower macular and peripapillary VDs, and thinner RNFL [14,16]. Compared with studies conducted in China, our population had AL similar to that of moderate myopia defined in these studies, with higher macular VD in our group, lower peripapillary VD, and thinner GCC and peripapillary RNFL, which were lower and thinner than those of their high-myopia groups [15,17,20]. The dynamic range of VD was decreased by myopia, but using peripapillary VD to differentiate between the various stages of glaucoma severity is feasible. However, the simultaneous presence of myopia and open-angle glaucoma resulted in a greater level of microvascular attenuation than with either pathology alone [22]. The values of reduction related to glaucoma may have been overestimated. Considering the effect of myopia, VD may be more valuable in following glaucoma progression in each individual than comparing data between individuals in clinical practice, and different baseline values of parameters should not be neglected.

According to the vascular theory of glaucoma, neural structure loss is a consequence of reduced ocular blood flow. Ischemia may damage the neural tissues [42,43]. On the contrary, the destruction of the neural tissue in glaucoma may lead to microvascular reduction through decreased metabolic demand [44]. The possible reasons why some studies failed to demonstrate this link might because of big variation of cross-sectional design. Longitudinal studies perhaps still cannot clarify whether neural tissue loss or vessel loss is the primary event since these events can be interdependent.

There are some limitations to our study. First, our scan size was only 3×3 mm^2, and a larger macular scan size (6×6 mm^2) was reported to have a higher diagnostic accuracy [26,45]. A larger scan size of macular VD may help us understand more macular microvascular changes in the early stages of glaucoma. Second, the small sample size of the PPG group in this study may have induced selection bias in our population. Moreover, most systemic factors did not show differences between the control and glaucoma patients. Further studies with more participants may provide different results. Finally, since this was a cross-sectional study, the interindividual variability of measurements and disease progression could not be discussed. Longitudinal studies will help elucidate the pattern of microvascular damage in the various stages of glaucoma.

5. Conclusions

In conclusion, the current study showed that peripapillary VD was significantly different between the healthy and PPG groups and the early-, moderate-, and late-stage glaucoma subgroups. Our results revealed that peripapillary VD measurement is helpful in differentiating the various stages of glaucoma severity, even in a myopic population.

Supplementary Materials: The following are available online at https://www.mdpi.com/article/10.3390/jcm10235490/s1, Table S1 : Demographics and Characteristics of the Control and Glaucoma groups, Table S2 : Demographics, Characteristics and Ocular Data of the Control and Glaucoma groups after Gender and Age Matching, Table S3 : Demographics, Clinical Characteristics and Ocular Data after Gender and Age Matching for Groups of Glaucomatous Subjects and Control Subjects, Table S4 : One Way Analysis of OCTA parameters and OCT measurement among the glaucoma severity groups, Table S5 : Comparison of advanced or terminal glaucoma with OCTA parameters and OCT measurement.

Author Contributions: Conceptualization, M.-L.K.; methodology, M.-L.K.; software, F.-Y.S.; validation, F.-Y.S.; formal analysis, F.-Y.S.; investigation, K.-I.H.; resources, M.-L.K.; data curation, F.-Y.S.; writing—original draft preparation, C.-K.K.; writing—review and editing, M.-L.K.; visualization, C.-K.K.; supervision, M.-L.K.; project administration, M.-L.K.; funding ac-quisition, M.-L.K. All authors have read and agreed to the published version of the manuscript.

Funding: This research received no external funding.

Institutional Review Board Statement: The study was conducted according to the guidelines of the Declaration of Helsinki, and approved by the Institutional Review Board of the NATIONAL TAIWAN UNIVERSITY HOSPITAL HSIN-CHU BRANCH, TAIWAN (IRB no. NTUHHCB 108-025-E).

Informed Consent Statement: Informed consent was obtained from all subjects involved in the study.

Data Availability Statement: The data presented in this study are available in supplementary materials.

Acknowledgments: We thank the staff of the Department of Medical Research, National Taiwan University Hsin-Chu Branch for their assistance in study design, statistical analysis.

Conflicts of Interest: The authors declare no conflict of interest.

References

1. GBD 2019 Blindness and Vision Impairment Collaborators; Vision Loss Expert Group of the Global Burden of Disease Study. Causes of blindness and vision impairment in 2020 and trends over 30 years, and prevalence of avoidable blindness in relation to VISION 2020: The Right to Sight: An analysis for the Global Burden of Disease Study. *Lancet Glob. Health* **2021**, *9*, e144–e160. [CrossRef]
2. Tham, Y.-C.; Li, X.; Wong, T.Y.; Quigley, H.A.; Aung, T.; Cheng, C. Global prevalence of glaucoma and projections of glaucoma burden through 2040: A systematic review and meta-analysis. *Ophthalmology* **2014**, *121*, 2081–2090. [CrossRef] [PubMed]
3. Garway-Heath, D.F.; Crabb, D.P.; Bunce, C.; Lascaratos, G.; Amalfitano, F.; Anand, N.; Azuara-Blanco, A.; Bourne, R.R.; Broadway, D.C.; A Cunliffe, I.; et al. Latanoprost for open-angle glaucoma (UKGTS): A randomised, multicentre, placebo-controlled trial. *Lancet* **2015**, *385*, 1295–1304. [CrossRef]
4. Werner, A.C.; Shen, L.Q. A Review of OCT Angiography in Glaucoma. *Semin. Ophthalmol.* **2019**, *34*, 279–286. [CrossRef] [PubMed]
5. Van Melkebeke, L.; Barbosa-Breda, J.; Huygens, M.; Stalmans, I. Optical Coherence Tomography Angiography in Glaucoma: A Review. *Ophthalmic Res.* **2018**, *60*, 139–151. [CrossRef]
6. Yarmohammadi, A.; Zangwill, L.M.; Diniz-Filho, A.; Saunders, L.J.; Suh, M.H.; Wu, Z.; Manalastas, P.I.C.; Akagi, T.; Medeiros, F.A.; Weinreb, R.N. Peripapillary and Macular Vessel Density in Patients with Glaucoma and Single-Hemifield Visual Field Defect. *Ophthalmology* **2017**, *124*, 709–719. [CrossRef] [PubMed]
7. Jia, Y.; Wei, E.; Wang, X.; Zhang, X.; Morrison, J.C.; Parikh, M.; Lombardi, L.H.; Gattey, D.M.; Armour, R.L.; Edmunds, B.; et al. Optical Coherence Tomography Angiography of Optic Disc Perfusion in Glaucoma. *Ophthalmology* **2014**, *121*, 1322–1332. [CrossRef] [PubMed]
8. Shin, J.W.; Lee, J.; Kwon, J.; Choi, J.; Kook, M.S. Regional vascular density–visual field sensitivity relationship in glaucoma according to disease severity. *Br. J. Ophthalmol.* **2017**, *101*, 1666–1672. [CrossRef]
9. Yarmohammadi, A.; Zangwill, L.M.; Diniz-Filho, A.; Suh, M.H.; Yousefi, S.; Saunders, L.J.; Belghith, A.; Manalastas, P.I.C.; Medeiros, F.A.; Weinreb, R.N. Relationship between Optical Coherence Tomography Angiography Vessel Density and Severity of Visual Field Loss in Glaucoma. *Ophthalmology* **2016**, *123*, 2498–2508. [CrossRef]
10. Chen, H.S.-L.; Liu, C.-H.; Wu, W.-C.; Tseng, H.-J.; Lee, Y.-S. Optical Coherence Tomography Angiography of the Superficial Microvasculature in the Macular and Peripapillary Areas in Glaucomatous and Healthy Eyes. *Investig. Opthalmol. Vis. Sci.* **2017**, *58*, 3637–3645. [CrossRef]
11. Ucak, T.; Icel, E.; Yilmaz, H.; Karakurt, Y.; Tasli, G.; Ugurlu, A.; Bozkurt, E. Alterations in optical coherence tomography angiography findings in patients with high myopia. *Eye (Lond.)* **2020**, *34*, 1129–1135. [CrossRef] [PubMed]
12. Yang, Y.; Wang, J.; Jiang, H.; Yang, X.; Feng, L.; Hu, L.; Wang, L.; Lü, F.; Shen, M. Retinal Microvasculature Alteration in High Myopia. *Investig. Opthalmol. Vis. Sci.* **2016**, *57*, 6020–6030. [CrossRef] [PubMed]

13. Milani, P.; Montesano, G.; Rossetti, L.; Bergamini, F.; Pece, A. Vessel density, retinal thickness, and choriocapillaris vascular flow in myopic eyes on OCT angiography. *Graefe's Arch. Clin. Exp. Ophthalmol.* **2018**, *256*, 1419–1427. [CrossRef] [PubMed]
14. Min, C.H.; Al-Qattan, H.M.; Lee, J.Y.; Kim, J.-G.; Yoon, Y.H.; Kim, Y.J. Macular Microvasculature in High Myopia without Pathologic Changes: An Optical Coherence Tomography Angiography Study. *Korean J. Ophthalmol.* **2020**, *34*, 106–112. [CrossRef] [PubMed]
15. Li, Y.; Miara, H.; Ouyang, P.; Jiang, B. The Comparison of Regional RNFL and Fundus Vasculature by OCTA in Chinese Myopia Population. *J. Ophthalmol.* **2018**, *2018*, 1–10. [CrossRef] [PubMed]
16. Sung, M.S.; Lee, T.H.; Heo, H.; Park, S.W. Clinical features of superficial and deep peripapillary microvascular density in healthy myopic eyes. *PLoS ONE* **2017**, *12*, e0187160. [CrossRef]
17. He, J.; Chen, Q.; Yin, Y.; Zhou, H.; Fan, Y.; Zhu, J.; Zou, H.; Xu, X. Association between retinal microvasculature and optic disc alterations in high myopia. *Eye (Lond.)* **2019**, *33*, 1494–1503. [CrossRef] [PubMed]
18. Cheng, D.; Chen, Q.; Wu, Y.; Yu, X.; Shen, M.; Zhuang, X.; Tian, Z.; Yang, Y.; Wang, J.; Lu, F.; et al. Deep perifoveal vessel density as an indicator of capillary loss in high myopia. *Eye (Lond.)* **2019**, *33*, 1961–1968. [CrossRef]
19. Hassan, M.; Sadiq, M.A.; Halim, M.S.; Afridi, R.; Soliman, M.K.; Sarwar, S.; Agarwal, A.; Do, D.V.; Nguyen, Q.D.; Sepah, Y.J. Evaluation of macular and peripapillary vessel flow density in eyes with no known pathology using op-tical coherence tomography angiography. *Int. J. Retin. Vitr.* **2017**, *3*, 27. [CrossRef] [PubMed]
20. Wu, Q.; Chen, Q.; Lin, B.; Huang, S.; Wang, Y.; Zhang, L.; Lin, H.; Wang, J.; Lu, F.; Shen, M. Relationships among retinal/choroidal thickness, retinal microvascular network and visual field in high my-opia. *Acta Ophthalmol.* **2020**, *98*, e709–e714.
21. Al-Sheikh, M.; Phasukkijwatana, N.; Dolz-Marco, R.; Rahimi, M.; Iafe, N.A.; Freund, K.B.; Sadda, S.R.; Sarraf, D. Quantitative OCT Angiography of the Retinal Microvasculature and the Choriocapillaris in Myopic Eyes. *Investig. Opthalmol. Vis. Sci.* **2017**, *58*, 2063–2069. [CrossRef]
22. Suwan, Y.; Fard, M.A.; Geyman, L.S.; Tantraworasin, A.; Chui, T.Y.; Rosen, R.B.; Ritch, R. Association of Myopia With Peripapillary Perfused Capillary Density in Patients With Glaucoma: An Op-tical Coherence Tomography Angiography Study. *JAMA Ophthalmol.* **2018**, *136*, 507–513. [CrossRef]
23. Haarman, A.E.G.; Enthoven, C.A.; Tideman, J.W.L.; Tedja, M.S.; Verhoeven, V.J.M.; Klaver, C.C.W. The Complications of Myopia: A Review and Meta-Analysis. *Investig. Opthalmol. Vis. Sci.* **2020**, *61*, 49. [CrossRef] [PubMed]
24. Benavente-Pérez, A.; Hosking, S.L.; Logan, N.S.; Broadway, D.C. Ocular blood flow measurements in healthy human myopic eyes. *Graefe's Arch. Clin. Exp. Ophthalmol.* **2010**, *248*, 1587–1594. [CrossRef]
25. Wang, Y.; Xin, C.; Li, M.; Swain, D.L.; Cao, K.; Wang, H.; Wang, N. Macular vessel density versus ganglion cell complex thickness for detection of early primary open-angle glaucoma. *BMC Ophthalmol.* **2020**, *20*, 1–9. [CrossRef] [PubMed]
26. Hood, D.C. Improving our understanding, and detection, of glaucomatous damage: An approach based upon optical co-herence tomography (OCT). *Prog. Retin. Eye Res.* **2017**, *57*, 46–75. [CrossRef] [PubMed]
27. Moghimi, S.; Bowd, C.; Zangwill, L.M.; Penteado, R.C.; Hasenstab, K.; Hou, H.; Ghahari, E.; Manalastas, P.I.C.; Proudfoot, J.; Weinreb, R.N. Measurement Floors and Dynamic Ranges of OCT and OCT Angiography in Glaucoma. *Ophthalmology* **2019**, *126*, 980–988. [CrossRef]
28. Phillips, M.J.; Dinh-Dang, D.; Bolo, K.; Burkemper, B.; Lee, J.C.; LeTran, V.H.; Chang, B.R.; Grisafe, D.J.; Chu, Z.; Zhou, X.; et al. Steps to Measurement Floor of an Optical Microangiography Device in Glaucoma. *Am. J. Ophthalmol.* **2021**, *231*, 58–69. [CrossRef]
29. Mikelberg, F.S.; Drance, S.M. The Mode of Progression of Visual Field Defects in Glaucoma. *Am. J. Ophthalmol.* **1984**, *98*, 443–445. [CrossRef]
30. Chen, M.-J.; Yang, H.-Y.; Chang, Y.-F.; Hsu, C.-C.; Ko, Y.-C.; Liu, C.J.-L. Diagnostic ability of macular ganglion cell asymmetry in Preperimetric Glaucoma. *BMC Ophthalmol.* **2019**, *19*, 12. [CrossRef]
31. Chang, P.-Y.; Wang, J.-Y.; Wang, J.-K.; Yeh, S.-C.; Chang, S.-W. Asymmetry analysis of optical coherence tomography angiography macular perfusion density measurements in preperimetric and perimetric glaucoma. *Sci. Rep.* **2020**, *10*, 14781. [CrossRef]
32. Hood, D.C.; Raza, A.; de Moraes, C.G.V.; Liebmann, J.M.; Ritch, R. Glaucomatous damage of the macula. *Prog. Retin. Eye Res.* **2013**, *32*, 1–21. [CrossRef]
33. Shakrawal, J.; Sihota, R.; Azad, S.; Kamble, N.; Dada, T. Circumpapillary optical coherence tomography angiography differences in perimetrically affected and unaffected hemispheres in primary open-angle glaucoma and the preperimetric fellow eye. *Indian J. Ophthalmol.* **2021**, *69*, 1120–1126. [CrossRef] [PubMed]
34. Hong, K.L.; Burkemper, B.; Urrea, A.L.; Chang, B.R.; Lee, J.C.; LeTran, V.H.; Chu, Z.; Zhou, X.; Xu, B.Y.; Wong, B.J.; et al. Hemiretinal Asymmetry in Peripapillary Vessel Density in Healthy, Glaucoma Suspect, and Glaucoma Eyes. *Am. J. Ophthalmol.* **2021**, *230*, 156–165. [CrossRef] [PubMed]
35. Lee, E.J.; Han, J.C.; Kee, C. Intereye comparison of ocular factors in normal tension glaucoma with asymmetric visual field loss in Korean population. *PLoS ONE* **2017**, *12*, e0186236. [CrossRef] [PubMed]
36. Lee, J.R.; Kim, S.; Lee, J.Y.; Back, S.; Lee, K.S.; Kook, M.S. Is Myopic Optic Disc Appearance a Risk Factor for Rapid Progression in Medically Treated Glaucomatous Eyes With Confirmed Visual Field Progression? *J. Glaucoma* **2016**, *25*, 330–337. [CrossRef]
37. Qiu, C.; Qian, S.; Sun, X.; Zhou, C.; Meng, F. Axial Myopia Is Associated with Visual Field Prognosis of Primary Open-Angle Glaucoma. *PLoS ONE* **2015**, *10*, e0133189. [CrossRef]
38. Lee, J.Y.; Sung, K.R.; Han, S.; Na, J.H. Effect of Myopia on the Progression of Primary Open-Angle Glaucoma. *Investig. Opthalmology Vis. Sci.* **2015**, *56*, 1775–1781. [CrossRef]

39. Naito, T.; Yoshikawa, K.; Mizoue, S.; Nanno, M.; Kimura, T.; Suzumura, H.; Umeda, Y.; Shiraga, F. Relationship between visual field progression and baseline refraction in primary open-angle glaucoma. *Clin. Ophthalmol.* **2016**, *10*, 1397–1403. [CrossRef]
40. Hou, H.; Moghimi, S.; Zangwill, L.M.; Shoji, T.; Ghahari, E.; Penteado, R.C.; Akagi, T.; Manalastas, P.I.C.; Weinreb, R.N. Macula Vessel Density and Thickness in Early Primary Open-Angle Glaucoma. *Am. J. Ophthalmol.* **2019**, *199*, 120–132. [CrossRef] [PubMed]
41. You, Q.S.; Chan, J.C.H.; Ng, A.L.K.; Choy, B.K.N.; Shih, K.C.; Cheung, J.J.C.; Wong, J.K.W.; Shum, J.W.H.; Ni, M.; Lai, J.S.M.; et al. Macular Vessel Density Measured with Optical Coherence Tomography Angiography and Its Associations in a Large Population-Based Study. *Investig. Opthalmol. Vis. Sci.* **2019**, *60*, 4830–4837. [CrossRef] [PubMed]
42. Flammer, J.; Orgül, S.; Costa, V.P.; Orzalesi, N.; Krieglstein, G.K.; Serra, L.M.; Renard, J.-P.; Stefánsson, E. The impact of ocular blood flow in glaucoma. *Prog. Retin. Eye Res.* **2002**, *21*, 359–393. [CrossRef]
43. Mansouri, K. Optical coherence tomography angiography and glaucoma: Searching for the missing link. *Expert Rev. Med. Devices* **2016**, *13*, 879–880. [CrossRef] [PubMed]
44. Akil, H.; Chopra, V.; Al-Sheikh, M.; Falavarjani, K.G.; Huang, A.S.; Sadda, S.R.; A Francis, B. Swept-source OCT angiography imaging of the macular capillary network in glaucoma. *Br. J. Ophthalmol.* **2017**, *102*, 515–519. [CrossRef] [PubMed]
45. Wan, K.; Lam, A.K.N.; Leung, C.K.-S. Optical Coherence Tomography Angiography Compared With Optical Coherence Tomography Macular Measurements for Detection of Glaucoma. *JAMA Ophthalmol.* **2018**, *136*, 866–874. [CrossRef]

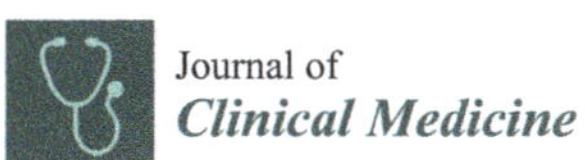

Journal of
Clinical Medicine

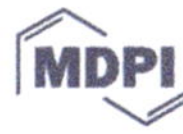

Article

Microvascular and Structural Alterations of the Macula in Early to Moderate Glaucoma: An Optical Coherence Tomography-Angiography Study

Mael Lever [1,2,*], **Moritz Glaser** [2], **Ying Chen** [1,2], **Christian Halfwassen** [1,2], **Jan Darius Unterlauft** [3], **Nikolaos E. Bechrakis** [1,2] and **Michael R. R. Böhm** [1,2]

[1]   Department of Ophthalmology, University Hospital Essen, 45147 Essen, Germany; ying.chen@uk-essen.de (Y.C.); christian.halfwassen@uk-essen.de (C.H.); nikolaos.bechrakis@uk-essen.de (N.E.B.); michael.boehm@uni-due.de (M.R.R.B.)
[2]   Achim Wessing Institute for Imaging in Ophthalmology, University Hospital Essen, 45147 Essen, Germany; moritz.glaser@uni-due.de
[3]   University Hospital of Ophthalmology, Inselspital, 3010 Bern, Switzerland; jandarius.unterlauft@insel.ch
*   Correspondence: mael.lever@uk-essen.de; Tel.: +49-(0)-201-723-2900

Abstract: In glaucoma, macular optical coherence tomography (OCT) typically shows a thinning of the three inner segments and OCT-angiography (OCTA) a reduction of the vascular density (VD). It is still unclear if glaucoma directly affects macular VD. This retrospective study included 31 glaucoma patients of early and moderate stage (GS1, GS2, Mills et al.) and 39 healthy individuals. Macular segments' thickness and superficial and deep plexus vascular density (VD) were obtained using spectral-domain OCT and OCTA, respectively. One-way analysis of variance (ANOVA) was used to compare healthy controls and glaucoma patients according to their glaucoma stage. Using correlation analyses, the association between glaucoma and either OCT or OCTA parameters was evaluated. A glaucoma stage-stratified linear regression analysis was then performed. Inner macular segment and whole retinal thickness were reduced in GS1 and GS2 patients compared to healthy controls (e.g., ganglion cell layer GCL: controls: 47.9 ± 7.4, GS1: 45.8 ± 5.1, GS2: 30.6 ± 9.4, ANOVA: $p < 0.0001$). Regarding OCTA-parameters, the VD of both segmentation levels was reduced in glaucoma patients, particularly when comparing GS2 patients with controls (superficial plexus: $p = 0.004$) and GS2 with GS1 ($p = 0.0008$). Linear regression revealed an association between these parameters and the presence of glaucoma (for superior plexus: $R^2 = 0.059$, $p = 0.043$). Finally, a correlation between macular segment thickness and VD was observed, but with a strength increasing with glaucoma severity (GCL and superior plexus VD: controls: $R^2 = 0.23$, GS1 $R^2 = 0.40$, GS2 $R^2 = 0.76$). Despite the glaucoma-independent correlation between macular segment thickness and VD, disease severity strengthens this correlation. This consideration suggests that glaucoma directly influences OCT and OCTA parameters individually.

Keywords: glaucoma; macula; macular segmentation; optical coherence tomography-angiography; vascular density; blood flow; biomarker

Citation: Lever, M.; Glaser, M.; Chen, Y.; Halfwassen, C.; Unterlauft, J.D.; Bechrakis, N.E.; Böhm, M.R.R. Microvascular and Structural Alterations of the Macula in Early to Moderate Glaucoma: An Optical Coherence Tomography-Angiography Study. *J. Clin. Med.* **2021**, *10*, 5017. https://doi.org/10.3390/jcm10215017

Academic Editors: Jose Javier Garcia-Medina and Maria Dolores Pinazo-Duran

Received: 30 September 2021
Accepted: 25 October 2021
Published: 28 October 2021

Publisher's Note: MDPI stays neutral with regard to jurisdictional claims in published maps and institutional affiliations.

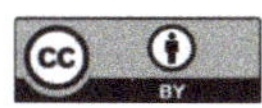

1. Introduction

Over the last two decades, advances in imaging techniques have led to significant changes to the diagnosis and management of ophthalmic conditions. Optical coherence tomography (OCT) is one of the most important of them. In glaucoma, OCT provides precise and objective structural measurements of the optic nerve head (ONH) and of the macula. These data have become crucial to assess the presence and the degree of severity of the disease. OCT measurements were shown to correlate with basic ophthalmologic glaucoma criteria like intraocular pressure (IOP) and ONH cupping, as well as ocular function like visual field perception [1]. While OCT is not recommended as a standalone glaucoma diagnostic tool, it greatly complements more subjective ophthalmologic parameters [2].

Initial research on OCT in glaucoma focused on ONH affection (e.g., peripapillary retinal nerve fiber (RNFL) thickness [3], cupping [4], and Bruch membrane opening [5]). More recent studies also identified macular changes that were useful for the management of glaucoma in adults [6] and children [7]. In particular, the thickness of the three innermost segments of the macula—the nerve fiber layer (NFL), ganglion cell layer (GCL), and inner plexiform layer (IPL), summarized as ganglion cell complex (GCC)—constitutes a reliable biomarker for assessing glaucoma severity and progression [8]. Compared to ONH, the macula presents structural advantages, which reduce possible measurement artifacts and enhance the reliability of the measurements [9]: the macula shows less interindividual variability than the peripapillary RNFL thickness [10], and it lacks blood vessels. These advantages justify the use of macular diagnostic tools for the management of glaucoma patients.

Finally, recent technical improvements to OCT technology led to the development of OCT-angiography (OCTA). In OCTA, up to 100,000 A-scans per second are performed to indirectly detect retinal blood flow [11]. Consecutive computation of the obtained data provides a precise evaluation of retinal and choroidal blood vessel density (VD) without the need for an intravenous dye as in fluoresceine angiography. The obtained three-dimensional representation of the ONH or macula allows for the VD quantification of a superficial and a deep vascular plexus, and measurements of associated parameters such as the surface of the foveal avascular zone (FAZ) [11]. In glaucoma patients, a reduction of the VD was first observed at the ONH [12] and later also at the macula [13]. The following research in glaucoma patients showed that VD quantification using OCTA is reproducible [14], can discriminate between glaucoma and healthy eyes [15,16], and correlates with disease progression [17] and visual function [18].

As already reported, both OCT and OCTA measure different structural characteristics of the macula, and thus a certain correlation between both diagnostic methods has been observed [16]. Yet, the pathophysiological mechanisms that lead to a reduction of VD in glaucoma are still unclear. To help determine if glaucoma has a direct effect on macular VD or indirectly through the reduction of macular thickness, we selected patients with early to moderate glaucoma and measured the alterations of macular segment thickness and OCTA parameters in comparison to healthy adults. These results were then used to analyze the correlation between both diagnostic parameters and to evaluate what individual effect glaucoma has on them.

2. Materials and Methods

2.1. Study Design

Retrospective chart analysis of patients from whom a macular OCT and OCTA was acquired between May and September 2019 at the Department of Ophthalmology of the University Hospital Essen, Germany. Patients of 18 to 85 years of age were included to the study based on the presence of early glaucoma (defined as stage 1 or stage 2 according to the Mills et al. [19] classification) or the absence of a retinal disease or optic nerve pathology other than glaucoma (healthy controls). Exclusion criteria were a history of ocular trauma or intraocular surgery (excluding uncomplicated cataract surgery), refractive errors > 3 diopters, advanced lens opacity/cataract, the presence of any systemic disease (in particular cardiovascular or neurologic), and current vasoactive systemic medication. Charts lacking data of best corrected visual acuity (BCVA), IOP, anterior segment examination, and/or fundoscopy were also excluded from the study. The eye with the best OCT image quality was selected for further analysis. This study was conducted in accordance with the 1964 Declaration of Helsinki and was approved by the ethics committee of the University Hospital Essen, Germany (approval number: 19-8840-BO).

2.2. Data Acquisition

A comprehensive ophthalmic examination was performed, including review of past medical history and current medication, determination of BCVA, slit-lamp examination of the anterior and posterior eye segment, and measurement of IOP (Goldmann applanation tonometer, Haag-Streit, Bern, Switzerland). For glaucoma patients, the examination also included an evaluation of the optic disc linear cup-to-disc ratio (CDR) and stereoscopic ONH photography, the measurement of the central corneal thickness (CCT; TX-20P tonometer, Canon Medical Systems, Zoetermeer, The Netherlands), and a visual field examination using 30-2 static automated perimetry (Twinfield 2, OCULUS Optikgeräte, Wetzlar, Germany).

Macular spectral domain-OCT and OCTA were obtained using a SPECTRALIS® HRA+OCT (Heidelberg Engineering, Heidelberg, Germany). Corneal curvature values (c-curve) were known for all patients. At least two consecutive examinations of sufficient image quality (quality score $\geq$ 20) were obtained. For macular OCT, 25 single horizontal axial scans centered to the fovea were acquired. Using the manufacturer's software, image segmentation was calculated to obtain individual retinal layer thicknesses: total retinal thickness (TRT), nerve fiber layer (NFL), ganglion cell layer (GCL), inner plexiform layer (IPL), inner nuclear layer (INL), outer plexiform layer (OPL), and outer nuclear layer (ONL) (Figure 1c). Additionally, the NFL, GCL, IPL, INL, OPL, and ONL segments were combined as inner retinal layers (IRL). Results of the semi-automated segmentation were inspected and corrected manually if necessary. Thickness results were divided into nine subfields using the 1, 2.22, 3.45 mm grid of the Early Treatment Diabetic Retinopathy Study (ETDRS) (Figure 1b). Thickness values of each subfield were exported using a software plug-in provided by the device manufacturer. For OCTA, the vessel density (VD) of the superficial (SVP) and deep vascular plexus (DVP), as well as the area of the foveal avascular zone (FAZ, in mm^2), were extracted and analyzed using the ImageJ software (Wayne Rasband, version 1.52e).

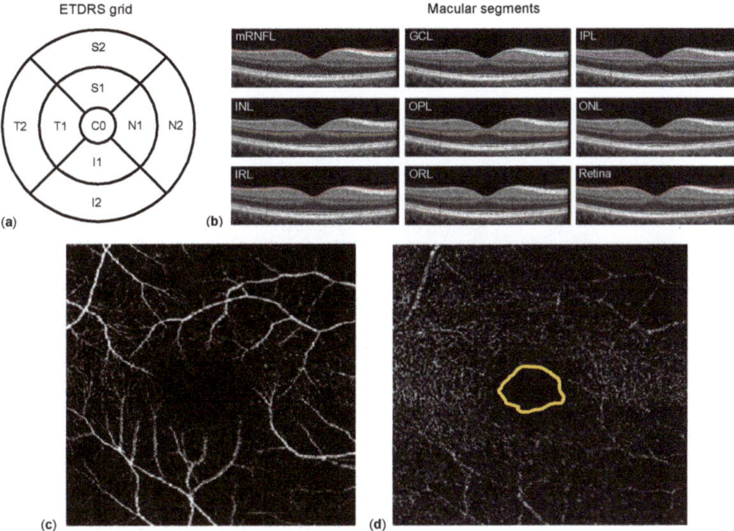

Figure 1. Methodology. (**a**) Representation of the Early Treatment Diabetic Retinopathy Study (ETDRS) grid 1, 2.22, 3.45 mm, which contains nine subfields (C0: center; S1 and S2 superior, N1 and N2 nasal, I1 and I2 inferior, and T1 and T2 temporal) and is used for thickness measurements. The macular segments (**b**) are separated semi-automatically by optical coherence tomography (OCT) software: nerve fiber layer (NFL), ganglion cell layer (GCL), inner plexiform layer (IPL), inner nuclear layer (INL), outer plexiform layer (OPL), outer nuclear layer (ONL)—together inner retinal layers (IRL)—and outer retinal layers (ORL). Example of the superior (**c**) and deep (**d**) vascular plexus of the macula obtained using OCT-angiography; the foveal avascular zone is located within the orange line in (**d**).

2.3. Statistical Methods

Numerical data were collected in Microsoft Excel (Microsoft, Redmond, WA, USA). Normal distribution was examined using the D'Agostino and Pearson normality test. Mean values were compared applying Student's *t*-test, or Mann–Whitney U test, when appropriate. One-way ANOVA was performed to compare multiple subgroups, and the Tukey method was applied for multiple comparison correction in post-hoc analyses. Correlation between parameters was evaluated calculating Pearson or Spearman correlation factors, when appropriate. The statistical analyses were performed using SAS Studio version 3.8 (SAS Institute Inc., Cary, NC, USA) and Prism 9.1 (GraphPad, La Jolla, CA, USA). In the results section of this article, dichotomous variables are presented as absolute and relative frequencies (*n*, %), continuous variables are presented as mean ± standard deviation (SD), and categoric variables as median ± interquartile range (IQR). In general, statistical significance was assumed for $p < 0.05$.

3. Results

3.1. Patients' Characteristics

Seventy patients aged 63.0 ± 13.1 years (range: 37–88 years) were included in this study. Age distribution was comparable among glaucoma patients (*n* = 31, 44%) and healthy controls (*n* = 39, 56%). Among the 31 glaucoma patients, disease severity was evaluated as stage 1 according to Mills et al. [19] in 22 cases (71%); stage 2 was identified in nine patients (29%). Male sex was slightly underrepresented in the whole study population (46%). This trend was also similar in the glaucoma and control subgroups. The median BCVA was 0.1 LogMAR (IQR: 0.1); 16% of glaucoma patients had a history of cataract surgery at the time of examination, and this was also the case for 12% of control participants. The overall mean IOP was 13.6 ± 3.0 mm Hg; in the control group, the mean IOP was 14.1 ± 3.2 mm Hg, compared to 12.7 ± 2.0 mm Hg in glaucoma patients. This difference is explained by the antiglaucomatous therapy in the glaucoma group, consisting of a median of 3 topical agents. Epidemiologic data are presented in Table 1.

Table 1. Epidemiologic and general ophthalmologic characteristics of patients.

Parameter	Value	*p*-Value [1]
Patients (*n*)	70	
Sex (male:female % (*n*))	46:54% (32:38)	
Glaucoma	45:55% (14:17)	
Healthy	46:54% (18:21)	
Eye (right:left % (*n*))	56:44% (39:31)	
Diagnosis (glaucoma: healthy % (*n*))	44:56% (31:39)	
Stage 1 (% of glaucoma (*n*))	71.0% (22)	
Stage 2 (% of glaucoma (*n*))	29.0% (9)	
Age (mean ± SD (y))	63.0 ± 13.1	
Glaucoma	63.8 ± 14.0	0.64
Glaucoma stage 1	64.7 ± 14.8	0.52
Glaucoma stage 2	61.8 ± 12.5	0.90
Healthy	62.4 ± 12.5	
BCVA (median ± IQR (LogMar))	0.1 ± 0.1	
Glaucoma	0.1 ± 0.2	0.23
Healthy	0.0 ± 0.1	
IOP (mean ± SD (mm Hg))	13.6 ± 3.0	
Glaucoma	12.7 ± 2.0	0.066
Healthy	14.1 ± 3.2	

Table 1. *Cont.*

Parameter	Value	*p*-Value [1]
Linear CDR * (median ± IQR)	0.7 ± 0.3	
Perimetry (MD) * (mean ± SD (dB))	2.0 ± 4.3	

[1] *p*-values of *t*-test (age, IOP, and BCVA) between the healthy controls and the respective glaucoma group. * Parameters displaying only data of the glaucoma group. Abbreviations: BCVA: best corrected visual acuity; IOP: intraocular pressure; CDR: cup-to-disc ratio (by fundoscopy and/or ONH photography); y: years; MD: mean deviation; dB: decibel; SD: standard deviation; and IQR: interquartile range.

3.2. Differences in Macular Segment Thickness between Glaucoma and Healthy

First, an analysis of the thickness of the whole macula and its segments was performed for all subfields of the ETDRS grid. To compare results of glaucoma stage 1 and 2 patients and healthy control participants, a one-way ANOVA was performed. The analysis revealed a statistically significant difference between the three groups for the GCL and IPL in all subfields but C0 (e.g., S2 subfield of GCL: controls: 47.9 ± 7.4, GS1: 45.8 ± 5.1, GS2: 30.6 ± 9.4, *p* < 0.0001). A similar observation appeared for measurements of the whole retina and the IRL (e.g., S2 subfield of whole retina: controls: 333.6 ± 18.8, GS1: 333.0 ± 18.0, GS2: 311.8 ± 28.7, *p* = 0.014). The post-hoc analysis returned statistically significant results for the comparison of the control and GS2 groups and of the GS1 and GS2 groups. Even though no such difference was present for the comparison of controls with GS1, a constant trend of GS1 patients having a slightly thinner GCL, IPL, IRL, and whole retina is visible. For measurements of the NFL, INL, OPL and ONL, as well as for ORL, no such difference could be discerned in our cohort (data not shown). Table 2 presents an excerpt of these measurements and ANOVA results. A graphical presentation of the results for the whole retina and for GCL is provided in Figure 2.

Table 2. Macular segment thickness differs between glaucoma patients and healthy controls. The table presents the mean thickness of selected macular segment sectors and the results of one-way ANOVA comparing thickness of each subfield in patients with glaucoma stage 1, stage 2, and healthy controls. The comparison of controls and glaucoma stage 1 patients almost never returned a statistically significant difference and thus is not presented here.

Macular Segment	Mean Thickness (µm) ± SD			ANOVA Summary		Adjusted *p*-Value	
	Controls	Glaucoma Stage 1 (GS1)	Glaucoma Stage 2 (GS2)	F	*p*-Value	Controls vs. GS2	GS1 vs. GS2
			Retina				
Inner superior (S1)	335.4 ± 20.0	337.2 ± 21.0	314.2 ± 20.5	4.54	0.014	0.018	0.016
Outer superior (S2)	333.6 ± 18.8	333.0 ± 18.0	311.8 ± 28.7	4.59	0.014	0.012	0.024
Inner inferior (I1)	337.0 ± 14.9	333.5 ± 20.9	301.8 ± 23.1	14.1	<0.0001	<0.0001	0.0001
Outer inferior (I2)	327.6 ± 8.7	327.5 ± 17.9	305.7 ± 17.9	5.57	0.0058	0.0054	0.010
			Ganglion cell layer				
Inner superior (S1)	47.6 ± 9.6	48.1 ± 9.8	31.1 ± 10.3	11.8	<0.0001	<0.0001	<0.0001
Outer superior (S2)	47.9 ± 7.4	45.8 ± 5.1	30.6 ± 9.4	23.3	<0.0001	<0.0001	<0.0001
Inner inferior (I1)	49.4 ± 7.2	44.5 ± 11.1	23.9 ± 12.2	27.7	<0.0001	<0.0001	<0.0001
Outer inferior (I2)	47.7 ± 5.9	45.8 ± 8.2	28.2 ± 9.1	28.1	<0.0001	<0.0001	<0.0001
			Inner plexiform layer				
Inner superior (S1)	39.8 ± 5.5	39.8 ± 5.1	30.1 ± 6.8	11.9	<0.0001	<0.0001	0.0001
Outer superior (S2)	38.3 ± 4.8	37.3 ± 4.1	27.7 ± 7.3	16.8	<0.0001	<0.0001	<0.0001
Inner inferior (I1)	40.3 ± 4.2	38.0 ± 6.1	27.4 ± 8.3	19.8	<0.0001	<0.0001	<0.0001
Outer inferior (I2)	37.7 ± 4.4	37.2 ± 5.2	27.2 ± 5.4	18.5	<0.0001	<0.0001	<0.0001

p-values of ANOVA (analysis of variance). Abbreviation: SD, standard deviation.

3.3. Macular Vasculature Differences between Glaucoma Patients and Healthy Controls

Regarding the macular vascular parameters provided by OCTA, no significant difference appeared when comparing all glaucoma patients and control group (Table 3). However, the separate analysis of stage 1 and stage 2 glaucoma patients using one-way

ANOVA returned statistical differences between the three groups. This was apparent for the vascular density (VD) of the superficial plexus ($p = 0.0011$) and of the deep plexus ($p = 0.0072$) (Table 4). The additional post-hoc analysis revealed a difference predominantly between controls and the GS2 group as well as between the GS1 and GS2 groups, but not between controls and GS1 (Figure 3).

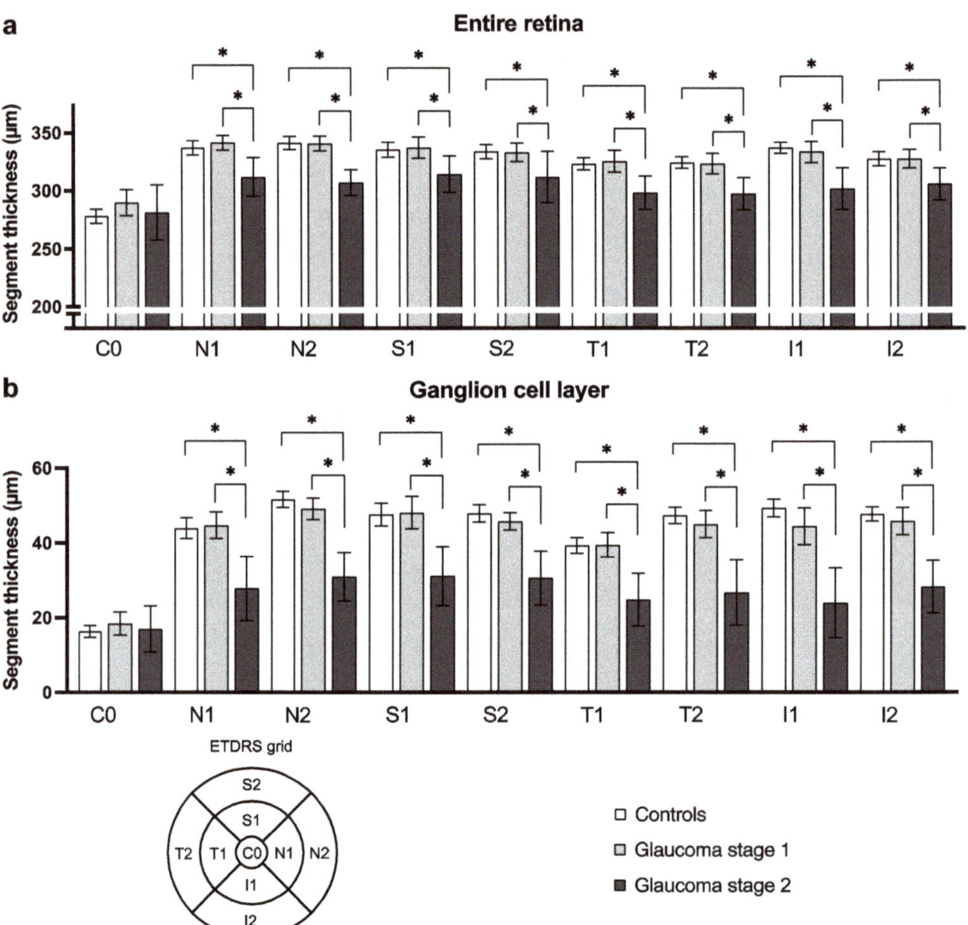

Figure 2. Retina and ganglion cell layer subfields' thickness differs between glaucoma patients and healthy controls. The figure depicts for exemplary purpose the mean thickness and 95% confidence interval of subfield thickness for the entire retina (**a**) and for the ganglion cell layer (**b**). Statistically significant results of one-way ANOVA comparing each subfield's mean thickness in patients with glaucoma stage 1, stage 2, and healthy controls are represented (* when $p < 0.05$). Abbreviations: subfields C0, center; S1, inner superior; S2, outer superior; N1, inner nasal; N2, outer nasal; I1, inner inferior; I2, outer inferior; T1, inner temporal; and T2, outer temporal, as shown in the ETDRS grid legend.

To evaluate if OCTA parameters correlate with the presence of glaucoma, we calculated the Spearman correlation factor between OCTA parameters and glaucoma stage. For all three parameters—FAZ area and VD of the superficial and deep plexus—no correlation was detected (data not shown). Further, we performed univariate linear regression analysis, which returned a weak association between the glaucoma stage and VD of both plexuses (superior plexus: $R^2 = 0.059$, deep plexus: $R^2 = 0.058$) (Table 5).

Table 3. OCTA parameters in glaucoma patients and healthy controls. The table displays the mean ± standard deviation and Students *t*-test (for SVP and DVP) and Mann–Whitney U results (for FAZ) of the foveal avascular zone area (FAZ) and vascular density (VD) of the macular superficial (SVP) and deep plexus (DVP) in glaucoma patients and healthy controls.

	Controls	Glaucoma	*p*-Value	Glaucoma Stage 1	Glaucoma Stage 2
FAZ area (mm^2)	0.28 ± 0.11	0.31 ± 0.16	0.37	0.29 ± 0.13	0.34 ± 0.23
Superior plexus VD (%)	27.0 ± 5.8	26.1 ± 8.6	0.58	29.0 ± 7.4	19.0 ± 7.4
Deep plexus VD (%)	25.8 ± 5.4	24.7 ± 6.4	0.42	26.7 ± 5.7	19.8 ± 5.7

Abbreviations: OCTA: optical coherence tomography-angiography.

Table 4. Summary of one-way ANOVA results for OCTA parameters between glaucoma patients and healthy controls. The table displays results of the one-way analysis of variance (ANOVA) comparing optical coherence tomography-angiography (OCTA) parameters of healthy controls and glaucoma patients of stage 1 (GS1) and stage 2 (GS2).

	F of ANOVA	*p*-Value	Mean Difference	95% CI	Adjusted *p*-Value
FAZ (mm^2)	0.84	0.44			
Controls vs. GS1			−0.015	−0.10 to 0.071	0.91
Controls vs. GS2			−0.064	−0.18 to 0.055	0.40
GS1 vs. GS2			−0.050	−0.18 to 0.078	0.62
Superior plexus (%)	7.8	**0.0011**			
Controls vs. GS1			−1.9	−6.1 to 2.3	0.52
Controls vs. GS2			8.0	2.2 to 13.8	**0.0040**
GS1 vs. GS2			9.9	3.8 to 16.1	**0.0008**
Deep plexus (%)	5.3	**0.0072**			
Controls vs. GS1			−0.85	−4.4 to 2.7	0.83
Controls vs. GS2			6.1	1.1 to 11.0	**0.0120**
GS1 vs. GS2			6.9	1.6 to 12.2	**0.0069**

p-Values are bold and underlined when statistically significant ($p < 0.05$). Abbreviation: FAZ: foveal avascular zone, 95% CI: 95% confidence interval of the mean difference.

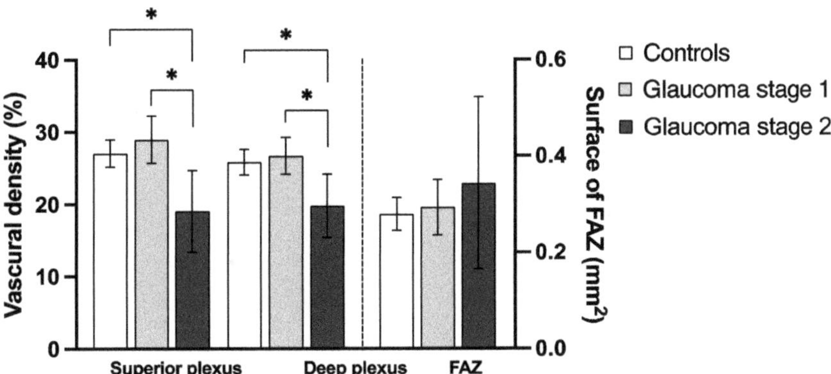

Figure 3. Superficial and deep vascular density of the macula differ between glaucoma patients and controls. This figure shows the comparison (mean and 95% confidence interval) of optical coherence tomography-angiography (OCTA) parameters between healthy controls (white bars) and glaucoma patients of stage 1 (light grey) and 2 (dark grey). Statistically significant results ($p < 0.05$) of one-way ANOVA are marked with an asterisk *. Abbreviation: FAZ, foveal avascular zone.

Table 5. Linear regression analysis between OCTA parameters and glaucoma stage. The table displays the results of univariate linear regression between the glaucoma stage and optical coherence tomography-angiography (OCTA) parameters: foveal avascular zone surface (FAZ) and vascular density of the macular superficial and deep plexus.

	Parameter Estimate	95% CI	R^2	*p*-Value
FAZ	0.78	−0.50 to 2.1	0.021	0.23
Superior plexus	−0.024	−0.048 to −0.00079	0.059	**0.043**
Deep plexus	−0.029	−0.058 to −0.00075	0.058	**0.045**

p-Values are bold and underlined when statistically significant ($p < 0.05$). Abbreviations: FAZ: foveal avascular zone, 95% CI: 95% confidence interval of the parameter estimate, and R^2: Tjur's pseudo R^2.

3.4. Correlation of Vascular Density and Macular Segment Thickness

Finally, to evaluate the strength of the association between macular segment thickness and VD of the superficial and deep plexuses, a correlation analysis between all subfields of all macular segments and the vascular density of the superior and deep plexus was performed. The parameters with the highest correlation factor in the entire cohort and in glaucoma stage 2 patients were selected for further regression modelling. Regarding the superior plexus, the T2 subfield of the GCL was selected (entire cohort: Pearson r = 0.67, 95% CI: 0.52–0.78; GS2: Pearson r = 0.87, 95% CI: 0.50–0.97). Regarding the deep plexus, the N2 subfield of IPL showed the highest correlation in both groups (entire cohort: Pearson r = 0.45, 95% CI: 0.24–0.62; GS2: Pearson r = 0.82, 95% CI: 0.33–0.96). A univariate linear regression analysis was performed using the selected parameter as independent variable. This analysis showed that the strengths of association between GCL thickness (T2 subfield) and vascular density increases with glaucoma severity. According to our results, an intermediate association is detectable in controls ($R^2 = 0.23$), as well as in GS1 patients ($R^2 = 0.40$), and a strong association in GS2 patients ($R^2 = 0.76$). Similarly, the strengths of association between IPL thickness (N2 subfield) and glaucoma increase with disease severity: R^2 is low — shows no association — in controls ($R^2 = 0.027$) and in GS1 patients ($R^2 = 0.097$) but high – shows a strong association – in GS2 patients ($R^2 = 0.66$). These results are presented in Table 6.

Table 6. Correlation between vascular density and macular segment thickness is strongest in glaucoma patients. The table presents the results of univariate linear regression analysis between either the outer temporal (T2) subfield of the ganglion cell layer (GCL) and the VD of the superficial plexus, or between the outer nasal (N2) subfield of the inner plexiform layer (IPL) and the VD of the deep plexus in optical coherence tomography-angiography.

	Parameter Estimate	95% CI	R^2
T2 of GCL → superficial plexus vascular density			
Controls	0.41	0.16 to 0.66	0.23
Glaucoma stage 1	0.57	0.24 to 0.89	0.40
Glaucoma stage 2	0.56	0.28 to 0.84	0.76
N2 of IPL → deep plexus vascular density			
Controls	0.19	−0.19 to 0.57	0.027
Glaucoma stage 1	0.43	−0.18 to 1.0	0.097
Glaucoma stage 2	0.74	0.27 to 1.0	0.66

Abbreviation: 95% CI, 95% confidence interval.

4. Discussion

The present study investigates the relation between macular segments' thickness as well as OCTA-assessed vascular density in the context of early or moderate glaucoma. The main findings of the study are:

- The vascular density of the deep and superficial plexus is reduced in glaucoma and correlates with the presence of glaucoma.

- Differences in macular vascular density are mainly detectable in GS2 but less so in GS1 eyes.
- The foveal avascular zone is not affected by glaucoma.
- Glaucoma severity directly influences the strength of association between macular inner segments' thickness and vascular density.

The study population analyzed in the present work is composed of healthy participants and patients with early or moderate glaucoma (as defined by Mills et al. [19]). Adult participants of a wide age range of 37 to 88 years were included, and the gender distribution was comparable between all subgroups. A comparison of the macular segments' thickness was performed between healthy controls and glaucoma patients, and between glaucoma stages. The present analysis showed a reduction of inner macular segment thickness (the GCL and IPL), in all ETDRS subfields except C0. This observation is consistent with recent reports about the glaucoma-induced loss of retinal ganglion cells located in the inner retinal layers [20] and the subsequent thinning of these layers. Similar observations were made in both adults [16,21] and children [7]. While macular diagnostics in glaucoma focuses mainly on the NFL, GCL, and IPL thickness (summarized as GCC, [21]), the presented one-way ANOVA also showed a thickness reduction of the entire retinal thickness and of the inner retinal layers (IRL). Additionally, the post-hoc analysis revealed a trend towards a thinning of the GCL and IPL between GS1 patients and controls. This difference is statistically significant between GS2 patients and controls as well as between GS2 and GS1 patients. These observations are in line with previous work stating that structural macular deterioration occurs early in glaucoma [22], even prior to detectable functional (perimetric) damage [23].

In most open-angle glaucoma patients, the glaucoma-induced structural retinal changes are explained by elevated IOP [24]. In addition to this, a vascular etiology for glaucoma progression was proposed [25]. This hypothesis is fueled by the possible occurrence and progression of glaucoma despite a seemingly acceptable IOP, which is qualified as normal tension glaucoma (NTG). The dysregulation of ocular blood flow observed in NTG patients is thought to be their leading pathophysiological mechanism [26]. Ocular blood flow monitoring never gained clinical relevance due to practicability reasons, high interindividual variability, and a lack of reproducible quantitative measurement methods. This trend changed with the development of OCT-angiography, which allows for a quantitative and objective, dye-free, and non-invasive method to measure blood flow at the optic nerve head [12]. Later, vascular density changes in glaucoma patients were also described at the macula [13]. The present study showed macular VD differences between early to moderate glaucoma patients and healthy individuals. Our analyses showed a clear reduction of VD in superficial and deep macular plexuses in GS2 patients compared to both controls and GS1 patients. While it may be unexpected that controls and GS1 patients show a similar VD, this lack of statistical difference could be explained by the relatively high mean age in our cohort or by a number of participants too low to detect a slight difference between both subgroups. Overall, our observations are in line with recent publications: while early studies described the decrease of the superficial plexus VD in glaucoma patients [13,15], newer investigations observed additional differences in the deep plexus [17,27]. The provided additional linear regression analyses returned a weak but statistically significant association between vascular density of both superficial and deep macular plexuses and glaucoma stage (no glaucoma, GS1, and GS2). This observation is similar to recent works studying the glaucoma diagnostic ability of macular OCTA measurements [16,28].

When studying macular OCTA parameters, FAZ area in our study population was also analyzed. FAZ area is known to increase in retinopathies involving ischemia (e.g., diabetic retinopathy) [29,30]. However, this does not seem to be the case in glaucoma. Accordingly, our results show no difference in FAZ size between healthy controls and glaucoma patients regardless of the disease stage. This was also observed recently by Lommatzsch et al. [31] for glaucoma patients with peripheral visual field defects, whereas patients with central VF defects (not present in our study) had an enlarged FAZ. This can be explained by the fact that the fovea only consists of photoreceptors, which are usually not directly affected in glaucoma. Additionally, the lacking difference between FAZ area in glaucomatous and healthy eyes is comparable to the lacking difference of C0 ETDRS-subfield thickness between these groups. In summary, the FAZ does not seem to be an informative biomarker for quantifying glaucomatous damage.

In the present study population, inner macular segment thickness and VD are both reduced in glaucoma patients compared the healthy controls. The fact that glaucoma leads to a reduced GCC thickness is well recognized [8], and a comparable effect of glaucoma on macular VD was also observed in the present study (Table 5) and described previously [18]. As these parameters both characterize a different aspect of the same anatomic region (i.e., the macula), it could be possible that glaucoma does not affect macular thickness and VD independently but rather influence one parameter (e.g., VD), leading to an indirect affection of the other parameter (e.g., macular thickness). To verify this hypothesis, a glaucoma stage-stratified quantification of the association between VD and inner macular thickness was performed. A notable strength of the present study population is its reduction of other potential confounders for macular parameters: the age and sex distribution are highly consistent between the control and glaucoma groups, and comorbidities knowingly altering retinal blood flow or macular thickness measurements by OCT(A) were excluded. Our analysis of the whole cohort returned a moderate correlation between GCL and IPL, and the macular VD. This suggests that a reduced VD correlates with a reduced macular segment thickness (and vice versa), which has been described previously in POAG [16] and NTG patients [18]. However, the glaucoma stage-stratified analysis revealed a stronger correlation between inner segment thickness and macular VD in GS2 patients than in GS1 patients or healthy controls: the goodness-of-fit of linear regression (R^2) increased along with disease severity. This allows one to postulate that glaucoma is causing a reduction of macular inner segment thickness and vascular density in addition to the physiological association between these two parameters. It is still unclear whether RGC loss (e.g., inner macular segment thinning) is the cause or the consequence of vascular density reduction, but the present analysis adds up to the common assumption that glaucoma severity is strongly associated with both inner macular thickness and VD.

The present study has several limitations that need to be discussed. First, it is unclear how topic antiglaucomatous medication affects ocular blood flow and OCTA measurements, which weakens the validity of comparisons of glaucoma patients and medication-naïve controls. Similarly, a possible vasoactive effect of phenylephrine used for pupil dilatation prior to OCTA measurements could also not be ruled out. Further, it must be noted that segmentation differences between devices of different manufacturers can affect the comparability of the present results with other studies. Another aspect influencing results reproducibility is the present use of 3×3 mm scans, as other scan sizes (6×6 mm or even 9×9 mm) might return different results. Finally, the relatively small size of the cohort analyzed here, the focus on early to moderate glaucoma, and absence of preperimetric patients do not allow for generalization of the present results, particularly for advanced glaucoma stages.

5. Conclusions

Using OCT and OCTA to identify and monitor the structural and vascular changes at the macula in glaucoma patients is gaining in clinical relevance. In the present study, an inner macular segment thinning is present in early to moderate glaucoma. Regarding OCTA-parameters, the vascular density of the superficial and deep plexuses is reduced compared to healthy controls, whereas no difference of the foveal avascular zone area is visible. Finally, a correlation between inner macular segment thickness and superficial and deep plexus vascular density is already present in healthy individuals. However, the strength of this association seems to be directly influenced by glaucoma severity, suggesting that glaucoma directly affects both diagnostic parameters.

Author Contributions: Conceptualization, M.G., Y.C., M.L. and M.R.R.B.; Data curation, M.G. and M.L.; Formal analysis, M.G., M.L. and M.R.R.B.; Funding acquisition, M.L., N.E.B. and M.R.R.B.; Investigation, M.G., Y.C., M.L., C.H. and M.R.R.B.; Methodology, M.L., M.G., Y.C. and M.R.R.B.; Project administration, M.G., M.L. and M.R.R.B.; Resources, N.E.B. and M.R.R.B.; Supervision, N.E.B. and M.R.R.B.; Validation, M.L., M.G., Y.C., C.H., J.D.U. and M.R.R.B.; Visualization, M.L., M.G. and M.R.R.B.; Writing—Original draft, M.L.; Writing—Review and editing, M.L., M.G., Y.C., C.H., J.D.U., N.E.B. and M.R.R.B. All authors have read and agreed to the published version of the manuscript.

Funding: The APC was funded by the Open Access Publication Fund of the University of Duisburg-Essen, 45147 Essen, Germany.

Institutional Review Board Statement: The study was conducted according to the guidelines of the Declaration of Helsinki and approved by the Ethics Committee of the University Hospital Essen, Germany (approval number: 19-8840-BO, 1 August 2019).

Informed Consent Statement: Patient consent was waived due to the retrospective design of the study.

Data Availability Statement: The data supporting the reported results can be provided by the corresponding author on reasonable request.

Acknowledgments: Heidelberg Engineering (Heidelberg, Germany) kindly provided the SPECTRALIS® HRA+OCT with OCTA module for the time of data acquisition.

Conflicts of Interest: The authors declare no conflict of interest. The funders had no role in the design of the study; in the collection, analyses, or interpretation of data; in the writing of the manuscript; or in the decision to publish the results.

References

1. Medeiros, F.A.; Zangwill, L.M.; Bowd, C.; Mansouri, K.; Weinreb, R.N. The structure and function relationship in glaucoma: Implications for detection of progression and measurement of rates of change. *Investig. Ophthalmol. Vis. Sci.* **2012**, *53*, 6939–6946. [CrossRef] [PubMed]
2. Lever, M.; Unterlauft, J.D.; Halfwassen, C.; Bechrakis, N.E.; Manthey, A.; Böhm, M.R.R. Individualized Significance of 24-Hour Intraocular Pressure Curves for Therapeutic Decisions in Primary Chronic Open-Angle Glaucoma Patients. *Clin. Ophthalmol.* **2020**, *14*, 1483–1494. [CrossRef] [PubMed]
3. Abe, R.Y.; Gracitelli, C.P.B.; Medeiros, F.A. The Use of Spectral-Domain Optical Coherence Tomography to Detect Glaucoma Progression. *Open Ophthalmol. J.* **2015**, *9*, 78–88. [CrossRef] [PubMed]
4. Yoshikawa, M.; Akagi, T.; Hangai, M.; Ohashi-Ikeda, H.; Takayama, K.; Morooka, S.; Kimura, Y.; Nakano, N.; Yoshimura, N. Alterations in the neural and connective tissue components of glaucomatous cupping after glaucoma surgery using swept-source optical coherence tomography. *Investig. Ophthalmol. Vis. Sci.* **2014**, *55*, 477–484. [CrossRef]
5. Enders, P.; Longo, V.; Adler, W.; Horstmann, J.; Schaub, F.; Dietlein, T.; Cursiefen, C.; Heindl, L.M. Analysis of peripapillary vessel density and Bruch's membrane opening-based neuroretinal rim parameters in glaucoma using OCT and OCT-angiography. *Eye* **2020**, *34*, 1086–1093. [CrossRef]
6. Unterlauft, J.D.; Rehak, M.; Böhm, M.R.R.; Rauscher, F.G. Analyzing the impact of glaucoma on the macular architecture using spectral-domain optical coherence tomography. *PLoS ONE* **2018**, *13*, e0209610. [CrossRef] [PubMed]
7. Lever, M.; Halfwassen, C.; Unterlauft, J.D.; Bechrakis, N.E.; Manthey, A.; Böhm, M.R.R. The Paediatric Glaucoma Diagnostic Ability of Optical Coherence Tomography: A Comparison of Macular Segmentation and Peripapillary Retinal Nerve Fibre Layer Thickness. *Biology* **2021**, *10*, 260. [CrossRef]
8. Renard, J.P.; Fénolland, J.R.; Giraud, J.M. Glaucoma progression analysis by Spectral-Domain Optical Coherence Tomography (SD-OCT). *J. Fr. Ophtalmol.* **2019**, *42*, 499–516. [CrossRef] [PubMed]
9. Sung, K.R.; Wollstein, G.; Kim, N.R.; Na, J.H.; Nevins, J.E.; Kim, C.Y.; Schuman, J.S. Macular assessment using optical coherence tomography for glaucoma diagnosis. *Br. J. Ophthalmol.* **2012**, *96*, 1452–1455. [CrossRef] [PubMed]
10. Oddone, F.; Lucenteforte, E.; Michelessi, M.; Rizzo, S.; Donati, S.; Parravano, M.; Virgili, G. Macular versus Retinal Nerve Fiber Layer Parameters for Diagnosing Manifest Glaucoma: A Systematic Review of Diagnostic Accuracy Studies. *Ophthalmology* **2016**, *123*, 939–949. [CrossRef] [PubMed]
11. Lommatzsch, A. OCT Angiography. *Klin. Monbl. Augenheilkd.* **2020**, *237*, 95–111. [CrossRef] [PubMed]
12. Jia, Y.; Morrison, J.C.; Tokayer, J.; Tan, O.; Lombardi, L.; Baumann, B.; Lu, C.D.; Choi, W.; Fujimoto, J.G.; Huang, D. [BOE]2012 Quantitative OCT angiography of optic nerve.pdf. Biomed. *Opt. Express* **2012**, *3*, 183–189.
13. Xu, H.; Kong, X.M. Study of retinal microvascular perfusion alteration and structural damage at macular region in primary open-angle glaucoma patients. *Zhonghua Yan Ke Za Zhi* **2017**, *53*, 98–103. [CrossRef] [PubMed]
14. Manalastas, P.I.C.; Zangwill, L.M.; Saunders, L.J.; Mansouri, K.; Belghith, A.; Suh, M.H.; Yarmohammadi, A.; Penteado, R.C.; Akagi, T.; Shoji, T.; et al. Reproducibility of optical coherence tomography angiography macular and optic nerve head vascular density in glaucoma and healthy eyes. *J. Glaucoma* **2017**, *26*, 851–859. [CrossRef] [PubMed]

15. Rao, H.L.; Pradhan, Z.S.; Weinreb, R.N.; Riyazuddin, M.; Dasari, S.; Venugopal, J.P.; Puttaiah, N.K.; Rao, D.A.S.; Devi, S.; Mansouri, K.; et al. A comparison of the diagnostic ability of vessel density and structural measurements of optical coherence tomography in primary open angle glaucoma. *PLoS ONE* **2017**, *12*, e0173930. [CrossRef] [PubMed]
16. Lommatzsch, C.; Rothaus, K.; Koch, J.M.; Heinz, C.; Grisanti, S. OCTA vessel density changes in the macular zone in glaucomatous eyes. *Graefes Arch. Clin. Exp. Ophthalmol.* **2018**, *256*, 1499–1508. [CrossRef]
17. Shoji, T.; Zangwill, L.M.; Akagi, T.; Saunders, L.J.; Yarmohammadi, A.; Manalastas, P.I.C.; Penteado, R.C.; Weinreb, R.N. Progressive Macula Vessel Density Loss in Primary Open-Angle Glaucoma: A Longitudinal Study. *Am. J. Ophthalmol.* **2017**, *182*, 107–117. [CrossRef]
18. Jeon, S.J.; Park, H.Y.L.; Park, C.K. Effect of Macular Vascular Density on Central Visual Function and Macular Structure in Glaucoma Patients. *Sci. Rep.* **2018**, *8*, 16009. [CrossRef]
19. Mills, R.P.; Budenz, D.L.; Lee, P.P.; Noecker, R.J.; Walt, J.G.; Siegartel, L.R.; Evans, S.J.; Doyle, J.J. Categorizing the stage of glaucoma from pre-diagnosis to end-stage disease. *Am. J. Ophthalmol.* **2006**, *141*, 24–30. [CrossRef]
20. Curcio, C.A.; Allen, K.A. Topography of ganglion cells in human retina. *J. Comp. Neurol.* **1990**, *300*, 5–25. [CrossRef]
21. Kim, N.R.; Lee, E.S.; Seong, G.J.; Kim, J.H.; An, H.G.; Kim, C.Y. Structure–Function Relationship and Diagnostic Value of Macular Ganglion Cell Complex Measurement Using Fourier-Domain OCT in Glaucoma. *Investig. Opthalmol. Vis. Sci.* **2010**, *51*, 4646. [CrossRef]
22. Hood, D.C.; Raza, A.S.; de Moraes, C.G.V.; Liebmann, J.M.; Ritch, R. Glaucomatous damage of the macula. *Prog. Retin. Eye Res.* **2013**, *32*, 1–21. [CrossRef]
23. Kuang, T.M.; Zhang, C.; Zangwill, L.M.; Weinreb, R.N.; Medeiros, F.A. Estimating lead time gained by optical coherence tomography in detecting glaucoma before development of visual field defects. *Ophthalmology* **2015**, *122*, 2002–2009. [CrossRef]
24. Kass, M.A.; Heuer, D.K.; Higginbotham, E.J.; Johnson, C.A.; Keltner, J.L.; Miller, J.P.; Parrish, R.K.; Wilson, M.R.; Gordon, M.O. The Ocular Hypertension Treatment Study. *Arch. Ophthalmol.* **2002**, *120*, 701. [CrossRef]
25. Cherecheanu, A.P.; Garhofer, G.; Schmidl, D.; Werkmeister, R.; Schmetterer, L. Ocular perfusion pressure and ocular blood flow in glaucoma. *Curr. Opin. Pharmacol.* **2013**, *13*, 36–42. [CrossRef]
26. Tobe, L.A.; Harris, A.; Hussain, R.M.; Eckert, G.; Huck, A.; Park, J.; Egan, P.; Kim, N.J.; Siesky, B. The role of retrobulbar and retinal circulation on optic nerve head and retinal nerve fibre layer structure in patients with open-angle glaucoma over an 18-month period. *Br. J. Ophthalmol.* **2015**, *99*, 609–612. [CrossRef] [PubMed]
27. Akil, H.; Huang, A.S.; Francis, B.A.; Sadda, S.R.; Chopra, V. Retinal vessel density from optical coherence tomography angiography to differentiate early glaucoma, pre-perimetric glaucoma and normal eyes. *PLoS ONE* **2017**, *12*, e0170476. [CrossRef] [PubMed]
28. Takusagawa, H.L.; Liu, L.; Ma, K.N.; Jia, Y.; Gao, S.S.; Zhang, M.; Edmunds, B.; Parikh, M.; Tehrani, S.; Morrison, J.C.; et al. Projection-Resolved Optical Coherence Tomography Angiography of Macular Retinal Circulation in Glaucoma. *Ophthalmology* **2017**, *124*, 1589–1599. [CrossRef] [PubMed]
29. Ragkousis, A.; Kozobolis, V.; Kabanarou, S.; Bontzos, G.; Mangouritsas, G.; Heliopoulos, I.; Chatziralli, I. Vessel Density around Foveal Avascular Zone as a Potential Imaging Biomarker for Detecting Preclinical Diabetic Retinopathy: An Optical Coherence Tomography Angiography Study. *Semin. Ophthalmol.* **2020**, *35*, 316–323. [CrossRef]
30. Shahlaee, A.; Samara, W.A.; Hsu, J.; Say, E.A.T.; Khan, M.A.; Sridhar, J.; Hong, B.K.; Shields, C.L.; Ho, A.C. In Vivo Assessment of Macular Vascular Density in Healthy Human Eyes Using Optical Coherence Tomography Angiography. *Am. J. Ophthalmol.* **2016**, *165*, 39–46. [CrossRef]
31. Lommatzsch, C.; Heinz, C.; Koch, J.M.; Heimes-Bussmann, B.; Hahn, U.; Grisanti, S. Does the Foveal Avascular Zone Change in Glaucoma? *Klin. Monbl. Augenheilkd.* **2020**, *237*, 879–888. [CrossRef]

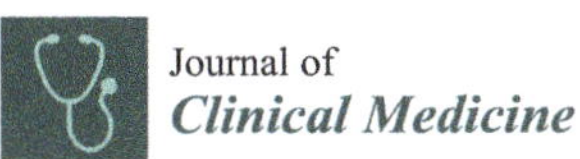

Journal of
Clinical Medicine

Article

Macular Structure–Function Relationships of All Retinal Layers in Primary Open-Angle Glaucoma Assessed by Microperimetry and 8 × 8 Posterior Pole Analysis of OCT

Jose Javier Garcia-Medina [1,2,3,4,5,*,†], Maurilia Rotolo [2,†], Elena Rubio-Velazquez [1], Maria Dolores Pinazo-Duran [4,5,6,‡] and Monica del-Rio-Vellosillo [7,‡]

[1] Department of Ophthalmology, General University Hospital Morales Meseguer, 30007 Murcia, Spain; erubiovelazquez@gmail.com
[2] Department of Ophthalmology, General University Hospital Reina Sofia, 30003 Murcia, Spain; rotolomaurilia@gmail.com
[3] Department of Ophthalmology and Optometry, University of Murcia, 30120 Murcia, Spain
[4] Ophthalmic Research Unit Santiago Grisolia, 46017 Valencia, Spain; pinazoduran@yahoo.es
[5] Red Temática de Investigación Cooperativa en Patología Ocular (OFTARED), Instituto de Salud Carlos III, 28029 Madrid, Spain
[6] Department of Ophthalmology, University of Valencia, 46010 Valencia, Spain
[7] Department of Anesthesiology, University Hospital Virgen de la Arrixaca, 30120 Murcia, Spain; monicadelriov@hotmail.com
* Correspondence: jj.garciamedina@um.es or josegarciam@yahoo.com
† J.J.G.-M. and M.R. equally contributed and shared the first authorship.
‡ M.D.P.-D. and M.d.-R.-V. shared the last authorship as senior authors.

Citation: Garcia-Medina, J.J.; Rotolo, M.; Rubio-Velazquez, E.; Pinazo-Duran, M.D.; del-Rio-Vellosillo, M. Macular Structure–Function Relationships of All Retinal Layers in Primary Open-Angle Glaucoma Assessed by Microperimetry and 8 × 8 Posterior Pole Analysis of OCT. *J. Clin. Med.* **2021**, *10*, 5009. https://doi.org/10.3390/jcm10215009

Academic Editor: Andrzej Grzybowski

Received: 28 September 2021
Accepted: 26 October 2021
Published: 28 October 2021

Publisher's Note: MDPI stays neutral with regard to jurisdictional claims in published maps and institutional affiliations.

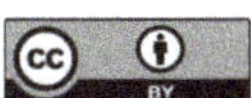

Abstract: Purpose: The aim of this study is too correlate the sensitivity and thickness values of intraretinal layers at macula in healthy eyes and primary open-angle glaucoma (POAG) eyes. Methods: The thickness of different intraretinal segmentations was estimated by means of optical coherence tomography (OCT) Spectralis (Heidelberg, Engineering, Inc., Heidelberg, Germany) with the posterior pole analysis program 8 × 8 in 91 eyes from 91 patients (60 with glaucoma and 31 healthy patients). Macular sensitivity was also measured with an MP-1 microperimeter (Nidek Instruments, Inc Padova, Italy) with a customized, 36-stimulus pattern adjusted to an anatomical correspondence with the OCT grid. Correlations were calculated by using Spearman's rho and the results were represented in color maps. Results: Significant structure–function correlations were much more frequent in the glaucoma group than in control group. In general terms, associations were positive for inner retinal layers but negative correlations were also found for the inner nuclear layer and outer retinal layer in glaucoma. Conclusions: In general terms, significant structure–function correlations for different intraretinal layers are higher and wider in POAG eyes than in healthy eyes. Inner and outer retinal layers behave differently in terms of the structure–function relationship in POAG as assessed by microperimetry and OCT.

Keywords: microperimetry; OCT; glaucoma; macula; structure; function; correlation; retina; inner; outer

1. Introduction

Glaucoma is a chronic and progressive neuropathy of the optic nerve characterized by retinal ganglion cell apoptosis [1]. This event is not only associated with optic nerve cupping due to retinal nerve fiber layer loss (dendrites of the retinal ganglion cells) but also with changes at different intraretinal layers of the macula as shown in our previous studies [2,3].

All these structural modifications are usually accompanied by functional losses that can be first observed as localized visual field (VF) defects or scotomas that can affect the macular region [4].

The structure–function relationship has been widely studied. However, most of the investigations have been functionally performed with standard automated perimetry (SAP) [5].

Microperimetry (MP) is a technology with theoretical benefits in relation to SAP such as automated eye tracking and more precise location of the stimulus on the retina [6]. However, few works have studied the macular structure–function relations in glaucoma using MP [7–10]. Plus, all of them have only structurally analyzed some of the inner retinal segmentations of the macula obtained by optical coherence tomography (OCT). Although glaucoma is primarily a disease of ganglion cells, in the light perception and early integration of visual stimuli all retinal layers participate, not only in inner retinal layers. Considering the structural changes detected by our group in glaucoma [2,3], we hypothesize that there could exist associations between thickness of all retinal layers with its anatomically corresponding sensitivity in glaucoma and, specifically, with such a precise technology as MP. To the best of our knowledge, we have not found any study in this sense. Thus, this is the purpose of the present work.

2. Materials and Methods

This is a prospective, observational, cross-sectional study. All the eyes included in the study were recruited from consecutive patients seen at the Glaucoma Clinic of General University Hospital Reina Sofia, Murcia, Spain. The investigation was approved by the institutional review board of the mentioned hospital. All participants signed an informed consent and the study was conducted in accordance with the tenets of the Declaration of Helsinki.

The inclusion criteria of glaucomatous group were as follow:

1. Caucasian race and age between 40 and 90 years;
2. Diagnosis of primary open-angle glaucoma (POAG) with threat to fixation according to our clinical records;
3. Refractive error of 3 dioptres or less of spherical equivalent and;
4. Best corrected visual acuity of 0.5 or better in the Snellen scale.

POAG diagnosis required:

1. Intraocular pressure > 21 mmHg in at least three different days;
2. Glaucomatous optic disc changes and/or characteristic glaucomatous SAP abnormalities, as judged by a glaucoma specialist (J.J.G.M.), and;
3. Open anterior chamber angle in gonioscopy.

Threat to fixation was defined as a depression of one or more of the four paracentral points with a $p < 1\%$ in the two previous reliable 30-2 SITA Fast VF tests [11]. SAPs were considered reliable when loss of fixation, false-positive and/or false-negative responses were under 20% and were obtained from clinical records in the past year.

Inclusion criteria for healthy group (controls) were the same that for glaucomatous group except for criterium number 2. Exclusion criteria for both groups were as follow:

1. Previous intraocular or refractive surgery, or laser procedure in the six months before the recruitment;
2. History of ocular trauma;
3. Use of ocular or systemic medications that could affect the VF;
4. Presence of other ophthalmic or systemic significant diseases (eyelid, corneal, lens or retinal disease, diabetes) that could influence microperimetry or OCT results.

Only one eye was selected per patient. When both eyes were eligible one of them was randomly chosen.

At the time of enrollment, an ophthalmic examination was performed that included the following tests, which were made in this order:

1. Autorefractometry;
2. Best Corrected Visual Acuity (BCVA), using decimal scale;
3. Intraocular pressure estimation using applanation tonometry.

Microperimetry and OCT examinations were performed in a subsequent visit if the patient was eligible.

Microperimetry was conducted with the MP-1 (Nidek Instruments Inc., Padova, Italia) using a customized pattern by the same examiner (M.R.) selecting a full-*threshold strategy* 4-2-1 decibels with a Goldmann III-size stimulus presented for 200 milliseconds and a 4 apostilb backgroud. The maximal sensitivity for each stimulus was 20 decibels.

This pattern consisted of 37 stimuli centered at the fovea and with the following features:

1. The nearest stimuli from vertical and horizontal main axes were located at 1.5 degrees from these axes;
2. The stimuli were separated 3 degrees from each.

The central stimulus (number 37), located in the intersection of the main vertical and horizontal axes, was not considered for the calculations (Figure 1).

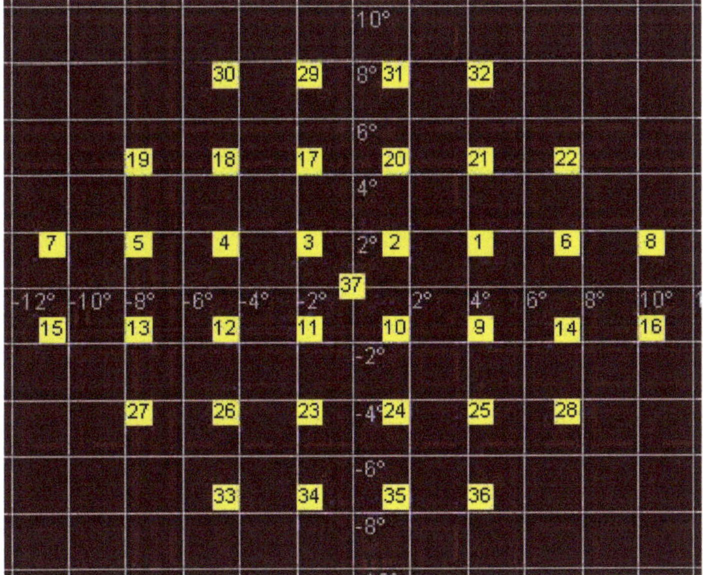

Figure 1. Customized pattern of microperimetry used in this study.

Then OCT examinations were performed using an 8 × 8 posterior pole algorithm with the device Spectralis (Heidelberg Engineering, Heidelberg, Germany; 6.0 software version). This algorithm estimates the thickness of the considered layer of 64 superpixels centered at the fovea. Each superpixel is 3 × 3 degrees wide. Alignment of the horizontal main axis according to the fovea—disc axis is automatically displayed in this algorithm (Figure 2).

In the present study, the 8 × 8 grids were horizontalized using a reference horizontal rectangle at zero degrees overlaying on the OCT interface by means of the software Overlay 2.1 (Collin Thomas Photography Ltd. London, UK, http://www.colinthomas.com/overlay (accessed on 25 October 2021)). (Figure 3).

Thus, using this customized pattern in microperimetry, we located each stimulus at the center of each superpixel of the horizontalized grid in the OCT 8 × 8 posterior pole grid to achieve the anatomical correspondence (Figure 4).

Only superpixels with a projected stimulus at the center were considered in this study. All maps were constructed as if all eyes were right ones (Figure 5).

Only reliable OCT examinations (with signal strength ≥ 20) were selected. All scans were checked by the same experienced operator (J.J.G.M.). If segmentation errors were detected, the examinations were considered unreliable and discarded.

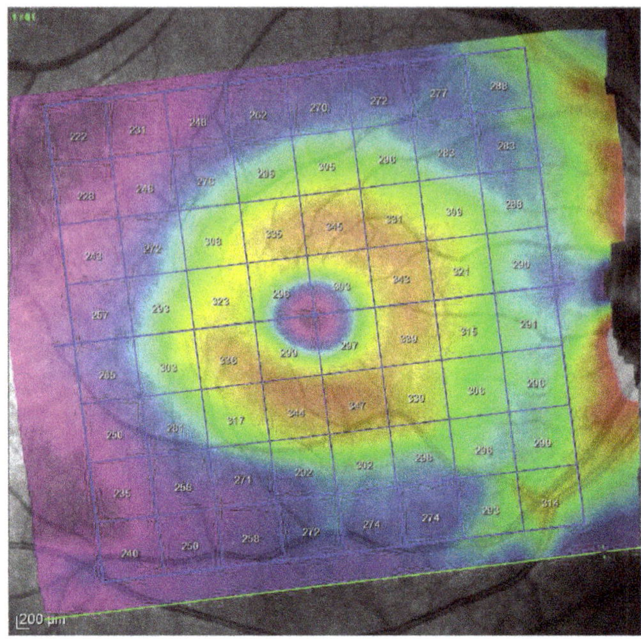

Figure 2. Posterior pole program analysis. Note the inclination of the grid automatically generated by the device.

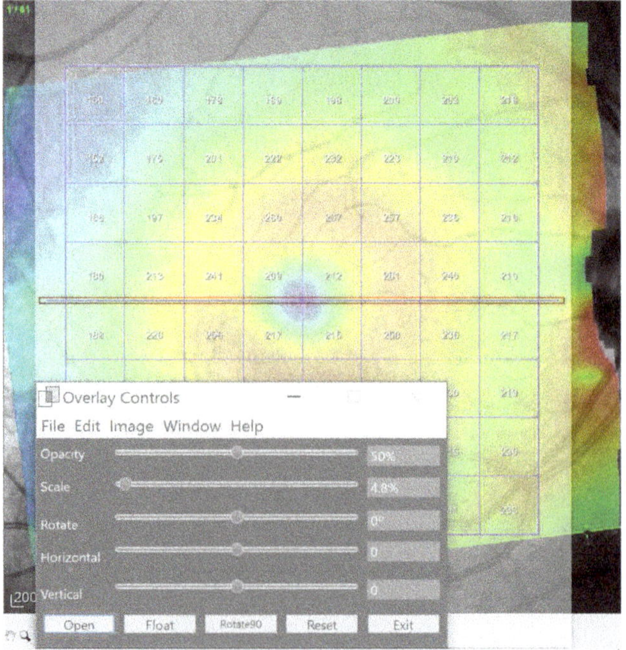

Figure 3. Horizontalization of the grid using a overlaid reference horizontal rectangles (red) by means of Overlay 2.1 software.

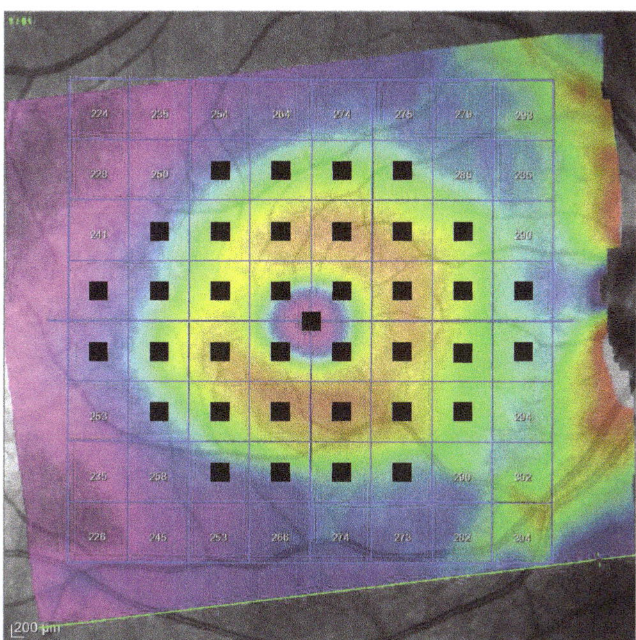

Figure 4. Horizontal OCT grid and microperimetry pattern.

8.1	8.2	8.3	8.4	8.5	8.6	8.7	8.8
7.1	7.2	7.3	7.4	7.5	7.6	7.7	7.8
6.1	6.2	6.3	6.4	6.5	6.6	6.7	6.8
5.1	5.2	5.3	5.4	5.5	5.6	5.7	5.8
4.1	4.2	4.3	4.4	4.5	4.6	4.7	4.8
3.1	3.2	3.3	3.4	3.5	3.6	3.7	3.8
2.1	2.2	2.3	2.4	2.5	2.6	2.7	2.8
1.1	1.2	1.3	1.4	1.5	1.6	1.7	1.8

Figure 5. Denomination of superpixels in 8 × 8 Posterior Pole Algorithm (right eye). Only the thickness of the superpixels represented in green (and its corresponding microperimetric sensitivities) were considered in this study. All eyes were represented as if they were all right eyes.

Spectralis OCT allows an automatic segmentation of different intraretinal layers (Figure 6) and estimation of thickness of the selected segmentation.

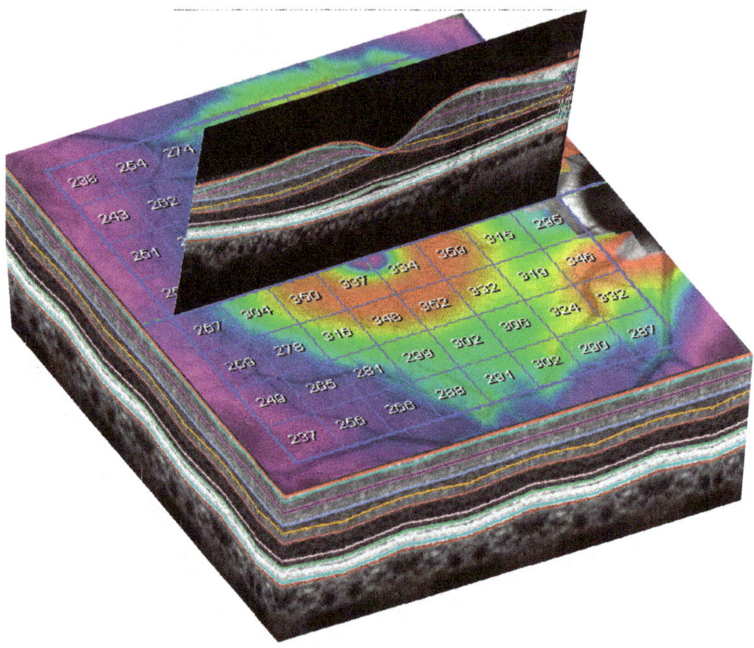

Figure 6. Three-dimensional (3D) representation of automatic segmentation of all retinal layers in a 8 × 8 grid.

In this study the thickness of the following automatic segmentations were considered at the macula: full retina, retina nerve fiber layer (mRNFL), ganglion cell layer(GCL), inner plexiform layer (IPL), inner nuclear layer (INL), outer plexiform layer (OPL), outer nuclear layer (ONL), outer retina, and retinal pigment epithelium (RPE). ONL and OPL thickness values were added (OPL + ONL) in order to avoid artefactual results due to Henle fibers orientation [12].

Statistical calculations were performed using SPSS software (IBM, version 22, Chicago, IL, USA). The sex and laterality of the eye were compared using Fisher's test between groups. All the continuous variables were assessed for normality with the Kolmogorov–Smirnov test. Age, clinical variables, all microperimetric results (in decibels), and many of the thickness OCT results (in microns) did not show a normal distribution. Thus, comparisons of mean age, BCVA, spherical equivalent, IOP, and vertical cupping between both groups were assessed by means of the Mann–Whitney test. Correlations between the sensitivity and thickness for each segmentation at each megapixel were calculated by Spearman's rank correlation coefficient. structure–function correlation maps were plotted for each considered segmentation. All were constructed as if all eyes were right eyes. The significance level was $p < 0.05$.

3. Results

Sixty eyes of 60 POAG patients and thirty-one eyes of 31 controls were finally selected. Demographic and clinical data are presented in Table 1.

Figure 7 sums up the structure function associations between full retina thickness and microperimetric sensitivity both in the control group and the glaucoma group. In the glaucoma group positive, several moderate–weak correlations were found in the superior and inferior hemisphere but not affecting the central area. There were only two positive correlations in the control group.

Table 1. Demographic and clinical data of this study. Significant results are indicated in bold.

Demographic and Clinical Data	Glaucoma Group	Control Group	Significance (Test)
Eyes and laterality	$n = 60$ Right eyes = 30 Left eyes = 30	$n = 31$ Right eyes = 15 Left eyes = 16	1 (Fisher's test)
Age (years)	73 (15)	67 (31)	0.07 (Mann–Whitney test)
Sex	29 men 32 women	9 men 22 women	0.11 (Fisher's test)
BCVA	0.9 (0.3)	1 (1.9)	0.07 (Mann–Whitney test)
IOP (mmHg)	20 (7)	17 (4)	0.004 (Mann–Whitney test)
Spherical equivalent	0.25 (4)	1 (2)	0.04 (Mann–Whitney test)
Vertical cupping	0.8 (0.3)	0.4 (0.2)	<0.001 (Mann–Whitney test)

Continuous variables are reported with median (interquartile range).

(a)

8.1	8.2	8.3	8.4	8.5	8.6	8.7	8.8
7.1	7.2	7.3 r=0.310 p=0.013	7.4 r=0.323 p=0.010	7.5 r=0.403 p=0.001	7.6 r=0.226 p=0.075	7.7	7.8
6.1	6.2 r=0.213 p=0.094	6.3 r=0.227 p=0.074	6.4 r=0.298 p=0.018	6.5 r=0.286 p=0.023	6.6 r=0.272 p=0.031	6.7 r=0.205 p=0.108	6.8
5.1 r=0.207 p=0.107	5.2 r=0.275 p=0.029	5.3 r=0.319 p=0.011	5.4 r=0.158 p=0.217	5.5 r=0.187 p=0.142	5.6 r=0.120 p=0.349	5.7 r=0.165 p=0.201	5.8 r=0.022 p=0.867
4.1 r=0.144 p=0.259	4.2 r=0.165 p=0.195	4.3 r=0.280 p=0.026	4.4 r=0.029 p=0.823	4.5 r=-0.034 p=0.791	4.6 r=0.055 p=0.668	4.7 r=0.089 p=0.494	4.8 r=0.277 p=0.032
3.1	3.2 r=0.027 p=0.833	3.3 r=0.172 p=0.178	3.4 r=0.261 p=0.038	3.5 r=0.386 P=0.002	3.6 r=0.260 p=0.040	3.7 r=0.349 p=0.005	3.8
2.1	2.2	2.3 r=0.181 p=0.157	2.4 r=0.158 p=0.215	2.5 r=0.259 p=0.041	2.6 r=0.174 p=0.176	2.7	2.8
1.1	1.2	1.3	1.4	1.5	1.6	1.7	1.8

(b)

8.1	8.2	8.3	8.4	8.5	8.6	8.7	8.8
7.1	7.2	7.3 r=-0.117 p=0.522	7.4 r=-0.067 p=0.717	7.5 r=-0.060 p=0.746	7.6 r=-0.257 p=0.155	7.7	7.8
6.1	6.2 r=0.116 p=0.533	6.3 r=0.122 p=0.512	6.4 r=0.160 p=0.381	6.5 r=0.085 p=0.645	6.6 r=0.199 p=0.276	6.7 r=0.019 p=0.917	6.8
5.1 r=0.197 p=0.281	5.2 r=0.189 p=0.299	5.3 r=0.107 p=0.560	5.4 r=-0.173 p=0.344	5.5 r=0.058 p=0.752	5.6 r=0.166 p=0.364	5.7 r=0.044 p=0.811	5.8 r=0.126 p=0.491
4.1 r=0.369 p=0.038	4.2 r=0.235 p=0.196	4.3 r=0.073 p=0.691	4.4 r=-0.238 p=0.189	4.5 r=-0.126 p=0.491	4.6 r=0.219 p=0.227	4.7 r=-0.079 p=0.668	4.8 r=-0.053 p=0.773
3.1	3.2 r=0.445 p=0.011	3.3 r=0.281 p=0.119	3.4 r=0.301 p=0.094	3.5 r=0.295 P=0.101	3.6 r=-0.094 p=0.607	3.7 r=-0.199 p=0.274	3.8
2.1	2.2	2.3 r=0.346 p=0.052	2.4 r=0.041 p=0.822	2.5 r=0.024 p=0.895	2.6 r=0.252 p=0.164	2.7	2.8
1.1	1.2	1.3	1.4	1.5	1.6	1.7	1.8

Figure 7. Color map of correlations for full retinal thickness in the glaucoma group (**a**) and control group (**b**). Green color indicates non-significant correlation. Blue color indicates significant positive correlation. Red color indicates significant negative correlation. Black color indicates OCT superpixels not considered in the calculations. r = Spearman's rho, *p* = significance.

mRNFL showed positive, weak–moderate correlations in the superior hemisphere and strong–moderate ones in the inferior hemisphere in the glaucoma group but none in the control group (Figure 8).

Figures 9 and 10 depict the correlations corresponding to GCL and IPL, respectively. In the glaucoma group, as it can be seen, difuse, positive, strong–moderate correlations were demonstrated in the field except for papillomacular bundle area. These correlations were stronger and more difuse for GCL than for IPL. In the control group, no significant association were found for GCL and scarce but negative ones were shown for IPL.

Figure 11 shows the completely different structure–function behavior for INL in both groups. While there were positive correlations in the glaucoma group, the control group showed negative correlations.

Figure 12 shows that barely any significant correlation was found in both groups when considering OPL + ONL.

Positive, ring-shape correlations for the glaucoma group were seen when considering inner retina (mRNFL + GCL + IPL + INL + OPL + ONL) and not affecting the to papillomacular bundle (Figure 13). Only three positive correlations were found in control the group.

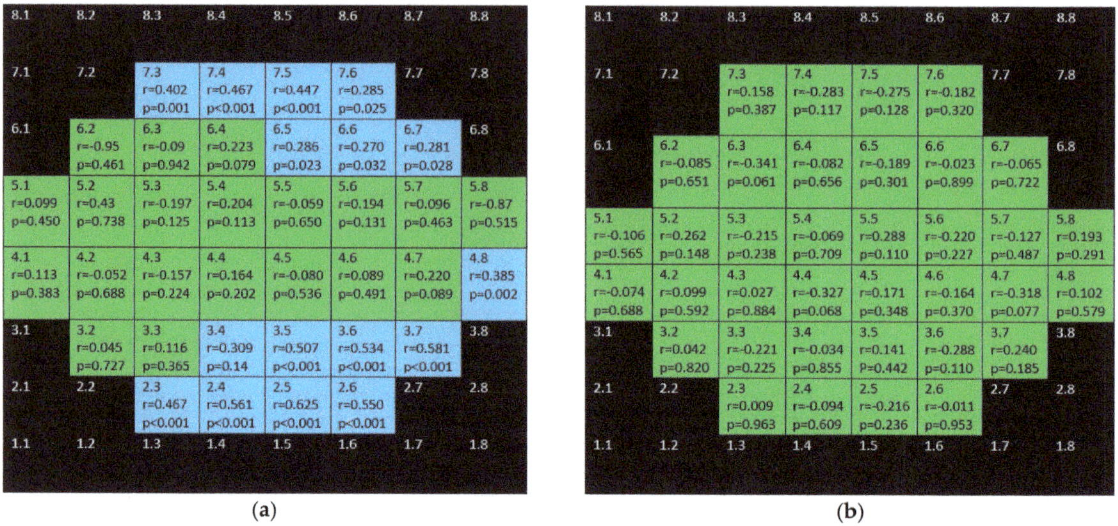

Figure 8 (a) — glaucoma group

8.1	8.2	8.3	8.4	8.5	8.6	8.7	8.8
7.1	7.2	7.3 r=0.402 p=0.001	7.4 r=0.467 p<0.001	7.5 r=0.447 p<0.001	7.6 r=0.285 p=0.025	7.7	7.8
6.1	6.2 r=-0.95 p=0.461	6.3 r=-0.09 p=0.942	6.4 r=0.223 p=0.079	6.5 r=0.286 p=0.023	6.6 r=0.270 p=0.032	6.7 r=0.281 p=0.028	6.8
5.1 r=0.099 p=0.450	5.2 r=0.43 p=0.738	5.3 r=-0.197 p=0.125	5.4 r=0.204 p=0.113	5.5 r=-0.059 p=0.650	5.6 r=0.194 p=0.131	5.7 r=0.096 p=0.463	5.8 r=-0.87 p=0.515
4.1 r=0.113 p=0.383	4.2 r=-0.052 p=0.688	4.3 r=-0.157 p=0.224	4.4 r=0.164 p=0.202	4.5 r=-0.080 p=0.536	4.6 r=0.089 p=0.491	4.7 r=0.220 p=0.089	4.8 r=0.385 p=0.002
3.1	3.2 r=0.045 p=0.727	3.3 r=0.116 p=0.365	3.4 r=0.309 p=0.14	3.5 r=0.507 p<0.001	3.6 r=0.534 p<0.001	3.7 r=0.581 p<0.001	3.8
2.1	2.2	2.3 r=0.467 p<0.001	2.4 r=0.561 p<0.001	2.5 r=0.625 p<0.001	2.6 r=0.550 p<0.001	2.7	2.8
1.1	1.2	1.3	1.4	1.5	1.6	1.7	1.8

(a)

Figure 8 (b) — control group

8.1	8.2	8.3	8.4	8.5	8.6	8.7	8.8
7.1	7.2	7.3 r=0.158 p=0.387	7.4 r=-0.283 p=0.117	7.5 r=-0.275 p=0.128	7.6 r=-0.182 p=0.320	7.7	7.8
6.1	6.2 r=-0.085 p=0.651	6.3 r=-0.341 p=0.061	6.4 r=-0.082 p=0.656	6.5 r=-0.189 p=0.301	6.6 r=-0.023 p=0.899	6.7 r=-0.065 p=0.722	6.8
5.1 r=-0.106 p=0.565	5.2 r=0.262 p=0.148	5.3 r=-0.215 p=0.238	5.4 r=-0.069 p=0.709	5.5 r=0.288 p=0.110	5.6 r=-0.220 p=0.227	5.7 r=-0.127 p=0.487	5.8 r=0.193 p=0.291
4.1 r=-0.074 p=0.688	4.2 r=0.099 p=0.592	4.3 r=0.027 p=0.884	4.4 r=-0.327 p=0.068	4.5 r=0.171 p=0.348	4.6 r=-0.164 p=0.370	4.7 r=-0.318 p=0.077	4.8 r=0.102 p=0.579
3.1	3.2 r=0.042 p=0.820	3.3 r=-0.221 p=0.225	3.4 r=-0.034 p=0.855	3.5 r=0.141 P=0.442	3.6 r=-0.288 p=0.110	3.7 r=0.240 p=0.185	3.8
2.1	2.2	2.3 r=0.009 p=0.963	2.4 r=-0.094 p=0.609	2.5 r=-0.216 p=0.236	2.6 r=-0.011 p=0.953	2.7	2.8
1.1	1.2	1.3	1.4	1.5	1.6	1.7	1.8

(b)

Figure 8. Color map of correlations for macular retinal nerve fiber layer in the glaucoma group (**a**) and control group (**b**). Green color indicates non–significant correlation. Blue color indicates significant positive correlation. Red color indicates significant negative correlation. Black color indicates OCT superpixels not considered in the calcula-tions. R = Spearman's rho, *p* = significance.

Figure 9 (a) — glaucoma group

8.1	8.2	8.3	8.4	8.5	8.6	8.7	8.8
7.1	7.2	7.3 r=0.508 p<0.001	7.4 r=0.540 p<0.001	7.5 r=0.557 p<0.001	7.6 r=0.353 p=0.005	7.7	7.8
6.1	6.2 r=0.501 p<0.001	6.3 r=0.444 p<0.001	6.4 r=0.485 p<0.001	6.5 r=0.333 p=0.008	6.6 r=0.282 p=0.025	6.7 r=0.371 p=0.003	6.8
5.1 r=0.353 p=0.005	5.2 r=0.507 p<0.001	5.3 r=0.532 p<0.001	5.4 r=0.341 p=0.007	5.5 r=0.285 p=0.025	5.6 r=-0.202 p=0.116	5.7 r=0.167 p=0.199	5.8 r=-0.003 p=0.984
4.1 r=0.316 p=0.012	4.2 r=0.455 p<0.001	4.3 r=0.581 p<0.001	4.4 r=0.431 p<0.001	4.5 r=0.261 p=0.040	4.6 r=0.077 p=0.550	4.7 r=-0.155 p=0.232	4.8 r=0.190 p=0.146
3.1	3.2 r=0.480 p<0.001	3.3 r=0.644 p<0.001	3.4 r=0.610 p<0.001	3.5 r=0.660 p<0.001	3.6 r=0.564 p<0.001	3.7 r=0.616 p<0.001	3.8
2.1	2.2	2.3 r=0.581 p<0.001	2.4 r=0.657 p<0.001	2.5 r=0.682 p<0.001	2.6 r=0.624 p<0.001	2.7	2.8
1.1	1.2	1.3	1.4	1.5	1.6	1.7	1.8

(a)

Figure 9 (b) — control group

8.1	8.2	8.3	8.4	8.5	8.6	8.7	8.8
7.1	7.2	7.3 r=0.020 p=0.915	7.4 r=0.070 p=0.703	7.5 r=0.047 p=0.798	7.6 r=-0.100 p=0.588	7.7	7.8
6.1	6.2 r=0.272 p=0.140	6.3 r=0.050 p=0.791	6.4 r=0.102 p=0.577	6.5 r=0.002 p=0.991	6.6 r=0.137 p=0.456	6.7 r=0.161 p=0.387	6.8
5.1 r=0.051 p=0.780	5.2 r=0.170 p=0.353	5.3 r=0.080 p=0.662	5.4 r=-0.027 p=0.883	5.5 r=0.001 p=0.994	5.6 r=0.106 p=0.564	5.7 r=0.083 p=0.653	5.8 r=0.163 p=0.372
4.1 r=0.211 p=0.247	4.2 r=0.127 p=0.487	4.3 r=0.079 p=0.669	4.4 r=-0.341 p=0.057	4.5 r=-0.166 p=0.365	4.6 r=0.214 p=0.240	4.7 r=0.032 p=0.864	4.8 r=-0.014 p=0.938
3.1	3.2 r=0.230 p=0.206	3.3 r=0.263 p=0.146	3.4 r=0.246 p=0.175	3.5 r=0.201 P=0.271	3.6 r=-0.021 p=0.910	3.7 r=-0.219 p=0.228	3.8
2.1	2.2	2.3 r=0.305 p=0.090	2.4 r=0.017 p=0.926	2.5 r=0.161 p=0.378	2.6 r=0.223 p=0.221	2.7	2.8
1.1	1.2	1.3	1.4	1.5	1.6	1.7	1.8

(b)

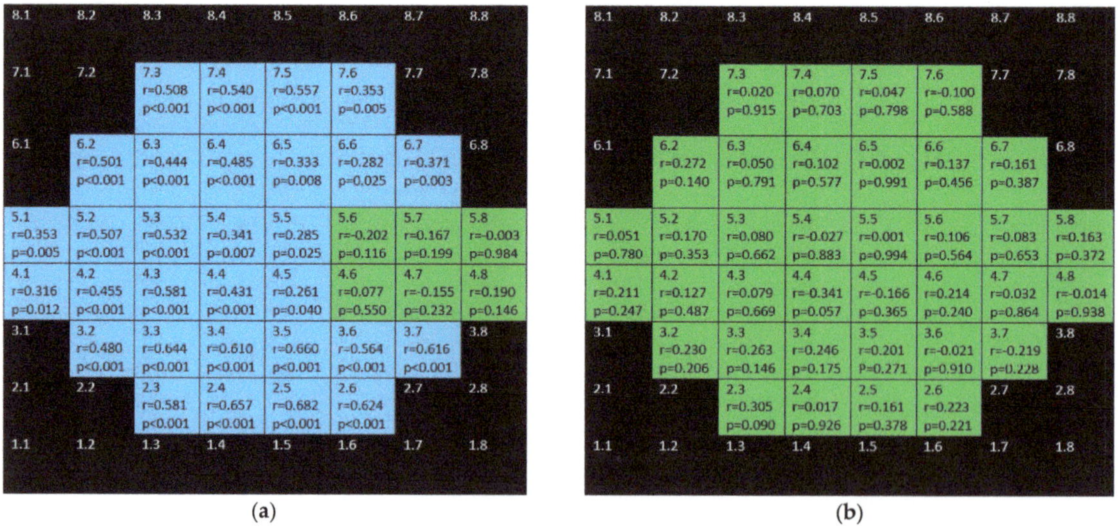

Figure 9. Color map of correlations for ganglion cell layer in the glaucoma group (**a**) and control group (**b**). Green color indicates non-significant correlation. Blue color indicates significant positive correlation. Red color indicates significant negative correlation. Black color indicates OCT superpixels not considered in the calculations. r = Spearman's rho, *p* = significance.

Figure 14 depicts that while there were significant, negative correlations for outer retina (including outer photoreceptors segments and RPE) in the inferior hemisphere of the glaucoma group, there was only one positive correlation in the control group.

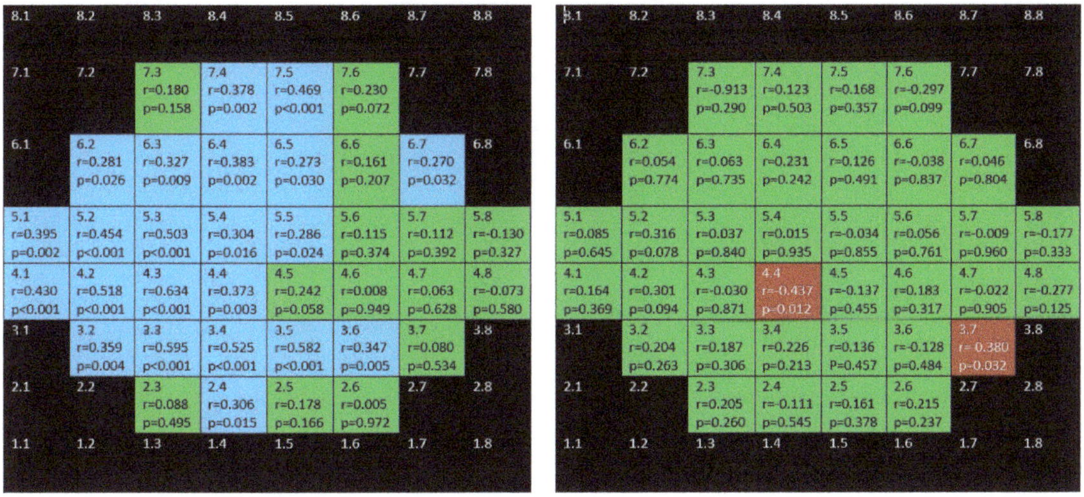

Figure 10 (a) — glaucoma group

8.1	8.2	8.3	8.4	8.5	8.6	8.7	8.8
7.1	7.2	7.3 r=0.180 p=0.158	7.4 r=0.378 p=0.002	7.5 r=0.469 p<0.001	7.6 r=0.230 p=0.072	7.7	7.8
6.1	6.2 r=0.281 p=0.026	6.3 r=0.327 p=0.009	6.4 r=0.383 p=0.002	6.5 r=0.273 p=0.030	6.6 r=0.161 p=0.207	6.7 r=0.270 p=0.032	6.8
5.1 r=0.395 p=0.002	5.2 r=0.454 p<0.001	5.3 r=0.503 p<0.001	5.4 r=0.304 p=0.016	5.5 r=0.286 p=0.024	5.6 r=0.115 p=0.374	5.7 r=0.112 p=0.392	5.8 r=-0.130 p=0.327
4.1 r=0.430 p<0.001	4.2 r=0.518 p<0.001	4.3 r=0.634 p<0.001	4.4 r=0.373 p=0.003	4.5 r=0.242 p=0.058	4.6 r=0.008 p=0.949	4.7 r=0.063 p=0.628	4.8 r=-0.073 p=0.580
3.1	3.2 r=0.359 p=0.004	3.3 r=0.595 p<0.001	3.4 r=0.525 p<0.001	3.5 r=0.582 p<0.001	3.6 r=0.347 p=0.005	3.7 r=0.080 p=0.534	3.8
2.1	2.2	2.3 r=0.088 p=0.495	2.4 r=0.306 p=0.015	2.5 r=0.178 p=0.166	2.6 r=0.005 p=0.972	2.7	2.8
1.1	1.2	1.3	1.4	1.5	1.6	1.7	1.8

(a)

Figure 10 (b) — control group

8.1	8.2	8.3	8.4	8.5	8.6	8.7	8.8
7.1	7.2	7.3 r=-0.913 p=0.290	7.4 r=0.123 p=0.503	7.5 r=0.168 p=0.357	7.6 r=-0.297 p=0.099	7.7	7.8
6.1	6.2 r=0.054 p=0.774	6.3 r=0.063 p=0.735	6.4 r=0.231 p=0.242	6.5 r=0.126 p=0.491	6.6 r=-0.038 p=0.837	6.7 r=0.046 p=0.804	6.8
5.1 r=0.085 p=0.645	5.2 r=0.316 p=0.078	5.3 r=0.037 p=0.840	5.4 r=0.015 p=0.935	5.5 r=-0.034 p=0.855	5.6 r=0.056 p=0.761	5.7 r=-0.009 p=0.960	5.8 r=-0.177 p=0.333
4.1 r=0.164 p=0.369	4.2 r=0.301 p=0.094	4.3 r=-0.030 p=0.871	4.4 r=-0.437 p=0.012	4.5 r=-0.137 p=0.455	4.6 r=0.183 p=0.317	4.7 r=-0.022 p=0.905	4.8 r=-0.277 p=0.125
3.1	3.2 r=0.204 p=0.263	3.3 r=0.187 p=0.306	3.4 r=0.226 p=0.213	3.5 r=0.136 P=0.457	3.6 r=-0.128 p=0.484	3.7 r=0.380 p=0.032	3.8
2.1	2.2	2.3 r=0.205 p=0.260	2.4 r=-0.111 p=0.545	2.5 r=0.161 p=0.378	2.6 r=0.215 p=0.237	2.7	2.8
1.1	1.2	1.3	1.4	1.5	1.6	1.7	1.8

(b)

Figure 10. Color map of correlations for inner plexiform layer in the glaucoma group (**a**) and control group (**b**). Green color indicates non-significant correlation. Blue color indicates significant positive correlation. Red color indicates significant negative correlation. Black color indicates OCT superpixels not considered in the calculations. r = Spearman's rho, *p* = significance.

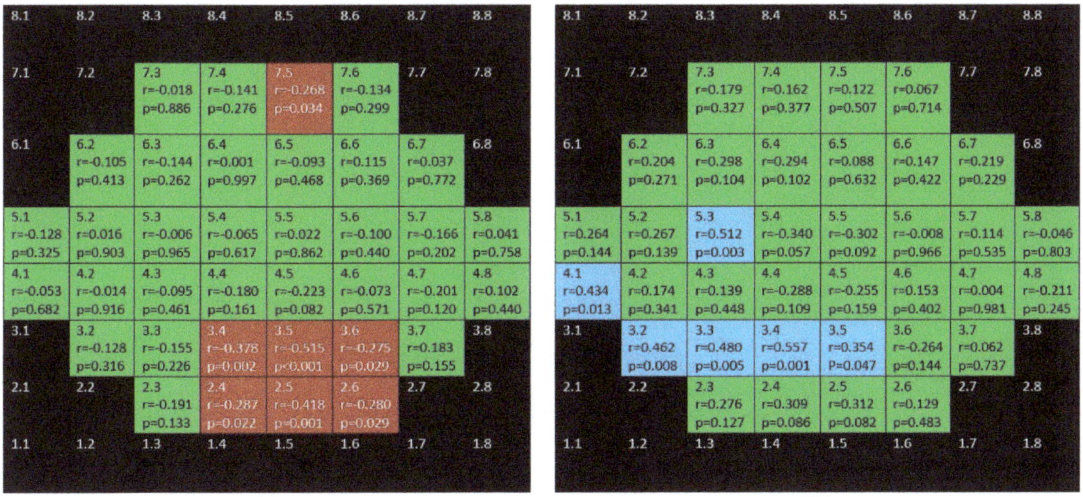

Figure 11 (a) — glaucoma group

8.1	8.2	8.3	8.4	8.5	8.6	8.7	8.8
7.1	7.2	7.3 r=-0.018 p=0.886	7.4 r=-0.141 p=0.276	7.5 r=-0.268 p=0.034	7.6 r=-0.134 p=0.299	7.7	7.8
6.1	6.2 r=-0.105 p=0.413	6.3 r=-0.144 p=0.262	6.4 r=0.001 p=0.997	6.5 r=-0.093 p=0.468	6.6 r=0.115 p=0.369	6.7 r=0.037 p=0.772	6.8
5.1 r=-0.128 p=0.325	5.2 r=0.016 p=0.903	5.3 r=-0.006 p=0.965	5.4 r=-0.065 p=0.617	5.5 r=0.022 p=0.862	5.6 r=-0.100 p=0.440	5.7 r=-0.166 p=0.202	5.8 r=0.041 p=0.758
4.1 r=-0.053 p=0.682	4.2 r=-0.014 p=0.916	4.3 r=-0.095 p=0.461	4.4 r=-0.180 p=0.161	4.5 r=-0.223 p=0.082	4.6 r=-0.073 p=0.571	4.7 r=-0.201 p=0.120	4.8 r=0.102 p=0.440
3.1	3.2 r=-0.128 p=0.316	3.3 r=-0.155 p=0.226	3.4 r=-0.378 p=0.002	3.5 r=-0.515 p<0.001	3.6 r=-0.275 p=0.029	3.7 r=0.183 p=0.155	3.8
2.1	2.2	2.3 r=-0.191 p=0.133	2.4 r=-0.287 p=0.022	2.5 r=-0.418 p=0.001	2.6 r=-0.280 p=0.029	2.7	2.8
1.1	1.2	1.3	1.4	1.5	1.6	1.7	1.8

(a)

Figure 11 (b) — control group

8.1	8.2	8.3	8.4	8.5	8.6	8.7	8.8
7.1	7.2	7.3 r=0.179 p=0.327	7.4 r=0.162 p=0.377	7.5 r=0.122 p=0.507	7.6 r=0.067 p=0.714	7.7	7.8
6.1	6.2 r=0.204 p=0.271	6.3 r=0.298 p=0.104	6.4 r=0.294 p=0.102	6.5 r=0.088 p=0.632	6.6 r=0.147 p=0.422	6.7 r=0.219 p=0.229	6.8
5.1 r=0.264 p=0.144	5.2 r=0.267 p=0.139	5.3 r=0.512 p=0.003	5.4 r=-0.340 p=0.057	5.5 r=-0.302 p=0.092	5.6 r=-0.008 p=0.966	5.7 r=0.114 p=0.535	5.8 r=-0.046 p=0.803
4.1 r=0.434 p=0.013	4.2 r=0.174 p=0.341	4.3 r=0.139 p=0.448	4.4 r=-0.288 p=0.109	4.5 r=-0.255 p=0.159	4.6 r=0.153 p=0.402	4.7 r=0.004 p=0.981	4.8 r=-0.211 p=0.245
3.1	3.2 r=0.462 p=0.008	3.3 r=0.480 p=0.005	3.4 r=0.557 p=0.001	3.5 r=0.354 P=0.047	3.6 r=-0.264 p=0.144	3.7 r=0.062 p=0.737	3.8
2.1	2.2	2.3 r=0.276 p=0.127	2.4 r=0.309 p=0.086	2.5 r=0.312 p=0.082	2.6 r=0.129 p=0.483	2.7	2.8
1.1	1.2	1.3	1.4	1.5	1.6	1.7	1.8

(b)

Figure 11. Color map of correlations for inner nuclear layer in the glaucoma group (**a**) and control group (**b**). Green color indicates non-significant correlation. Blue color indicates significant positive correlation. Red color indicates significant negative correlation. Black color indicates OCT superpixels not considered in the calculations. r = Spearman's rho, *p* = significance.

Finally, there are isolated correlations for RPE in both glaucoma and control group (Figure 15).

8.1	8.2	8.3	8.4	8.5	8.6	8.7	8.8
7.1	7.2	7.3 r=-0.009 p=0.944	7.4 r=-0.134 p=0.307	7.5 r=0.020 p=0.878	7.6 r=-0.069 p=0.600	7.7	7.8
6.1	6.2 r=-0.053 p=0.686	6.3 r=-0.029 p=0.826	6.4 r=-0.027 p=0.839	6.5 r=-0.081 p=0.537	6.6 r=-0.029 p=0.828	6.7 r=-0.053 p=0.690	6.8
5.1 r=0.143 p=0.245	5.2 r=-0.004 p=0.978	5.3 r=-0.149 p=0.275	5.4 r=-0.188 p=0.151	5.5 r=-0.149 p=0.256	5.6 r=-0.045 p=0.733	5.7 r=0.072 p=0.585	5.8 r=-0.018 p=0.890
4.1 r=-0.056 p=0.656	4.2 r=-0.151 p=0.251	4.3 r=-0.151 p=0.249	4.4 r=-0.277 p=0.081	4.5 r=-0.268 p=0.038	4.6 r=-0.073 p=0.580	4.7 r=-0.008 p=0.949	4.8 r=-0.083 p=0.530
3.1	3.2 r=-0.147 p=0.263	3.3 r=-0.208 p=0.110	3.4 r=-0.068 p=0.606	3.5 r=-0.156 P=0.211	3.6 r=-0.170 p=0.195	3.7 r=-0.082 p=0.534	3.8
2.1	2.2	2.3 r=-0.249 p=0.055	2.4 r=-0.187 p=0.153	2.5 r=-0.115 p=0.383	2.6 r=-0.146 p=0.268	2.7	2.8
1.1	1.2	1.3	1.4	1.5	1.6	1.7	1.8

(a)

8.1	8.2	8.3	8.4	8.5	8.6	8.7	8.8
7.1	7.2	7.3 r=0.149 p=0.417	7.4 r=-0.113 p=0.539	7.5 r=-0.067 p=0.716	7.6 r=-0.022 p=0.905	7.7	7.8
6.1	6.2 r=0.042 p=0.820	6.3 r=0.144 p=0.433	6.4 r=-0.110 p=0.548	6.5 r=0.123 p=0.504	6.6 r=-0.230 p=0.205	6.7 r=-0.053 p=0.772	6.8
5.1 r=0.270 p=0.135	5.2 r=0.66 p=0.720	5.3 r=0.109 p=0.553	5.4 r=-0.233 p=0.200	5.5 r=0.003 p=0.985	5.6 r=0.215 p=0.237	5.7 r=0.034 p=0.842	5.8 r=-0.135 p=0.460
4.1 r=0.417 p=0.017	4.2 r=0.096 p=0.601	4.3 r=0.017 p=0.928	4.4 r=-0.150 p=0.566	4.5 r=-0.013 p=0.943	4.6 r=-0.122 p=0.507	4.7 r=-0.233 p=0.200	4.8 r=0.119 p=0.516
3.1	3.2 r=-0.331 p=0.064	3.3 r=0.085 P=0.642	3.4 r=-0.062 P=0.736	3.5 r=0.164 P=0.369	3.6 r=0.071 p=0.700	3.7 r=-0.013 p=0.944	3.8
2.1	2.2	2.3 r=0.272 p=0.131	2.4 r=0.052 p=0.778	2.5 r=-0.096 p=0.620	2.6 r=0.320 p=0.075	2.7	2.8
1.1	1.2	1.3	1.4	1.5	1.6	1.7	1.8

(b)

Figure 12. Color map of correlations for outer plexiform layer + outer nuclear layer in the glaucoma group (**a**) and control group (**b**). Green color indicates non-significant correlation. Blue color indicates significant positive correlation. Red color indicates significant negative correlation. Black color indicates OCT superpixels not considered in the calculations. r = Spearman's rho, p = significance.

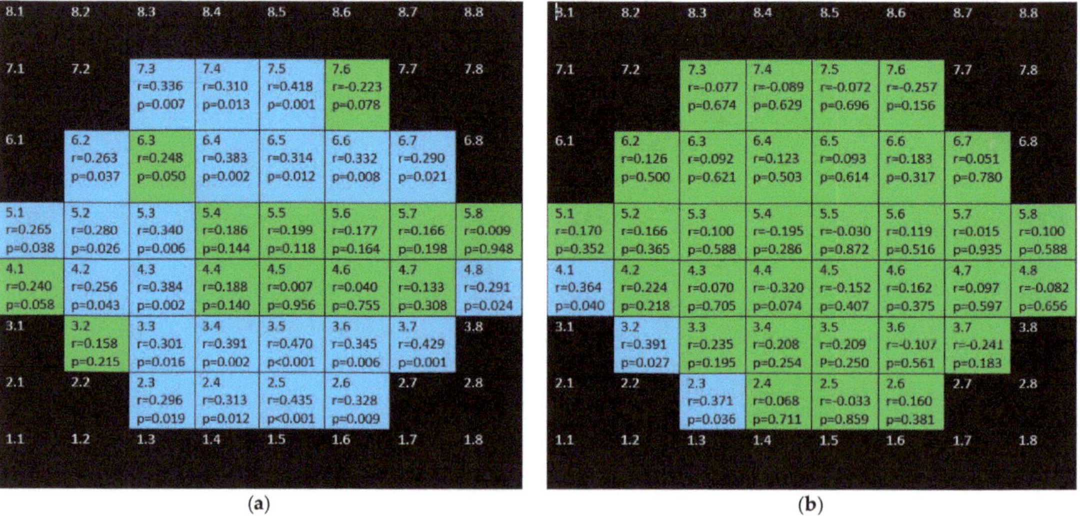

8.1	8.2	8.3	8.4	8.5	8.6	8.7	8.8
7.1	7.2	7.3 r=0.336 p=0.007	7.4 r=0.310 p=0.013	7.5 r=0.418 p=0.001	7.6 r=-0.223 p=0.078	7.7	7.8
6.1	6.2 r=0.263 p=0.037	6.3 r=0.248 p=0.050	6.4 r=0.383 p=0.002	6.5 r=0.314 p=0.012	6.6 r=0.332 p=0.008	6.7 r=0.290 p=0.021	6.8
5.1 r=0.265 p=0.038	5.2 r=0.280 p=0.026	5.3 r=0.340 p=0.006	5.4 r=0.186 p=0.144	5.5 r=0.199 p=0.118	5.6 r=0.177 p=0.164	5.7 r=0.166 p=0.198	5.8 r=0.009 p=0.948
4.1 r=0.240 p=0.058	4.2 r=0.256 p=0.043	4.3 r=0.384 p=0.002	4.4 r=0.188 p=0.140	4.5 r=0.007 p=0.956	4.6 r=0.040 p=0.755	4.7 r=0.133 p=0.308	4.8 r=0.291 p=0.024
3.1	3.2 r=0.158 p=0.215	3.3 r=0.301 p=0.016	3.4 r=0.391 p=0.002	3.5 r=0.470 p<0.001	3.6 r=0.345 p=0.006	3.7 r=0.429 p=0.001	3.8
2.1	2.2	2.3 r=0.296 p=0.019	2.4 r=0.313 p=0.012	2.5 r=0.435 p<0.001	2.6 r=0.328 p=0.009	2.7	2.8
1.1	1.2	1.3	1.4	1.5	1.6	1.7	1.8

(a)

8.1	8.2	8.3	8.4	8.5	8.6	8.7	8.8
7.1	7.2	7.3 r=-0.077 p=0.674	7.4 r=-0.089 p=0.629	7.5 r=-0.072 p=0.696	7.6 r=-0.257 p=0.156	7.7	7.8
6.1	6.2 r=0.126 p=0.500	6.3 r=0.092 p=0.621	6.4 r=0.123 p=0.503	6.5 r=0.093 p=0.614	6.6 r=0.183 p=0.317	6.7 r=0.051 p=0.780	6.8
5.1 r=0.170 p=0.352	5.2 r=0.166 p=0.365	5.3 r=0.100 p=0.588	5.4 r=-0.195 p=0.286	5.5 r=-0.030 p=0.872	5.6 r=0.119 p=0.516	5.7 r=0.015 p=0.935	5.8 r=0.100 p=0.588
4.1 r=0.364 p=0.040	4.2 r=0.224 p=0.218	4.3 r=0.070 p=0.705	4.4 r=-0.320 p=0.074	4.5 r=-0.152 p=0.407	4.6 r=0.162 p=0.375	4.7 r=0.097 p=0.597	4.8 r=-0.082 p=0.656
3.1	3.2 r=0.391 p=0.027	3.3 r=0.235 p=0.195	3.4 r=0.208 p=0.254	3.5 r=0.209 P=0.250	3.6 r=-0.107 p=0.561	3.7 r=-0.241 p=0.183	3.8
2.1	2.2	2.3 r=0.371 p=0.036	2.4 r=0.068 p=0.711	2.5 r=-0.033 p=0.859	2.6 r=0.160 p=0.381	2.7	2.8
1.1	1.2	1.3	1.4	1.5	1.6	1.7	1.8

(b)

Figure 13. Color map of correlations for inner retinal layer in the glaucoma group (**a**) and the control group (**b**). Green color indicates non-significant correlation. Blue color indicates significant positive correlation. Red color indicates significant negative correlation. Black color indicates OCT superpixels not considered in the calculations. R = Spearman´s rho, p = significance.

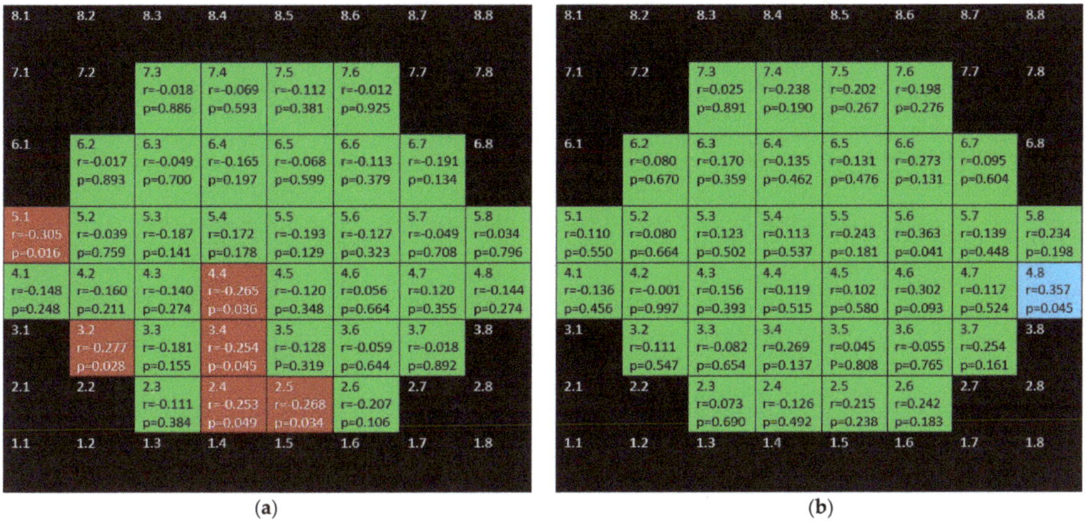

Figure 14. Color map of correlations for outer retina layer in the glaucoma group (**a**) and control group (**b**). Green color indicates non-significant correlation. Blue color indicates significant positive correlation. Red color indicates significant negative correlation. Black color indicates OCT superpixels not considered in the calculations. r = Spearman's rho, *p* = significance.

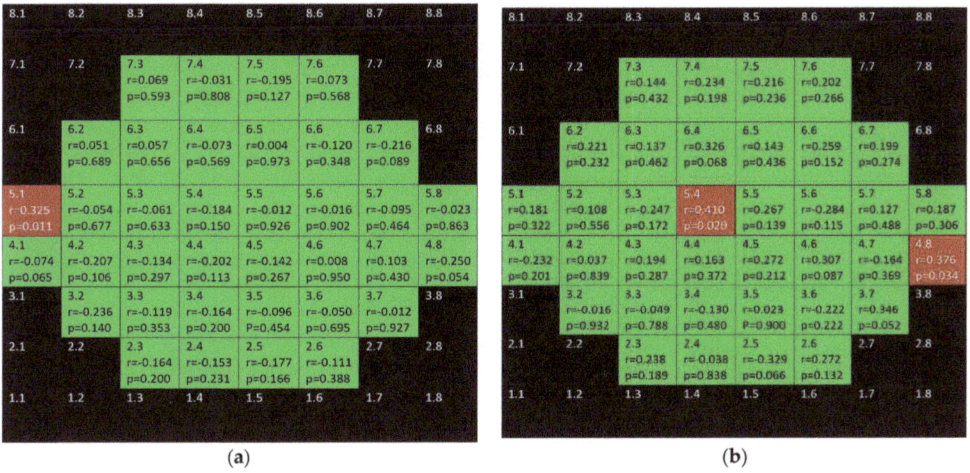

Figure 15. Color map of correlations for retinal pigment epithelium in the glaucoma group (**a**) and control group (**b**). Green color indicates non-significant correlation. Blue color indicates significant positive correlation. Red color indicates significant negative correlation. Black color indicates OCT superpixels not considered in the calculations. r = Spearman's rho, *p* = significance.

4. Discussion

This study dealt with the structure–function correlation of all retinal layers using OCT and MP. As mentioned in the introduction, a number of studies about the structure–function relationship have been performed by means of SAP [5]. SAP is a technique in which the projection of the stimulus on the retina can vary anatomically due to head misalignments and fixation losses. In contrast, MP is a technique that ensures that the projection of the stimulus is exactly at a specific anatomical point [6]. This is possible because MP has a real-time eye tracking system that stops the test until the eye is exactly oriented as it should be. This fact is controlled because the device continuously detects anatomical references that should be correctly positioned and only in this case does the examination go on. Plus, MP has been shown in some studies to have better ability to detect VF defects in comparison with SAP [13,14].

Only few studies have investigated macular structure–function correlation with MP in glaucoma. Some authors demonstrated that there were strong–moderate positive correlations between retinal sensitivity measured by microperimetry and ganglion cell layer + inner plexiform layer (GCLIPL) thickness in all the sectors and the sector average of the macular ellipsoid implemented in the Cirrus OCT device [7–9]. Zabel et.al. also found good positive correlations between the mean ganglion cell complex (mRNFL + GCL + IPL) thickness of the complete macula as determined by OCT and the average sensitivity threshold in a study aiming to correlate OCT angiography results and microperimetry results [10]. The results in this study are coincident with these mentioned studies in relation to ganglion cell-related layers showing positive, strong–moderate correlations. However, not only inner retinal layers are affected in glaucoma. Experimental studies [15,16] and human studies [2,3] have shown that outer retinal layers are also altered in glaucoma. However, to the best of our knowledge, the structure–function relationship for outer retinal layers has not been previously studied with MP.

In our study, they are remarkable the negative correlations found for outer retinal layer (photoreceptors + RPE) in the glaucoma group. This could be in relation to the changes found in these layers in our previous works [2,3] and these findings merit further investigation. Another noteworthy result in this study is the behavior of the structure–function relationship in the inner nuclear layer: while in the control group positive and moderate relationships were demonstrated, in the glaucoma group, the relationships found were also moderate but negative.

In general terms, the correlations found in this study were larger in glaucoma group than in the control group for almost all the considered retinal segmentations achieving the most intense associations for GCL and mRNFL and specially in the inferior hemisphere.

In this study we selected glaucomatous eyes with a threat to fixation in order to make sure that there was macular alteration in glaucomatous eyes. When scotomas progress towards the VF center in glaucoma, they may ultimately threaten fixation. Threat to fixation is considered an alarm sign in the management of patients with glaucoma because its progression may result in a significant decrease in vision-related quality of life [11,17–19]. However, threaten to fixation is not unusual in patients suffering from glaucoma. It has been described that threat to fixation is present at the diagnosis of glaucomain almost 60% of eyes [20].

This study presents several limitations to be considered. One was the relatively small size of the sample. Another one was the fact that the glaucoma group was made up of Caucasic patients suffering from POAG, so our results might not be extrapolated to other ethnic groups or to other types of glaucoma. Otherwise, each MP Goldmann III-size stimulus (circular light spot with a diameter of 43 degrees) [21] is projected at the center of a 3×3 degree OCT superpixel so the anatomical correspondence is not exact but it is representative of the studied area. Plus, it has been recently show that the MP-1 device has an overall bias in sensitivity values, as well as an eccentricity based measuring anomaly so our results may have been influenced by these facts [22]. Additionally, the fact that the strength of a correlation changes with the range of measurements being considered [23] could have induced, at least in part, the stronger correlations seen in the glaucoma group where both sensitivities and thicknesses change over a greater range. Finally, this is a cross-sectional study so, due to its nature, this investigation does not permit to study progressive changes of POAG.

5. Conclusions

In general terms, significant structure–function correlations for different intraretinal layers are higher and wider in POAG eyes than in healthy eyes and it is more marked for inner retinal layers as determined by using MP and OCT. Additionally, inner and outer retinal layers behave differently in terms of the structure–function relationship in POAG.

Author Contributions: Conceptualization and methodology, writing—original draft preparation: All authors; software J.J.G.-M., E.R.-V.; validation, formal analysis, and investigation: J.J.G.-M., M.d.-R.-V. and M.D.P.-D.; data curation J.J.G.-M.; critically reviewed the last draft of the paper: All authors.; supervision: J.J.G.-M., M.d.-R.-V. and M.D.P.-D. All authors have read and agreed to the published version of the manuscript.

Funding: This research received no external funding.

Institutional Review Board Statement: The study was conducted according to the guidelines of the Declaration of Helsinki, and approved by the Institutional Ethics Committee) of General University Hospital Reina Sofia (protocol number 0416, approved on January 2016).

Informed Consent Statement: Informed consent was obtained from all subjects involved in the study.

Conflicts of Interest: The authors declare no conflict of interest.

References

1. Weinreb, R.N.; Aung, T.; Medeiros, F.A. The Pathophysiology and Treatment of Glaucoma. *JAMA* **2014**, *311*, 1901–1911. [CrossRef] [PubMed]
2. García-Medina, J.; Del-Rio-Vellosillo, M.; Palazón-Cabanes, A.; Tudela-Molino, M.; Gómez-Molina, C.; Guardiola-Fernández, A.; Villegas-Pérez, M. Mapeo de los cambios de grosor en el glaucoma de las capas retinianas maculares segmentadas usando el programa de polo posterior de la tomografía de coherencia óptica de dominio espectral. *Archivos de la Sociedad Española de Oftalmología* **2018**, *93*, 263–273. [CrossRef] [PubMed]
3. Garcia-Medina, J.J.; Del-Rio-Vellosillo, M.; Palazon-Cabanes, A.; Pinazo-Duran, M.D.; Zanon-Moreno, V.; Villegas-Perez, M.P. Glaucomatous Maculopathy: Thickness Differences on Inner and Outer Macular Layers between Ocular Hypertension and Early Primary Open-Angle Glaucoma Using 8×8 Posterior Pole Algorithm of SD-OCT. *J. Clin. Med.* **2020**, *9*, 1503. [CrossRef]
4. Kitazawa, Y.; Yamamoto, T. Glaucomatous visual field defects: Their characteristics and how to detect them. *Clin. Neurosci. (New York N.Y.)* **1997**, *4*, 279–283.
5. Torres, L.A.; Hatanaka, M. Correlating Structural and Functional Damage in Glaucoma. *J. Glaucoma* **2019**, *28*, 1079–1085. [CrossRef] [PubMed]
6. Talib, M.; Jolly, J.; Boon, C.J.F. Measuring Central Retinal Sensitivity Using Microperimetry. *Methods Mol. Biol.* **2018**, *1715*, 339–349. [PubMed]
7. Sato, S.; Hirooka, K.; Baba, T.; Tenkumo, K.; Nitta, E.; Shiraga, F. Correlation Between the Ganglion Cell-Inner Plexiform Layer Thickness Measured With Cirrus HD-OCT and Macular Visual Field Sensitivity Measured With Microperimetry. *Investig. Opthalmol. Vis. Sci.* **2013**, *54*, 3046–3051. [CrossRef]
8. Rao, H.L.; Januwada, M.; Hussain, R.S.M.; Pillutla, L.N.; Begum, V.U.; Chaitanya, A.; Senthil, S.; Garudadri, C.S. Comparing the Structure–Function Relationship at the Macula With Standard Automated Perimetry and Microperimetry. *Investig. Opthalmol. Vis. Sci.* **2015**, *56*, 8063–8068. [CrossRef]
9. Akar, S.; Tekeli, O.; Ozturker, Z.K. Macular Integrity Assessment Microperimeter, Humphrey Field Analyzer and Optical Coherence Tomography in Glaucoma Practice: A Correlation Study. *Can. J. Ophthalmol.* **2021**, S0008418221002556. [CrossRef]
10. Zabel, K.; Zabel, P.; Kaluzna, M.; Lamkowski, A.; Jaworski, D.; Wietlicka-Piszcz, M.; Kaluzny, J.J. Correlation of retinal sensitivity in microperimetry with vascular density in optical coherence tomography angiography in primary open-angle glaucoma. *PLoS ONE* **2020**, *15*, e0235571. [CrossRef]
11. Zhang, L.; Drance, S.M.; Douglas, G.R. Automated perimetry in detecting threats to fixation. *Ophthalmology* **1997**, *104*, 1918–1920. [CrossRef]
12. Lujan, B.J.; Roorda, A.; Croskrey, J.A.; Dubis, A.M.; Cooper, R.F.; Bayabo, J.K.; Duncan, J.L.; Antony, B.J.; Carroll, J. Directional optical coherence tomography provides accurate outer nuclear layer and henle fibre layer measurements. *Retina* **2015**, *35*, 1511–1520. [CrossRef]
13. Orzalesi, N.; Miglior, S.; Lonati, C.; Rosetti, L. Microperimetry of localized retinal nerve fiber layer defects. *Vis. Res.* **1998**, *38*, 763–771. [CrossRef]
14. Lima, V.C.; Prata, T.; De Moraes, C.G.V.; Kim, J.; Seiple, W.; Rosen, R.B.; Liebmann, J.M.; Ritch, R. A comparison between microperimetry and standard achromatic perimetry of the central visual field in eyes with glaucomatous paracentral visual-field defects. *Br. J. Ophthalmol.* **2009**, *94*, 64–67. [CrossRef]

15. Vidal-Sanz, M.; Valiente-Soriano, F.J.; Ortín-Martínez, A.; Nadal-Nicolás, F.M.; Jiménez-López, M.; Salinas-Navarro, M.; Alarcón-Martínez, L.; García-Ayuso, D.; Avilés-Trigueros, M.; Agudo-Barriuso, M.; et al. Retinal neurodegeneration in experimental glaucoma. *Prog. Brain Res.* **2015**, *220*, 1–35. [CrossRef] [PubMed]
16. Kumar, S.; Ramakrishnan, H.; Viswanathan, S.; Akopian, A.; Bloomfield, S.A. Neuroprotection of the Inner Retina Also Prevents Secondary Outer Retinal Pathology in a Mouse Model of Glaucoma. *Investig. Opthalmol. Vis. Sci.* **2021**, *62*, 35. [CrossRef] [PubMed]
17. Membrey, W.L.; Poinoosawmy, D.P.; Bunce, C.; Fitzke, F.W.; A Hitchings, R. Comparison of visual field progression in patients with normal pressure glaucoma between eyes with and without visual field loss that threatens fixation. *Br. J. Ophthalmol.* **2000**, *84*, 1154–1158. [CrossRef] [PubMed]
18. McKean-Cowdin, R.; Wang, Y.; Wu, J.; Azen, S.P.; Varma, R. Impact of Visual Field Loss on Health-Related Quality of Life in Glaucoma: The Los Angeles Latino Eye Study. *Ophthalmology* **2008**, *115*, 941–948.e1. [CrossRef]
19. Sawada, H.; Fukuchi, T.; Abe, H. Evaluation of the relationship between quality of vision and the visual function index in Japanese glaucoma patients. *Graefe's Arch. Clin. Exp. Ophthalmol.* **2011**, *249*, 1721–1727. [CrossRef]
20. Peters, D.; Bengtsson, B.; Heijl, A. Threat to Fixation at Diagnosis and Lifetime Risk of Visual Impairment in Open-Angle Glaucoma. *Ophthalmology* **2015**, *122*, 1034–1039. [CrossRef] [PubMed]
21. Swanson, W.H. Stimulus Size for Perimetry in Patients With Glaucoma. *Investig. Opthalmol. Vis. Sci.* **2013**, *54*, 3984. [CrossRef] [PubMed]
22. Xu, L.; Wu, Z.; Guymer, R.H.; Anderson, A.J. Investigating the discrepancy between MAIA and MP-1 microperimetry results. *Ophthalmic Physiol. Opt.* **2021**, *41*, 1231–1240. [CrossRef] [PubMed]
23. Bland, J.M.; Altman, D. Statistical methods for assessing agreement between two methods of clinical measurement. *Lancet* **1986**, *327*, 307–310. [CrossRef]

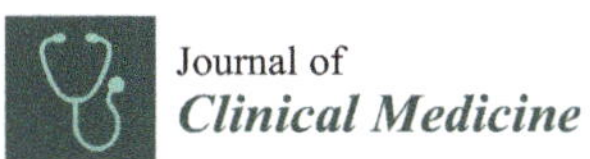

Journal of
Clinical Medicine

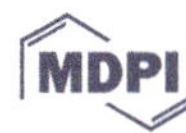

Article

Is Saffron Able to Prevent the Dysregulation of Retinal Cytokines Induced by Ocular Hypertension in Mice?

José A. Fernández-Albarral [1,†], Miguel A. Martínez-López [2,†], Eva M. Marco [3], Rosa de Hoz [1,4], Beatriz Martín-Sánchez [2], Diego San Felipe [2], Elena Salobrar-García [1,4], Inés López-Cuenca [1], María D. Pinazo-Durán [5], Juan J. Salazar [1,4], José M. Ramírez [1,6], Meritxell López-Gallardo [2,*] and Ana I. Ramírez [1,4,*]

1   Instituto de Investigaciones Oftalmológicas Ramón Castroviejo, Grupo UCM 920105, Universidad Complutense de Madrid, 28040 Madrid, Spain; joseaf08@ucm.es (J.A.F.-A.); rdehoz@med.ucm.es (R.d.H.); elenasalobrar@med.ucm.es (E.S.-G.); inelopez@ucm.es (I.L.-C.); jjsalazar@med.ucm.es (J.J.S.); ramirezs@med.ucm.es (J.M.R.)
2   Departamento de Fisiología, Facultad de Medicina, Grupo UCM 951579, Universidad Complutense de Madrid, 28040 Madrid, Spain; miguma19@ucm.es (M.A.M.-L.); beatrm14@ucm.es (B.M.-S.); diesanfe@ucm.es (D.S.F.)
3   Departamento de Genética, Facultad de CC. Biológicas, Fisiología y Microbiología, Grupo UCM 951579, Universidad Complutense de Madrid, 28040 Madrid, Spain; emmarco@bio.ucm.es
4   Departamento de Inmunología, Facultad de Óptica y Optometría, Oftalmología y ORL, IdISSC, Universidad Complutense de Madrid, 28040 Madrid, Spain
5   Ophthalmic Research Unit "Santiago Grisolía"—FISABIO and Cellular and Molecular Ophthalmobiology Unit, University of Valencia, 46017 Valencia, Spain; dolores.pinazo@uv.es
6   Departamento de Inmunología, Facultad de Medicina, Oftalmología y ORL, IdISSC, Universidad Complutense de Madrid, 28040 Madrid, Spain
*   Correspondence: mlopezga@ucm.es (M.L.-G.); airamirez@med.ucm.es (A.I.R.)
†   These authors should be considered as joint first authors.

Citation: Fernández-Albarral, J.A.; Martínez-López, M.A.; Marco, E.M.; de Hoz, R.; Martín-Sánchez, B.; San Felipe, D.; Salobrar-García, E.; López-Cuenca, I.; Pinazo-Durán, M.D.; Salazar, J.J.; et al. Is Saffron Able to Prevent the Dysregulation of Retinal Cytokines Induced by Ocular Hypertension in Mice? *J. Clin. Med.* **2021**, *10*, 4801. https://doi.org/10.3390/jcm10214801

Academic Editor: Fumi Gomi

Received: 24 August 2021
Accepted: 18 October 2021
Published: 20 October 2021

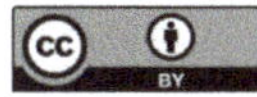

Abstract: Cytokine- and chemokine-mediated signalling is involved in the neuroinflammatory process that leads to retinal ganglion cell (RGC) damage in glaucoma. Substances with anti-inflammatory properties could decrease these cytokines and chemokines and thus prevent RGC death. The authors of this study analysed the anti-inflammatory effect of a hydrophilic saffron extract standardized to 3% crocin content, focusing on the regulation of cytokine and chemokine production, in a mouse model of unilateral laser-induced ocular hypertension (OHT). We demonstrated that following saffron treatment, most of the concentration of proinflammatory cytokines (IL-1β, IFN-γ, TNF-α, and IL-17), anti-inflammatory cytokines (IL-4 and IL-10), Brain-derived Neurotrophic Factor (BDNF), Vascular Endothelial Growth Factor (VEGF), and fractalkine were unaffected in response to laser-induced OHT in both the OHT eye and its contralateral eye. Only IL-6 levels were significantly increased in the OHT eye one day after laser induction compared with the control group. These results differed from those observed in animals subjected to unilateral OHT and not treated with saffron, where changes in cytokine levels occurred in both eyes. Therefore, saffron extract regulates the production of proinflammatory cytokines, VEGF, and fractalkine induced by increasing intraocular pressure (IOP), protecting the retina from inflammation. These results indicate that saffron could be beneficial in glaucoma by helping to reduce the inflammatory process.

Keywords: cytokines; BDNF; VEGF; fractalkine; glaucoma; ocular hypertension; microglia; saffron; crocin; retinal glial cells

1. Introduction

Glaucoma is a neurodegenerative disease in which there is an irreversible loss of retinal ganglion cells (RGCs), leading to blindness [1]. Intraocular pressure (IOP) is one of the main risk factors for this pathology and the one on which the main current treatments are based [2]. However, IOP control often fails to prevent the progression of the disease, so new factors that could be related to glaucomatous neurodegeneration, such as neuroinflammation, are being discovered [3,4].

In the course of the inflammatory process, retinal glial cells, both microglia and macroglia (Müller cells and astrocytes), can be activated and release factors that can be neuroprotective in some cases and neurodegenerative in others [5–7]. Activated microglia can be found along two extreme activation phenotypes, M1 and M2. The M2 phenotype releases neurotrophic factors (neurotrophins, Glial cell line-derived Neurotrophic Factor (GDNF), Brain-derived Neurotrophic Factor (BDNF), etc. and anti-inflammatory cytokines (TGFβ, IL-4, IL-10, etc.) that help control inflammation and promote neuronal survival. However, the M1 phenotype releases proinflammatory mediators (nitric oxide and reactive oxygen species) and proinflammatory cytokines (IL-1β, IL-6, IFN-γ, TNF-α, etc.). Therefore, if this phenotype becomes chronic, it can promote the neurodegenerative process [5,8,9].

In previous studies, we analysed microglial activation [9–13] and the expression of different proinflammatory cytokines (IL-1β, IL-6, IL-17, IFN-γ, TNF-α), anti-inflammatory cytokines (IL-4 and IL-10), BDNF, VEGF, and fractalkine (CX3CL1) [14] in a mouse model of glaucoma at different time points (1, 3, 5, 7, and 15 days) after ocular hypertension (OHT) induction. In this model, we found that the highest microglial activation, as measured by increased cell number, increased number of vertical processes, increased soma size, retraction of the processes, and downregulation of P2RY12 (which is a sensitive marker of the switch from resting to activated microglia [15]), occurred at 3 and 5 days after OHT induction [11]. This peak of microglial activation seemed to overlap with an increased expression of pro-inflammatory cytokines (IL-6 and IFN-γ), anti-inflammatory (IL-4 and IL-10) cytokines, VEGF, fractalkine, and BDNF, which showed greater expression at 1, 3, and 5 days after OHT induction [14]. Higher inflammation was found to occur at these time points, and RGC loss was thereafter triggered; at 3 days after OHT induction, we observed a decrease in the expression of the RGCs marker Brn3a, and from 5 and 7 days onwards, the neurodegenerative process became evident [14,16]. Therefore, 1, 3, and 5 days after OHT induction (especially after 1 and 3 days) would be the ideal time points to analyse whether a substance has anti-inflammatory effects in this murine glaucoma model. Accordingly, we analysed the possible beneficial effect of saffron extracts on the neuroinflammatory and neurodegenerative process in this model of glaucoma, as saffron has important anti-inflammatory, antiapoptotic, and antioxidant properties [17–20]. The therapeutic activity of saffron may be due to its content in carotenoids, such as crocetin, crocin, and safranal, which are saffron's main bioactive components, with crocetin being the major component responsible for its therapeutic properties [21–24]. Different mechanisms of action have been attributed to crocetin including a reduction of proinflammatory molecules and protection against oxidative damage. Crocetin's anti-inflammatory properties could be due to its capacity to modulate the proinflammatory cytokines' release from glial cells (IL-6, IL-1β among others); to its ability to block TNF-α expression by microglia, to DNA fragmentation avoidance and thus cell death; to its capacity to modulate the expression of adhesion molecules; to reduce mRNA of some proinflammatory enzymes; and to modulate the NF-κB inflammatory pathway [25–31]. With regard to its antioxidant properties, crocetin, together with other carotenoids contained in the saffron extract, is able to modulate the expression of genes related to the redox cells system, to inhibit the proteins, and DNA and RNA synthesis; to modify stress markers in the endoplasmic reticulum system; to reduce telomerase activity; and to counteract oxidative stress via tRNA–crocetin union and suppression of the activation of NF-κB through activation of the nuclear factor erythroid 2-related factor 2 (Nrf2) signal related to the modulation of oxidative stress [24,26,32–35].

We found that at day 3 after OHT induction, animals treated with saffron extracts showed a decrease in the morphological signs of microglial activation and partially reversed the downregulation of P2RY12. Furthermore, they prevented the death of RGCs 7 days after OHT induction, indicating that saffron extracts were able to produce an anti-inflammatory and neuroprotective effect against the damage caused by increased IOP [36]. However, the effects of this saffron extract on the release of different inflammatory mediators with anti-inflammatory or proinflammatory properties to promote the protection of RGCs are currently unknown. Therefore, the purpose of the present work was to analyse whether the administration of saffron extracts in a laser-induced OHT model at 1 and 3 days after OHT induction, in which we found increased cytokine expression in OHT eyes, causes changes in the expression of proinflammatory cytokines (IL-1β, IL-6, IL-17, IFN-γ, and TNF-α), anti-inflammatory cytokines (IL-4 and IL-10), BDNF, VEGF, and fractalkine using multiplex and immunohistochemical techniques.

2. Materials and Methods

2.1. Animals

The study was performed on male Swiss mice weighing 40–45 g and aged 12–16 weeks, obtained from Charles River Laboratories (Barcelona, Spain). The animals were kept in the animal house of the Faculty of Medicine of the Universidad Complutense de Madrid (Spain). The animals were placed in cages in which the light intensity varied between 9 and 12 lux and the light/dark cycles were 12 h. The animals were fed a standard diet and had free access to it and water. The experimental protocols complied with all of the ethical guidelines endorsed by Spanish law and the Guidelines for Humane Endpoints for Animals Used in Biomedical Research. The study was approved by the Ethics Committee for Animal Research of Complutense University (Madrid, Spain) and the Directorate General of Agriculture and Food, Ministry of Economy and Employment of the Community of Madrid (approval ID number: ES280790000086, 1 April 2016). Finally, the procedures also followed institutional guidelines, the European Union regulations for the use of animals in research, and the Association for Research in Vision and Ophthalmology (ARVO) statement for the use of animals in ophthalmic and vision research.

2.2. Experimental Groups

The animals were divided into three study groups: (i) a naïve age-matched control group that received saffron extract (saffron-naïve group; SNG) and (ii) two groups of laser-treated animals that were photocoagulated with laser in the left eye to provoke an OHT and that were treated with saffron extract. These groups were sacrificed 1 (saffron laser-induced group sacrificed on day 1, SLG1d) and 3 days (saffron laser-induced group sacrificed on day 3, SLG3d) after OHT induction. In the laser groups, both saffron OHT eyes (SOHT) and their normotensive saffron-contralateral eyes (S-contralateral) were analysed.

2.3. Treatment with Saffron

The company Pharmactive Biotech Products S.L. (Madrid, Spain) was responsible for supplying the hydrophilic stigma extracts of saffron (Crocus sativus L.) that were marketed under the saffron ® EYE brand (Pharmactive Biotech Products S.L., Madrid, Spain) [37,38]. These extracts were standardised to 3.14% total crocin and contain dextrin as a carrier. They were prepared by a proprietary method and analysed by high performance liquid chromatograph (HPLC) (Agilent Technologies 1220, Hewlett-Packard-Strasse, Waldbronn, Germany) [37]. The extract was in powder form and was stored in the dark until use. The dose selected and the time of administration was the same as that used in a previous work [36]. The dose was 60 mg/kg b.w. per day, which contained a total amount of crocin of 1.8 mg. Saffron extract was administered for 15 days in the SNG and 15 days before OHT induction in the laser groups. The administration of saffron extract was maintained after laser treatment until the day of animal sacrifice: 1 day (SL1d) and 3 days (SL3d). At the beginning of the study, in order to calculate the proportion of extract per kilogram of body weight, the animals were weighed. To ensure that the animals received their exact dose, the extract was diluted in water and administered by gavage (0.01 mL/g b.w.).

2.4. Anaesthetics

To avoid animal suffering, surgical procedures were performed after the intraperitoneal administration of a general anaesthetic consisting of a mixture of medetomidine

(0.26 mg/kg; Medetor®, Virbac España S.A., Barcelona, Spain) and ketamine (75 mg/kg; Anesketin®, Dechra Veterinary Products SLU, Barcelona, Spain). After the procedure, an ointment containing tobramycin (Tobrex®; Alcon, Barcelona, Spain) was administered on to the eyes to prevent eye drying and infection. Subsequently, the animals were returned to their cages for recovery from anaesthesia. An overdose of sodium pentobarbital (Dolethal Vetoquinol®, Especialidades Veterinarias, Alcobendas, Madrid, Spain) was used for the sacrifice of the animals. For the measurement of IOP, the animals were given inhalational anaesthesia of 2% isoflurane in oxygen (ISOFLO Isoflurane 100% *w/w*, Zoetis SL, Alcobendas, Madrid, Spain).

2.5. Laser Treatment and Measurement of IOP

A laser treatment was performed to induce an OHT. For this purpose, the left eyes of previously anaesthetised animals were treated with a diode laser according to previously described protocols [39,40]. Briefly, the laser beam was applied directly, without any lens, on the episcleral and limbal veins, so that 55–76 burns were performed. The used parameters were: a spot size of 50–100 μm, a duration of 0.5 s, and a power of 0.3 W. IOP was measured in both eyes of all of the experimental groups using a rebound tonometer (Tono-Lab, Tiolat, OY, Helsinki, Finland) [41,42]. IOP was measured after the administration of anaesthesia and always at the same time point (around 9 a.m.) to avoid changes due to circadian rhythms [43]. Six consecutive IOP measurements were performed and averaged each time. In the control group (SNG), IOP was measured before sacrifice. In the SLGs, IOP was measured before laser induction. In the SLG1d group, IOP was also measured on day 1 after laser induction, and in the SLG3d group, it was measured on days 1, 2, and 3 after laser induction.

2.6. Multiplexed Immunoassay Study

2.6.1. Protein Assay

For the multiplex immunoassay, animals were sacrificed with an overdose of sodium pentobarbital, after which the retinas were removed and frozen. As in previous studies [14], three retinas were pooled to perform the assay because of the small amount of protein obtained per mouse retina. Thus, four samples per experimental group were assayed, each one coming from three pooled retinas from eyes from the same experimental group. Retinas were homogenized on ice with a lysis buffer (MILLIPLEX MAP Lysis buffer for Multiplexing, Merck KGaA, Darmstadt, Germany) at a ratio of 1: 3 (*w/v*) and then frozen overnight at -70 °C. The following day, the samples were centrifuged (12,000× *g* for 5 min at 4 °C), and the supernatants were collected and processed again in the same way. These last supernatants were aliquoted to analyse the protein concentration by using the Bradford protein assay (Bio-RadDye Reagent Concentrate, Bio-Rad Laboratories, Irvine, CA, USA), which was then measured by a Multiskan reader (Thermo Fisher Technologies, Madrid, Spain). The obtained protein concentration was suitable for immunoassay.

2.6.2. Multiplexed Magnetic Bead Immunoassay

Using two multiplexed magnetic bead immunoassay kits (MILLIPLEX MAP Mouse Cytokine/Chemokine Magnetic Bead Panel; MILLIPLEX MAP Myokine Magnetic Bead Panel, Merck KGaA, Darmstadt, Germany), based on Luminex© technology, we measured the cytokines and myokines chosen for the study in duplicate. Briefly, the followed protocol used magnetic beads (25 μL) that were conjugated with the specific antibodies for the different cytokines/myokines (IFN-γ, IL-1β, IL-4, IL-6, IL-10, IL-17, TNF-α, VEGF, BDNF, and then fractalkine (CX3CL1)) were incubated together with the tissue samples (25 μL) under agitation overnight at 4 °C. After this, the wells were washed three times using a wash buffer. They were then incubated with a biotinylated antibody for 1 h at room temperature. The beads were then incubated for 30 min at room temperature with streptavidin-PE (phycoerythrin), which is a reporter molecule that completes the reaction on the surface of each microsphere. The samples were then washed three times, and the detection component included in the immunoassay kit was added. After immunoassay completion, the samples were analysed using the Bio-Plex suspension array system 200, and the mean fluorescence intensity was measured using Bio-Plex Manager Software 4.1 (Bio-Rad Laboratories, Irvine, CA, USA).

2.6.3. Immunostaining

In order to locate the cells that expressed the factors and cytokines detected in the multiplex assay, we performed an immunohistochemical analysis. As Fernández-Albarral et al. (2021) described [14], each animal was anaesthetised, then transcardially perfused by first employing a 0.9% saline solution and then 4% paraformaldehyde (PFA 4%) in a 0.1 M phosphate buffer. Then, eyes were dissected and fixed for 24 h at 4 °C in PFA. After 24 h, corneas and lenses were removed, and the optical cups containing the retina stood overnight at 4 °C in PFA again. The next day, each eye was washed in phosphate-buffered saline (PBS), pH 7.2, for 30 min. This procedure was repeated 3 times, and then each eye stood in PBS with 11% sucrose at 4 °C for 24 h in order to start the cryoprotection process. Then, the eyes passed to 33% sucrose PBS at 4 °C for 48 h. After the cryoprotection process was finished, the eyes were embedded in a tissue-freezing medium (Tissue-Tek® O.C.T.TM Compound, Sakura Finetek Spain, Barcelona, Spain). During the inclusion, the eye anatomical references were noted to keep track of each part of the retinas. The samples were frozen at −30 °C till they were later used and processed.

For immunostaining techniques, optical cups with retinas were frozen sectioned using a Leica CM-3050 cryostat (Leica Biosystems, Heidelberger, Germany) in 16-μm-thick serial sagittal sections from the nasal to temporal retina. Tissue sections were collected onto gelatine-coated slides (two sections per slide), air-dried, and stored at −30 °C until use. We selected those retinas (OHT and/or contralateral) and time points where the expression of cytokines and factors analysed by multiplex were greatest.

In the present study, we employed primary antibodies (Table 1) against IL-1β, IL-4, IL-6, IL-10, IL-17, INF-Y, fractalkine, TNF-α, and BDNF, which were co-located with Iba-1, a microglial marker; Glial fibrillary Acidic Protein (GFAP), a macroglial marker, and NF-200 (200 kD neurofilament), an RGC axon marker. Each secondary antibody was conjugated with a determined fluorochrome, as indicated in Table 1, which allowed for their detection during a double-labelling fluorescent immunohistochemistry study.

Slides were allowed to dry at room temperature for 60 min in order to increase the adhesion of the slices to the slides. All washes were conducted in PBS, pH 7.2, containing 0.1% Triton X-100, which constituted the washing buffer (WB); incubations were performed in WB with 1% universal serum and the antibody in the desired concentration. After three washes in WB, sections were incubated overnight at 4 °C with the primary antibodies (see Table 1), then rinsed three times in WB, and incubated for 2 h at room temperature with the secondary antibodies, except for Iba-1 (not needed). The details and dilutions of all of the primary and secondary antibodies used are presented in Table 1.

After incubations, sections were washed three more times with WB, then cover-slipped with a Vectashield Vibrance Antifade® mounting medium with DAPI (Ref. H-1800; Vector Laboratories, Burlingame, CA, USA).

Immunostaining batches contained slides of every animal from every experimental group (n = 4 per experimental group) as well as an internal control (omitting the primary antibody) to check the specificity of the immunoreaction and to rule out nonspecific binding. Three different batches were run for each primary antibody.

Table 1. Antibodies employed for the immunostaining analysis and their corresponding concentrations.

Colour	Primary Antibody	Conc.	Secondary Antibody	Conc.
GREEN	Rabbit polyclonal anti-IL-1β (ref. ab9722, Abcam plc) [44]	1:250	Goat anti-rabbit Alexa Fluor 488 (ref. ab150077, Abcam plc)	1:150
	Rabbit polyclonal anti-IL-6 (ref. ab208113, Abcam plc) [45]	1:200		
	Rabbit polyclonal anti-IL-17 (ref. ab79056, Abcam plc) [46]	1:300		
	Rabbit polyclonal anti-IFNγ (ref. ab9657, Abcam plc) [47]	1:300		
	Rabbit monoclonal anti-BDNF (ref. ab213323, Abcam plc) [44]	1:250		
	Rabbit monoclonal anti-VEGF receptor 1 (ref. ab32152, Abcam plc) [48]	1:200		
	Rabbit polyclonal anti-CX3CL1 (ref. ab25088, Abcam plc) [49]	1:500		
	Rabbit polyclonal anti-TNFα (ref. ab9739, Abcam plc) [50]	1:300		
	Rat monoclonal anti-IL-4 (ref. ab11524, Abcam plc) [51]	1:250	Goat anti-rat Alexa Fluor 488 (ref. ab150165, Abcam plc)	1:150
	Rat monoclonal anti-IL-10 (ref. ab189392, Abcam plc) [52]	1:200		
RED	Rabbit polyclonal anti-Iba1 Red Fluorochrome 635 conjugated (ref. 5100756, Wako Chemicals GmbH) [53]	1:200		
	Chicken polyclonal anti-GFAP (ref. AB5541, Sigma-Aldrich) [54]	1:200	Goat anti-chicken IgY (H+L) Alexa Fluor 594 (ref. A-11042, Invitrogen)	1:300
	Rabbit polyclonal anti-NF-200 (ref. N4142, Sigma-Aldrich) [55]	1:150	Donkey anti-rabbit IgG1 Alexa Fluor 594 (ref. A21207, Invitrogen)	1:800

Antibodies used in the study: interleukin 1 beta (IL-1β), interleukin 6 (IL-6), interleukin 17 (IL-17), interferon gamma (IFN-γ), brain-derived neurotrophic factor (BDNF), vascular endothelial growth factor (VEGF), fractalkine (CX3CL1), tumour necrosis factor alpha (TNF-α), interleukin 4 (IL-4), and interleukin 10 (IL-10); also included are the antibodies used to identify microglial cells (Iba-1), axons (NF-200 KDa), and macroglia (GFAP). The colour (green/red) indicates how the immunostaining is labelled.

Immunostained slides were observed under a Zeiss Axio Imager M.2 fluorescence microscope (Carl Zeiss AG, Oberkochen, Germany) associated with the Apotome-2 module (Carl Zeiss AG, Oberkochen, Germany) and AxioCam 503 Mono high-resolution camera (Carl Zeiss AG, Oberkochen, Germany). The microscope was equipped with a Zeiss 10 filter set for Alexa Fluor 488, a Zeiss 64 filter set for Alexa Fluor 594, and a 49 filter set for Alexa Fluor 405. Taken images were analysed using ZEN2 software (Carl Zeiss AG, Oberkochen, Germany). All lighting conditions and magnifications were kept constant during the capture process. Figures were prepared using Adobe Photoshop CS4 Extended 10.0 (Adobe Systems, San Jose, CA, USA).

2.7. Statistical Analysis

The results obtained both in the IOP measurements and the multiplex analysis were analysed using SPSS version 25 (IBM, Armonk, NY, USA) and were reported as the mean (±standard deviation; SD). If the results followed a normal distribution and equal variances, we performed an ANOVA and then a post-hoc Bonferroni comparison analysis in order to establish significant differences between experimental groups.

If data did not follow a normal distribution and were not homoscedastic, they were transformed (only for IL-6, IL-17, and BDNF analysis). Outliers were deleted according to the SPSS program [56]. Otherwise, non-parametric analyses—in particular, Kruskal–Wallis analysis followed by Mann–Whitney comparisons as a post-hoc—were performed. Only *p*-values under 0.05 were considered statistically significant.

3. Results

3.1. Intraocular Pressure

Eyes that had undergone OHT induction (saffron OHT eyes) had significant differences in IOP compared with SNG and saffron-contralateral eyes. (all $p < 0.001$; Figure 1). At all of the analysed time points, the contralateral eyes had an IOP similar to that of the naïve eyes ($p > 0.05$; Figure 1).

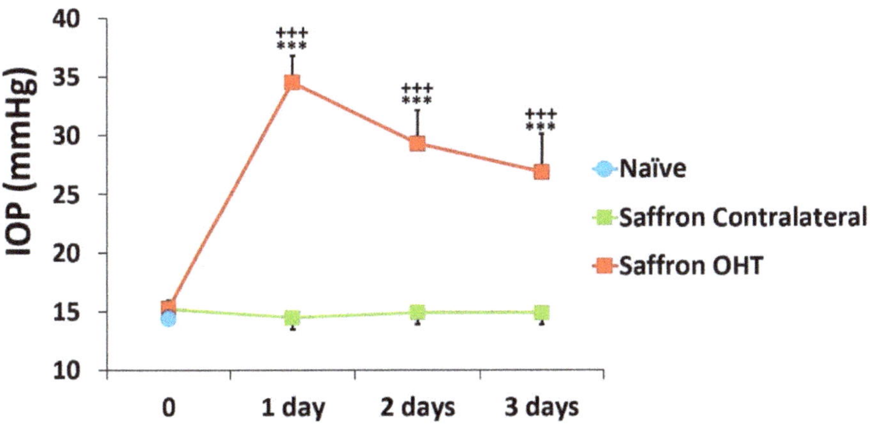

Figure 1. Intraocular pressure (IOP) values after laser-induced ocular hypertension (OHT) in 1, 2, and 3 days after laser OHT induction in saffron-naïve eyes, saffron ocular hypertension eyes (Saffron OHT), and saffron-contralateral eyes (saffron-contralateral). Statistical significance indicators: *** $p < 0.001$ vs. saffron-naïve; +++ $p < 0.001$ vs. saffron-contralateral.

3.2. Multiplex Analysis

Among the measured proinflammatory cytokines, 1 and 3 days after OHT induction, no significant differences were found in IL-1β expression between saffron OHT and saffron contralateral eyes compared to saffron-naïve eyes. Thus, retinal IL-1β levels were not affected by the laser OHT induction (Figure 2).

Regarding the IL-6 content, 1 day after OHT laser induction, a significant increase in its expression was observed in saffron OHT eyes compared to saffron contralateral eyes and saffron-naïve eyes (all $p < 0.05$). No significant differences were observed for IL-6 expression 3 days after OHT laser induction. Thus, retinal IL-6 expression was significantly higher exclusively 1 day after the laser induction in the saffron OHT eyes; cytokine levels were then returned to normal values 3 days post-laser treatment (Figure 3).

The analysis of IFN-γ levels showed no significant differences after experimental OHT induction. IFN-γ levels were not affected by the laser induction at any of the time-points considered (Figure 4). Similarly, the analysis of IL-17 levels showed no significant differences after laser induction in comparison to saffron-naïve eyes. Retinal IL-17 levels were not affected by the experimental OHT induction in the saffron OHT eyes and neither in saffron-contralateral eyes (Figure 5).

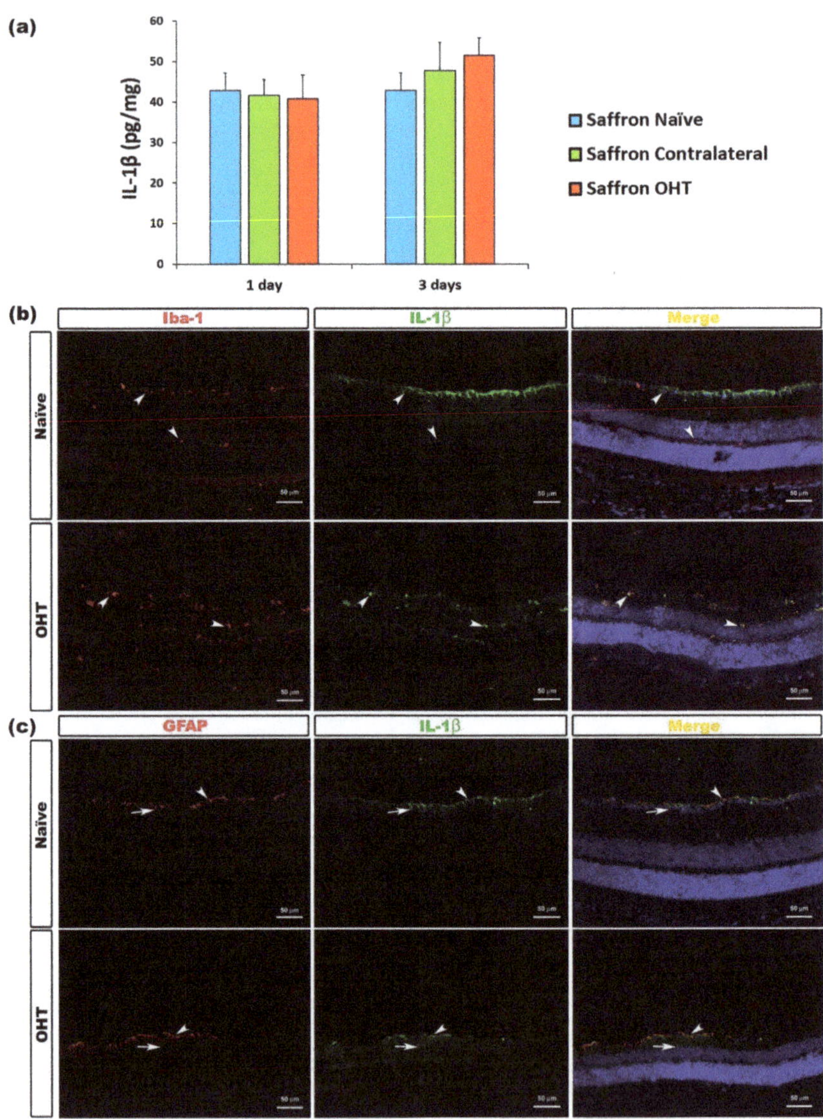

Figure 2. IL-1β levels at 1 and 3 days after laser-induced ocular hypertension (OHT). (**a**) The IL-1β values obtained in the multiplex assay. The histogram shows the mean levels (± SD) of IL-1β (pg/mg) at days 1 and 3 after laser OHT induction, in saffron ocular hypertension eyes (saffron OHT), saffron-contralateral eyes (saffron-contralateral), and naïve eyes. (**b**,**c**) Immunohistochemical study of IL-1β expression in naïve and saffron OHT eyes three days after unilateral laser-induced OHT. Retinal sections were immunolabeled with antibodies to IL-1β (green), Iba-1 (red in (**b**)), or GFAP (red in (**c**)). The merge section is denoted with the colour yellow. (**b**) The arrowhead shows the co-expression of Iba-1 and IL-1β. (**c**) Arrowhead (astrocytes) and arrow (Müller cells) indicate the co-expression of GFAP and IL-1β. Abbreviations: OHT (ocular hypertension); IL-1β (interleukin 1 beta); Iba-1 (ionized calcium-binding adaptor molecule); GFAP (glial fibrillary acidic protein).

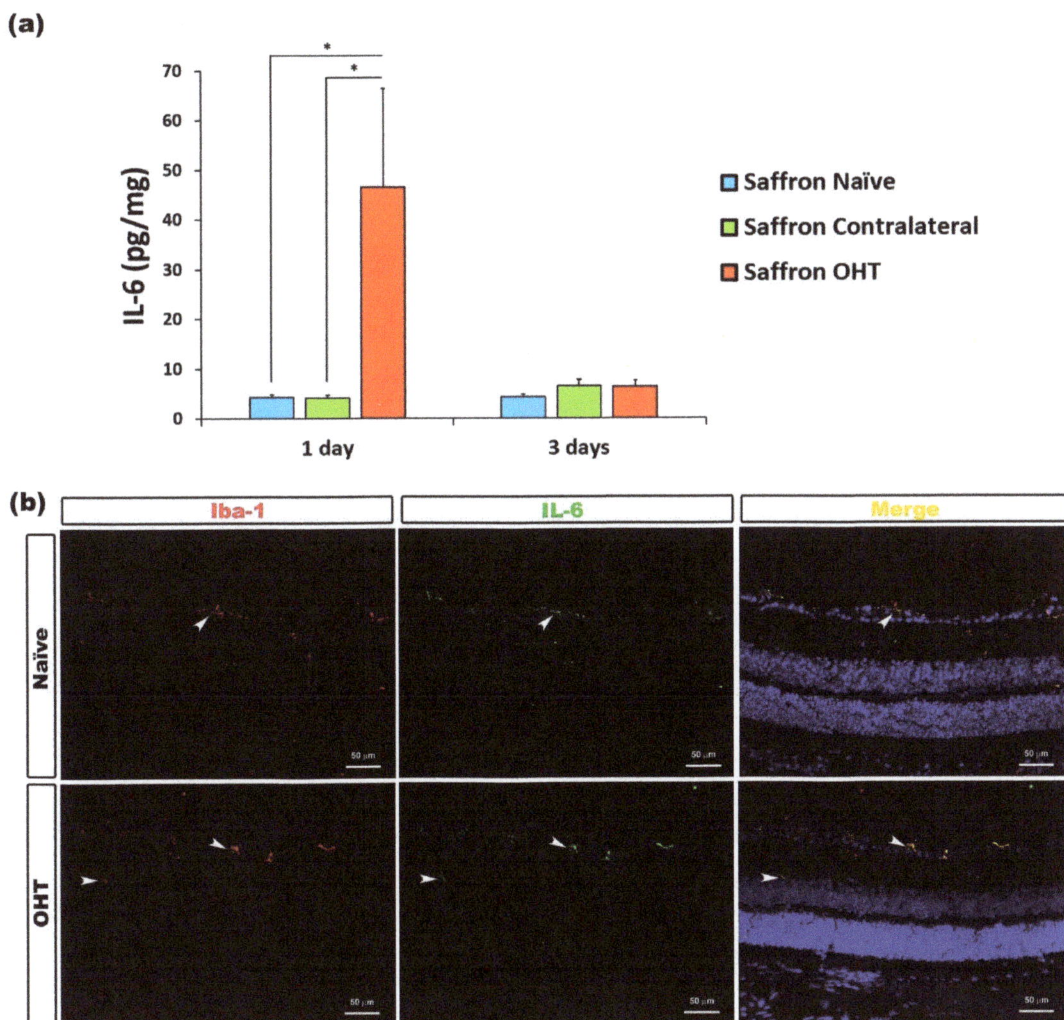

Figure 3. IL-6 levels at 1 and 3 days after laser-induced ocular hypertension (OHT). (**a**) The IL-6 values obtained in the multiplex assay. The histogram shows the mean levels (±SD) of IL-6 (pg/mg) at days 1 and 3 after laser OHT induction in saffron ocular hypertension eyes (saffron OHT), saffron-contralateral eyes (saffron-contralateral), and saffron-naïve eyes. Statistical significance indicators: * $p < 0.05$. (**b**) Immunohistochemical study of IL-6 expression in saffron OHT eyes one day after unilateral laser-induced OHT. Retinal sections were immunolabeled with antibodies to IL-6 (green) and Iba-1 (red). Merge is denoted by the colour yellow. The arrowhead shows the co-expression of Iba-1 and IL-6 in saffron OHT and saffron-naïve eyes. Abbreviations: OHT (ocular hypertension); IL-6 (interleukin 6); Iba-1 (ionized calcium-binding adaptor molecule).

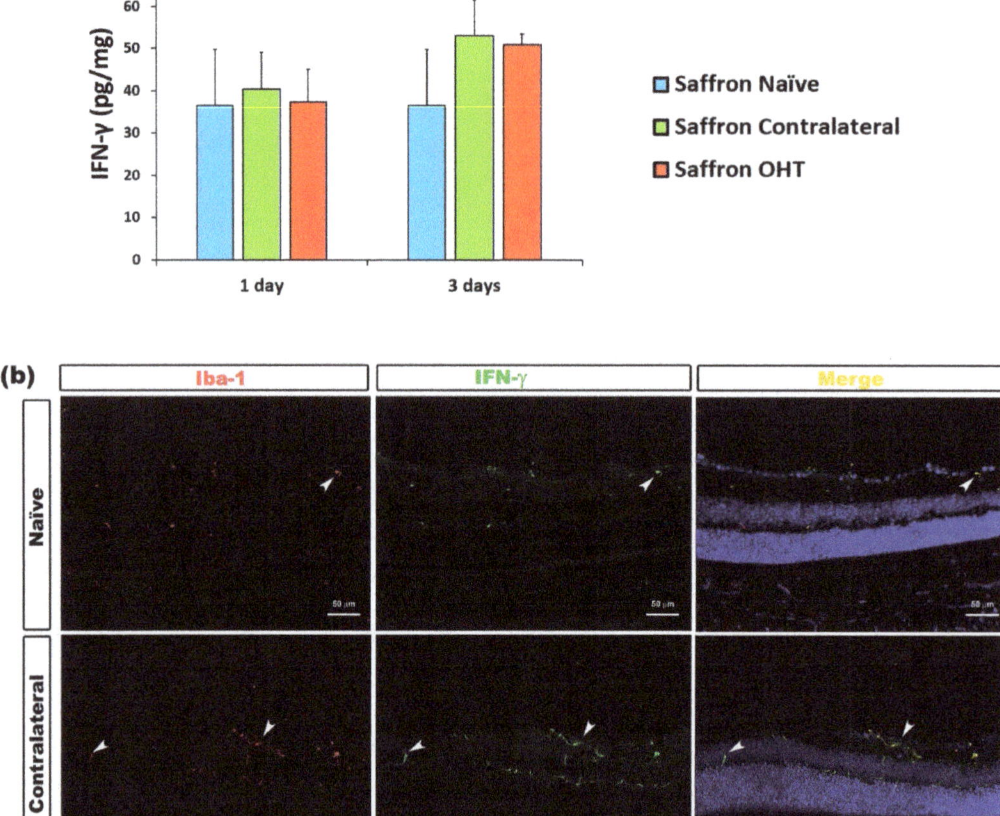

Figure 4. IFN-γ levels at 1 and 3 days after laser-induced ocular hypertension (OHT). (**a**) The IFN-γ values obtained in the multiplex assay. The histogram shows the mean levels (±SD) of IFN-γ (pg/mg) at days 1 and 3 after laser OHT induction in saffron ocular hypertension eyes (saffron OHT), saffron-contralateral eyes (saffron-contralateral), and saffron-naïve eyes. (**b**) Immunohistochemical study of IFN-γ expression in saffron-contralateral eyes three days after unilateral laser-induced OHT. Retinal sections were immunolabeled with antibodies to IFN-γ (green) and Iba-1 (red). Merge is denoted with the colour yellow. The arrowhead shows the co-expression of Iba-1 and IFN-γ in saffron-contralateral and saffron-naïve eyes. Abbreviations: OHT (ocular hypertension); IFN-γ (interferon-γ); Iba-1 (ionized calcium-binding adaptor molecule).

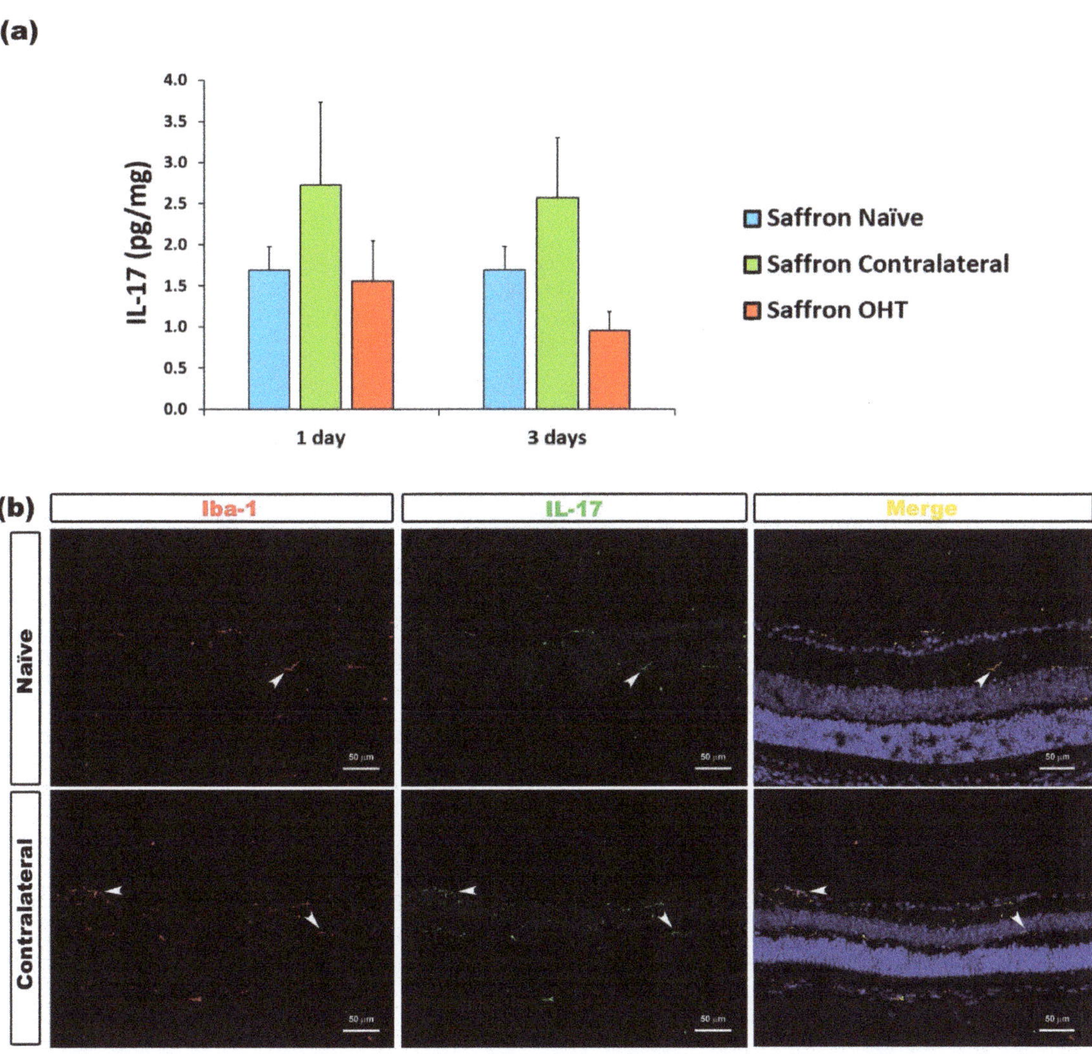

Figure 5. IL-17 levels at 1 and 3 days after laser-induced ocular hypertension (OHT). (**a**) The IL-17 values obtained in the multiplex assay. The histogram shows the mean levels (±SD) of IL-17 (pg/mg) at days 1 and 3 after laser OHT induction in saffron ocular hypertension eyes (saffron OHT), saffron-contralateral eyes (saffron-contralateral), and naïve eyes. (**b**) Immunohistochemical study of IL-17 expression in saffron-contralateral eyes one day after unilateral laser-induced OHT. Retinal sections were immunolabeled with antibodies to IL-17 (green) and Iba-1 (red). Merge is denoted by the colour yellow. The arrowhead shows the co-expression of Iba-1 and IL-17 in saffron-contralateral and saffron-naïve eyes. Abbreviations: OHT (ocular hypertension); IL-17 (interleukin-17); Iba-1 (ionized calcium-binding adaptor molecule).

Regarding TNF-α levels, 1 and 3 days after OHT induction, no significant changes were found in its expression neither in saffron OHT eyes nor in saffron contralateral eyes when compared to saffron-naïve eyes. Retinal TNF-α levels were not affected by the experimental OHT induction (Figure 6).

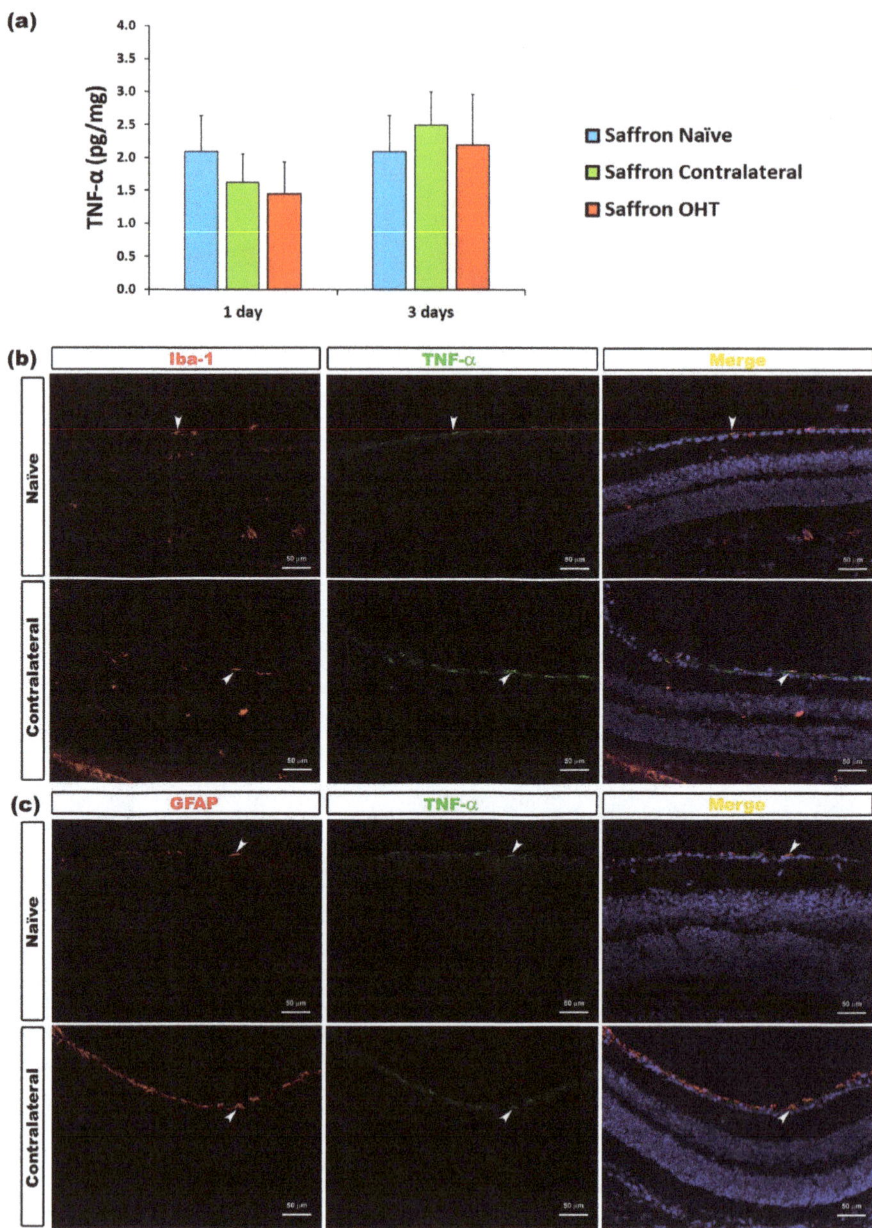

Figure 6. TNF-α levels at 1 and 3 days after laser-induced ocular hypertension (OHT). (**a**) The TNF-α values obtained in the multiplex assay. The histogram shows the mean levels (±SD) of TNF-α (pg/mg) at days 1 and 3 after laser OHT induction in saffron ocular hypertension eyes (saffron OHT) and saffron-contralateral eyes (saffron-contralateral) as well as in saffron-naïve eyes. (**b**) Immunohistochemical study of TNF-α expression in saffron-contralateral eyes three days after unilateral laser-induced OHT. Retinal sections were immunolabeled with antibodies to TNF-α (green) and Iba-1 (red in (**b**)), or GFAP (red in (**c**)). Merge is denoted by the colour yellow. (**b**) The arrowhead shows the co-expression of Iba-1 and TNF-α. (**c**) The arrowhead shows the co-expression of GFAP and TNF-α. Abbreviations: OHT (ocular hypertension); TNF-α (tumour necrosis factor-α); Iba-1 (ionized calcium-binding adaptor molecule); GFAP (glial fibrillary acidic protein).

The analysis of the anti-inflammatory cytokines showed that 1 and 3 days after OHT induction, IL-4 expression was not significantly affected by the laser treatment in saffron-treated eyes, neither in OHT nor in their contralateral eyes, compared to saffron-naïve eyes (Figure 7).

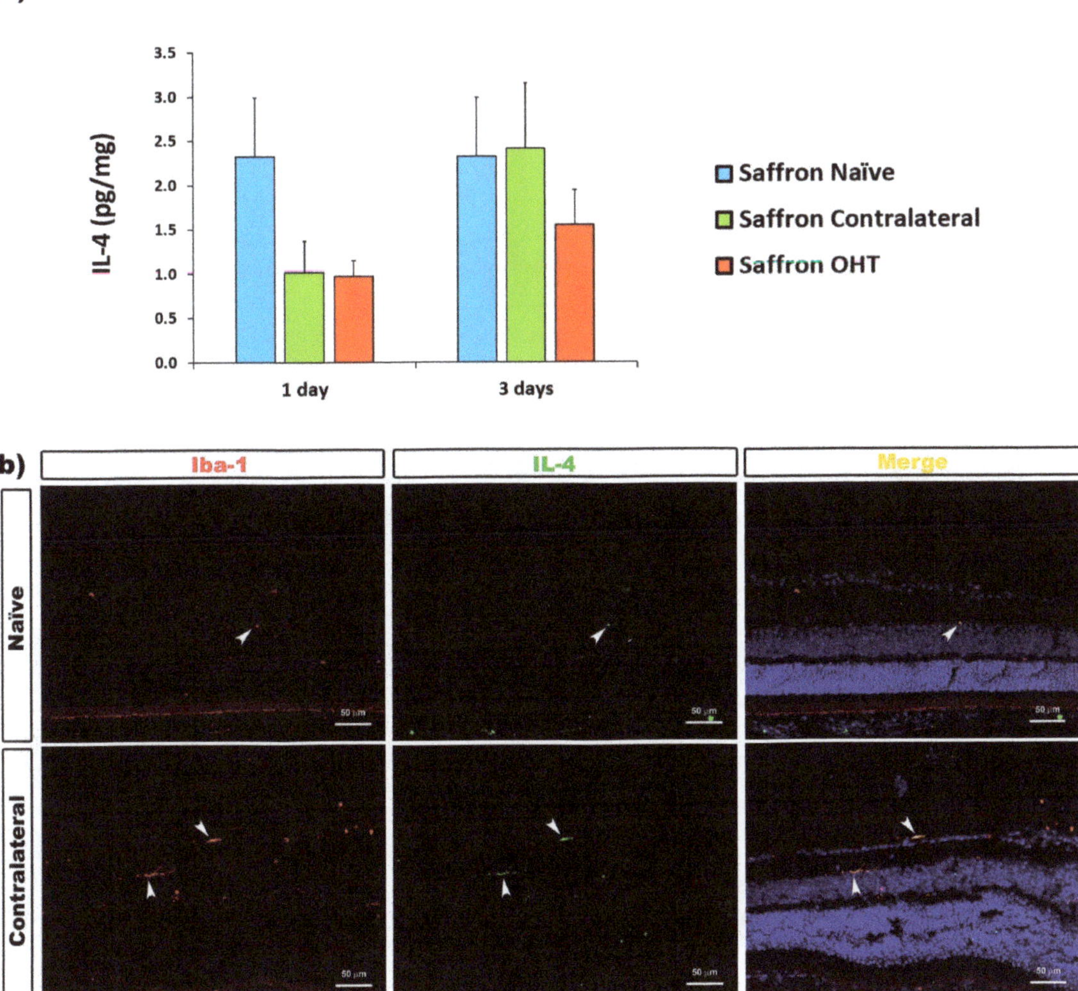

Figure 7. IL-4 levels at 1 and 3 days after laser-induced ocular hypertension (OHT). (**a**) The IL-4 obtained in the multiplex assay. The histogram shows the mean levels (±SD) of IL-4 (pg/mg) at days 1 and 3 after laser OHT induction in saffron ocular hypertension eyes (saffron OHT) and saffron-contralateral eyes (saffron-contralateral) as well as in naïve eyes. (**b**) Immunohistochemical study of IL-4 expression in saffron-contralateral eyes three days after unilateral laser-induced OHT. Retinal sections were immunolabeled with antibodies to IL-4 (green) and Iba-1 (red). Merge is denoted by the colour yellow. The arrowhead shows the co-expression of Iba-1 and IL-4 in saffron-contralateral and saffron-naïve eyes. Abbreviations: OHT (ocular hypertension); IL-4 (interleukin- 4); Iba-1 (ionized calcium-binding adaptor molecule).

Regarding IL-10, at all time-points studied after OHT induction, no significant differences were found. IL-10 expression was not altered in saffron OHT and saffron contralateral eyes compared to saffron-naïve eyes; retinal IL-10 levels were not affected by the laser treatment in saffron-treated animals (Figure 8).

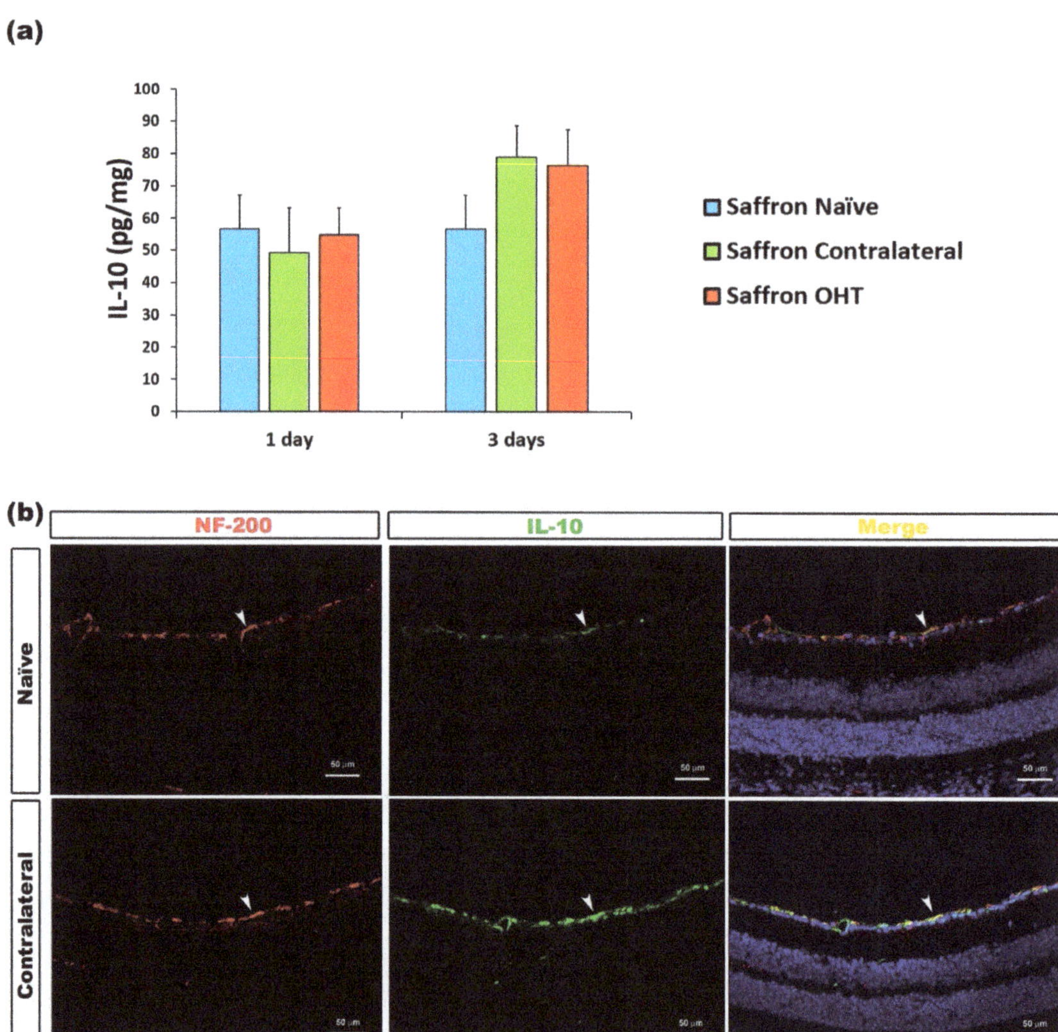

Figure 8. IL-10 levels at 1 and 3 days after laser-induced ocular hypertension (OHT). (**a**) The IL-10 values obtained in the multiplex assay. The histogram shows the mean levels (±SD) of IL-10 (pg/mg) at days 1 and 3 after laser OHT induction in saffron ocular hypertension eyes (saffron OHT) and saffron-contralateral eyes (saffron-contralateral) as well as in naïve eyes. (**b**) Immunohistochemical study of IL-10 expression in saffron-contralateral eyes three days after unilateral laser-induced OHT. Retinal sections were immunolabeled with antibodies to IL-10 (green) and NF-200 (red). Merge is denoted by the colour yellow. The arrowhead shows the co-expression of Iba-1 and IL-10 in saffron-contralateral and saffron-naïve eyes. Abbreviations: OHT (ocular hypertension); IL-10 (interleukin-10); NF-200 (neurofilament-200 KDa).

Regarding the analysed neurotrophic factors, BDNF levels showed no significant changes among the saffron groups after experimental OHT induction. Retinal BDNF levels were not affected by the laser treatment at 1 or 3 days post OHT laser-induction (Figure 9).

(a)

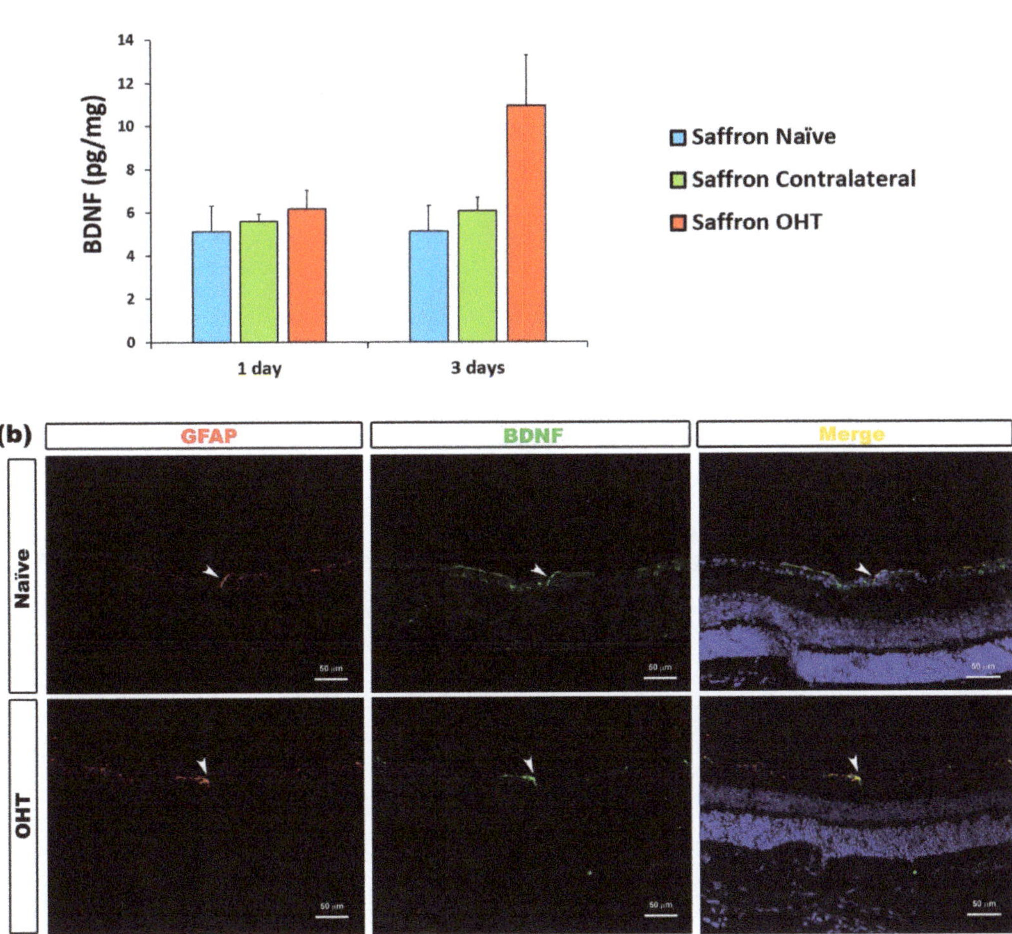

Figure 9. BDNF levels at 1 and 3 days after laser-induced ocular hypertension (OHT). (**a**) The BDNF values obtained in the multiplex assay. The histogram shows the mean levels (± SD) of BDNF (pg/mg) at days 1 and 3 after laser OHT induction in saffron ocular hypertension eyes (saffron OHT), saffron-contralateral eyes (saffron-contralateral), and naïve eyes. (**b**) Immunohistochemical study of BDNF expression in saffron OHT eyes three days after unilateral laser-induced OHT. Retinal sections were immunolabeled with antibodies to BDNF (green) and GFAP (red). Merge is denoted by the colour yellow. The arrowhead shows the co-expression of GFAP and BDNF in saffron OHT and saffron-naïve eyes. Abbreviations: OHT (ocular hypertension); BDNF (brain-derived neurotrophic factor); GFAP (glial fibrillary acidic protein).

The analysis of VEGF expression rendered no significant differences between saffron-naïve eyes and saffron OHT and saffron-contralateral eyes after laser treatment. Retinal VEGF levels were not affected by the experimental OHT induction in these saffron-treated animals (Figure 10).

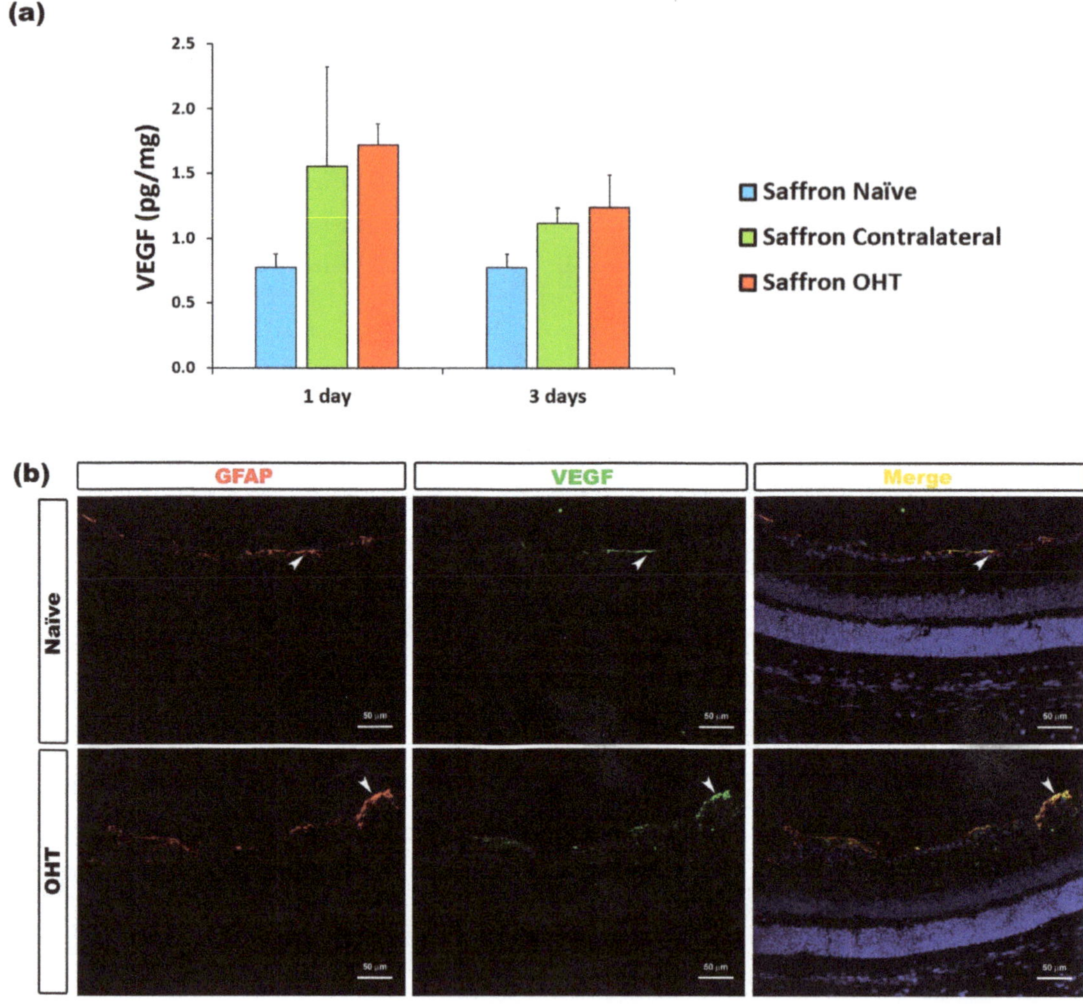

Figure 10. VEGF levels at 1 and 3 days after laser-induced ocular hypertension (OHT). (**a**) The VEGF values obtained in the multiplex assay. The histogram shows the mean levels (±SD) of VEGF (pg/mg) at days 1 and 3 after laser OHT induction in saffron ocular hypertension eyes (saffron OHT) and saffron-contralateral eyes (saffron-contralateral) as well as in saffron-naïve eyes. (**b**) Immunohistochemical study of VEGF expression in saffron OHT eyes one day after unilateral laser-induced OHT. Retinal sections were immunolabeled with antibodies to VEGF (green) and GFAP (red). Merge is denoted by the colour yellow. The arrowhead shows the co-expression of GFAP and VEGF in saffron OHT and saffron-naïve eyes. Abbreviations: OHT (ocular hypertension); VEGF (vascular endothelial growth factor); GFAP (glial fibrillary acidic protein).

The analysis of the content of the microglial activator factor fractalkine (Figure 11) 1 and 3 days after OHT induction revealed no significant differences between experimental groups. Retinal fractalkine levels were not affected by the laser treatment at any day post-laser among the saffron-treated animals.

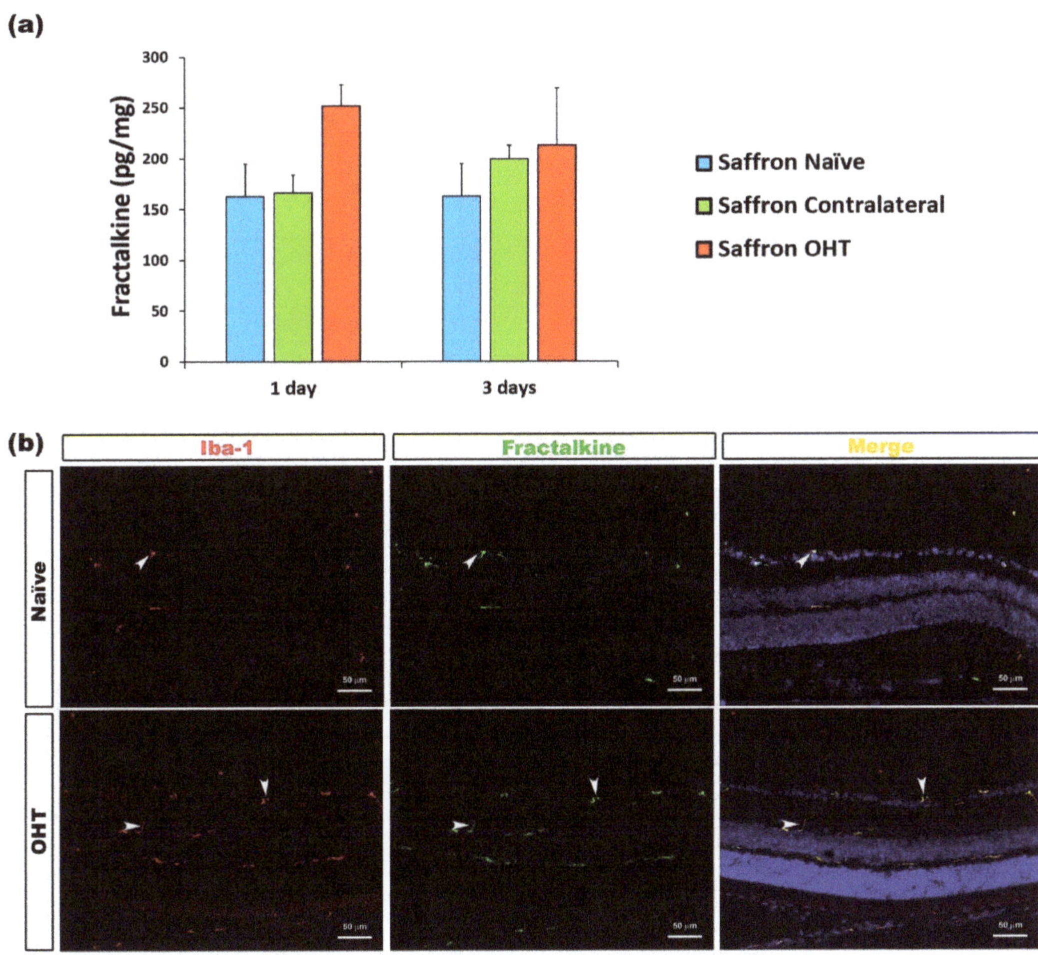

Figure 11. Fractalkine levels at 1 and 3 days after laser-induced ocular hypertension (OHT). (**a**) The fractalkine values obtained in the multiplex assay. The histogram shows the mean levels (±SD) of fractalkine (pg/mg) at days 1 and 3 after laser OHT induction in saffron ocular hypertension eyes (saffron OHT) and saffron-contralateral eyes (saffron-contralateral) as well as in saffron-naïve eyes. (**b**) Immunohistochemical study of fractalkine expression in saffron OHT eyes one day after unilateral laser-induced OHT. Retinal sections were immunolabeled with antibodies to fractalkine (green) and Iba-1 (red). Merge is denoted by the colour yellow. The arrowhead shows the co-expression of Iba-1 and fractalkine in saffron OHT and saffron-naïve eyes. Abbreviations: OHT (ocular hypertension); Iba-1 (ionized calcium-binding adaptor molecule).

3.3. Cytokine Colocalizations with Different Cell Populations

The results obtained in the immunohistochemical assay demonstrated that all of the pro- and anti-inflammatory cytokines as well as BDNF, VEGF, and fractalkine, colocalized with specific retinal cell populations (see Table 2).

Table 2. Co-location of cytokines with specific cell types.

Cytokine	Co-Expression Cell Type	Figures
IL-1β	Microglia and Macroglia (astrocytes and Müller cells)	Figure 2
IL-6	Microglia	Figure 3
INF-γ	Microglia	Figure 4
IL-17	Microglia	Figure 5
TNF-α	Microglia and Astrocytes	Figure 6
IL-4	Microglia	Figure 7
IL-10	Axons of retinal ganglion cells	Figure 8
BDNF	Macroglia (astrocytes and Müller cells)	Figure 9
VEGF	Macroglia (astrocytes and Müller cells)	Figure 10
Fractalkine	Microglia	Figure 11

The table represents the cells showing the expression of the different cytokines and factors used in this study: interleukin 1 beta (IL-1β), interleukin 6 (IL-6), interleukin 17 (IL-17), interferon gamma (IFN-γ), brain-derived neurotrophic factor (BDNF), vascular endothelial growth factor (VEGF), fractalkine (CX3CL1), tumour necrosis factor alpha (TNF-α), interleukin 4 (IL-4), and interleukin 10 (IL-10).

4. Discussion

In the present study, we demonstrated that following saffron treatment, most of the previously observed changes in the concentration of proinflammatory (IL-1β, IFN-γ, IL-6, and IL-17) cytokines, anti-inflammatory cytokines (IL-4 and IL-10), BDNF, VEGF, and fractalkine in response to laser-induced OHT [14] were absent. Among all of the analysed pro- and anti-inflammatory cytokines, only IL-6 levels were significantly increased in the OHT eye one day after the surgery compared with the naïve control group, although to a much lesser extent. These augmented IL-6 levels returned to normal at day 3 after laser treatment, an effect that might have been related to the changes in IOP. Moreover, the immunofluorescent study allowed us to confirm that the cytokines were located on the same cellular subtypes within the retina, which was in agreement to a previous study that characterized the temporal profile of neuroinflammation in the same experimental model of glaucoma [14]. Specifically, IL-1β, IL-6, IFN-γ, IL-17, TNF-α, IL-4, and fractalkine colocalize with microglia; IL-1β, TNF-α, VEGF, and BDNF colocalize with macroglia; and IL-10 colocalizes with axons of RGCs. Since the saffron extract used in this study is commercialized, as saffron ® EYE with 3.14% of crocin, results could be replicated in future experiments, and its underlying mechanisms further investigated, as well as its potential therapeutic application.

In a previous study, using this experimental model of glaucoma, we were able to prevent RGC death and the associated neuroinflammation (focused on morphological signs of microglial activation and on the expression of P2RY12) following the oral administration of saffron at the same dosage as that used in the current study [36]. Recently, we better characterized the temporal profile of the neuroinflammatory damage, focusing on both the morphological signs of microglial activation [11] and the cytokine expression profile [14] induced in both the OHT and contralateral eye in this animal model of glaucoma. Therefore, in the present research, which was designed as an extension of these three previous studies, we aimed to further investigate the anti-inflammatory properties of saffron in glaucoma while focusing on the cytokine expression profile. This research was performed 1 and 3 days after laser-induced OHT since previous studies had detected microglial activation one day after surgery, and the peak of microglial activation was described on day 3 after lasering [11]. In addition, these two days after OHT induction were also selected as in our previous study because these were the days on which the greatest variation in cytokine expression occurred in both OHT and contralateral eyes [14].

In the previous study [14], we demonstrated that this model of laser-induced OHT led to a loss of cytokine homeostasis in the retina. Similar changes in cytokine levels have also been observed in the heritable DBA/2J model of glaucoma in response to activation of retinal glial cells [57]. Moreover, another natural compound, a Chinese herb extract containing Triptolide, has been shown to exert anti-inflammatory effects in DBA/2J mice, mostly by reducing microglial activation and proinflammatory factors, such as TNF-α, probably due to modulation of NF-κB [58]. Thus, herbal extracts with anti-inflammatory properties, such as saffron, may be effective in the management of glaucomatous eyes not only in our laser-induced OHT murine model, but also in other genetic and/or interventional models. Future studies will evaluate the efficacy of this saffron extract in additional and complimentary animal models.

It has been found that saffron suppresses the secretion of proinflammatory cytokines, such as TNF-α, IL-1β, IL-6, and IFNγ, among others, decreasing inflammation in different organs or systems (such as the nervous system [59–63], respiratory system [64,65], gastrointestinal system [66,67], cardiovascular system [68,69], and urogenital system [70,71]), as observed in various experimental models and in vitro experiments. In the present study, the oral administration of saffron seems to prevent and/or revert the release of these cytokines, possibly as a result of the previously reported decrease in microglial activation [36].

In the current study, no significant differences were observed in IL-1β levels between all groups treated with saffron. However, in the previous study, performed on untreated saffron mice [14], a significant decrease in IL-1β levels was detected in the OHT at 1 day, but an increase in its content in both contralateral (1 day) and contralateral (3 days) eyes was also detected. Discrepant results have been previously reported when using a similar model of laser-induced OHT in which only a modest IL-1β mRNA upregulation, not IL-1β immunolabeling, was observed in the retina. Three hypotheses were then proposed to explain such discrepancies: (i) the absence of mRNA translation and an overly fast protein degradation; (ii) an expression restricted to isolated cells; or (iii) an insufficient amount of protein that did not allow for its detection through the employed assay [72]. The reported downregulation of IL-1β in OHT at 1 day was explained by the actions of IL-4 and IL-10 [14]. IL-4 and IL-10 polarize the M2 microglial phenotype and downregulate the production of IL-1β, following a negative feedback model in order to control the inflammatory response [73]. The results of Chidlow et al. (2012) [72] and Fernández-Albarral et al. (2021) [36] are contradictory to those obtained in this work, but our model demonstrated that either the changes produced by OHT were reversed by saffron treatment or that OHT did not affect the retinal content of IL-1β in the saffron-treated groups. Following the approach of Chidlow et al. (2012) [72], IL-1β expression may have not been high enough to be detected. However, after comparing our results with those obtained by Fernández-Albarral et al. (2021) [14] and considering the possible relationship between the anti-inflammatory cytokines IL-4 with IL-1β, we can state that since our treatment lowered IL-1β levels, a compensatory response of IL-4 might not be further required, thus explaining the absence of significant differences detected in these anti-inflammatory cytokines compared with the control group. Our current results may reinforce this association since in the saffron-treated animals, OHT did not affect the IL-1β retinal content and IL-4 levels did not change.

TNF-α levels did not differ in any group with respect to the control one, and a comparison could not be established with the previous non-saffron model, since no detectable concentration was found in the previously performed multiplex immunoassay. However, TNF-α regulation seemed to follow the same route as the one previously described for IL-1β, which is evidence indicating the preventive role of saffron in neuroinflammation and microglial activation, thus avoiding the release of proinflammatory cytokines and the need for a compensatory anti-inflammatory cytokine release [36,72,73]. Another possible approach could be the one previously stated by Chidlow et al. (2012) [72]: the absence of mRNA translation and an overly fast protein degradation; an expression by isolated cells; or an insufficient amount of protein that did not allow for its detection through the employed assay.

In the present study, as previously indicated, only IL-6 levels were significantly increased in the OHT eye at 1 day. This result further corroborates the increase in IL-6 levels observed in the prior study following OHT on saffron-free animals, despite the reported increase in that study being around 20 times higher (716.28 pg/mg) than among saffron-treated animals (46.53 pg/mg). Thus, saffron once again seems to counteract the effects induced by OHT. This cytokine is one of the main causes of RGC death in glaucoma models, leading to massive optic nerve degeneration that provokes a loss in visual acuity, as Echevarría et al. (2017) [74] demonstrated in a microbead glaucoma mouse model. However, IL-6 has also been proposed to have a neuroprotective effect; in particular, in an in vitro model of increased IOP, IL-6 was reported to counteract the proapoptotic effects of other factors [75]. The relationship between IOP elevation and IL-6 secretions was confirmed in both Fernández-Albarral et al. (2021) [14] and the current study, in which the highest expression of IL-6 occurred 1 day after OHT induction. However, in this study, we observed that despite the fact that pressure values remained elevated 3 days after laser induction, saffron was able to regulate IL-6 values.

IFN-γ showed no significant differences in the present study, but in the study of Fernández-Albarral et al. (2021) [14], it significantly increased in OHT eyes at 3 day. IFN-γ is directly related to microglial activation, polarizing it into the M1 phenotype and inducing the production of IL-1β, IL-6, TNF-α, reactive oxygen species (ROS), and nitric oxide (NO) [76], all of them being part of the inflammatory response. The capacity of saffron to prevent an increase in IFN-γ levels may underlie its ability to reduce microglial activation [14] and, thus (indirectly), its capacity to diminish the production and release of proinflammatory mediators. Its potential action on IFN-γ may be key for the anti-inflammatory properties of saffron.

IL-17 can induce neuroinflammation by recruiting T-helper-17 lymphocytes, which are highly related to the inflammatory response in autoimmune pathologies [77]. As expected, in our current study, non-significant changes in IL-17 levels were detected in both experimental groups, although in our previous study in untreated saffron animals, a downregulation of IL-17 content was detected in OHT eyes 1 and 3 days after surgery. We previously hypothesised this IL-17 decrease is caused by the counteracting effect of some anti-inflammatory cytokines, such as IL-4 and IL-10 [36]. In the present study, no elevations of IL-4 or IL-10 levels were detected, and no changes in IL-17 levels were expected.

In our previous study, we showed an upregulation of BDNF in OHT eyes 1 and 3 days after laser treatment [14], probably due to the fact that BDNF is mainly released after a significant RGC loss. BDNF participates in RGC survival by inhibiting apoptosis, as demonstrated in a rat OHT model [78]. In the current study, BDNF levels were not changed. As microglial activation may have been downregulated thanks to the saffron treatment, the glaucoma-related massive RGC death might not have occurred, thus making BDNF release unnecessary.

In our previous study, in untreated saffron animals, VEGF levels were significantly increased in OHT at 1 day (54.35 pg/mg); however, the VEGF values obtained in the present work in the saffron-treated animals were much lower (1.72 pg/mg). The increased expression of VEGF is associated with an augmentation of vascular permeability and the attraction of phagocytic cells [79]. VEGF directly participates in vasculogenesis, increasing its levels around damaged tissue. The excessive IOP may have exerted damaging effects, or even a disruption of the blood–retinal barrier (BRB), caused by a direct increase in the surrounding VEGF levels [80]. In the current study, no significant differences were observed in VEGF levels in any experimental group, suggesting that saffron may have protected BRB integrity, avoiding damage and/or disruption and thus avoiding the infiltration of hazardous substances and/or specific, potentially harmful cell populations to the retina. Future studies focused on the integrity of the BRB would be of great interest to elucidate whether saffron is able to prevent damage (if the BRB is intact) or counteract the already induced neuroinflammatory response (if the BRB is damaged).

No significant differences were found regarding fractalkine levels. As previously stated, fractalkine is a chemokine secreted by neurons that directly induce the proliferation, activation, and migration of microglia [81,82]. Microglia seems to co-locate with fractalkine because of the fractalkine–receptor (CXCR1) interaction since CXCR1 is located on microglial cells, so fractalkine may remain on the microglial surface. Sokolowski et al. (2014) [83] proposed that apoptotic neurons release fractalkine as a "find me" signal, stimulating the migration of microglial processes towards the apoptotic neurons in order to eliminate debris. In our previous analysis, fractalkine levels were higher in OHT at 1 day, possibly as an initial response to neuronal damage that enhanced early microglial activation and migration [14]. Upon fractalkine increase and consequent microglial activation on OHT at 1 day, microglial cells may remain active through additional signals from the cellular environment (mainly astroglia and Müllers cells) and not just by fractalkine. This may explain the decrease in fractalkine levels in OHT eye at 3 days and contralateral eye at 1 and 3 days, which may not imply a lack of microglial activation. In the current work, saffron prevented the appearance of fractalkine changes, thus suggesting a neuroprotective role for saffron that may initially prevent neuronal apoptosis and subsequent posterior fractalkine release. The maintenance of fractalkine homeostasis gives support to our main hypothesis of a reduction of the inflammatory response, since under normal fractalkine levels, microglial cells might not become active, cytokine release may not occur, and RGC survival might therefore be enhanced.

It is worth mentioning that saffron-dried stigmas have been used in traditional medicine for a long time, but Zeinali et al. (2019) [31] questioned how the saffron affects the immune response, explaining its antioxidant, antiapoptotic, and anti-inflammatory properties with its radical scavenging properties. Saffron acts as a transcription inhibitor for TNF-α, IFN-Y, IL-1β, IL-6, and IL-17, and it downregulates inflammatory enzymes, such as myeloperoxidase, cyclooxygenase-2 (COX-2), inducible nitric oxide synthase (INOS), phospholipase A2, and prostanoids. These authors reviewed different models of inflammation and proposed that saffron may reduce the production of inflammatory mediators by blocking Toll-like receptors (such as TLR2) or their subsequent activation cascade, which leads to the production of inflammatory cytokines and chemokines, enzymes, and growth factors. Saffron blocks the NF-kB pathway, which produces IL-1, IL-2, IFN-Y, COX-2, iNOS, and TNF-α, inflammatory mediators related to carcinogenesis [84,85]. In particular, crocin has been reported to reduce the mRNA expression of TNF-α, IFN-Y, IL-1β, and IL-6, as well as iNOS and COX-2, in the mucosa [85]. Crocin can also inhibit the MAPK pathway, as it was found to block the synthesis of TNF-α, IL-1β, IL-6, and iNOS in the intervertebral discs in an LPS rat model [86]. Moreover, different neuroinflammation models focused on the study of microglia have also demonstrated the anti-inflammatory effects of saffron. Pretreatment with crocin is able to reduce the production of NO, TNF-α, and IL-1β by repressing NF-κB activity [62]. Crocetin was found to decrease the expression of inflammatory cytokines (IL-1β, IL-6, IL-10, TNF-α, iNOS, and COX-2) in BV2 microglial cells [87]. Crocin prevents NF-κB activation and decreases NO, TNF-α, IL-1β, and ROS expression in brain microglial cells after LPS stimulation [27]. All of these previously stated studies reinforce our main hypothesis, since the blocking of the MAPK and NF-kB routes can regulate the production of the above-mentioned inflammatory mediators in different tissues and animal models that can be compared with our OHT-induced glaucoma model. It is important to consider that our study may have certain limitations, such as the limited number of Inflammatory markers evaluated, which would require new studies with a broader and more unbiased proteomic approach in which the mechanistic aspects associated with saffron extracts could be defined.

5. Conclusions

In conclusion, this study demonstrates that saffron extract standardized to 3.14% crocin content is effective in regulating the production of proinflammatory cytokines, VEGF, and fractalkine induced by increased IOP, thus protecting the retina from its related damage. In addition, it highlights the relevance of anti-inflammatory treatment to control the inflammatory process generated after ocular hypertension. Saffron extracts could be beneficial as coadjuvant therapies in the treatment of glaucoma, thus helping to decrease the inflammatory process that occurs in this pathology.

Author Contributions: Conceptualization, J.A.F.-A., E.M.M., M.D.P.-D., J.J.S., J.M.R., M.L.-G. and A.I.R.; Data curation, J.A.F.-A., M.A.M.-L., B.M.-S., D.S.F., I.L.-C. and A.I.R.; Formal analysis, J.A.F.-A., M.A.M.-L., E.M.M., R.d.H., B.M.-S., D.S.F., E.S.-G., I.L.-C., M.D.P.-D., J.J.S., J.M.R., M.L.-G. and A.I.R.; Funding acquisition, R.d.H., J.J.S., J.M.R., M.L.-G. and A.I.R.; Investigation, J.A.F.-A., E.M.M., M.A.M.-L.; R.d.H., B.M.-S., I.L.-C., J.J.S., J.M.R., M.L.-G. and A.I.R.; Methodology, J.A.F.-A., M.A.M.-L., E.M.M., R.d.H., D.S.F., E.S.-G., M.D.P.-D., J.M.R., M.L.-G. and A.I.R.; Project administration, J.J.S., J.M.R. and M.L.-G.; Resources, E.M.M., R.d.H., J.J.S., J.M.R., M.L.-G. and A.I.R.; Software, J.A.F.-A.; Supervision, A.I.R.; Validation, M.D.P.-D., J.J.S., J.M.R. and A.I.R.; Visualization, J.A.F.-A., M.A.M.-L., E.S.-G. and I.L.-C.; Writing—original draft, J.A.F.-A., M.A.M.-L., M.L.-G. and A.I.R.; Writing—review & editing, J.A.F.-A., M.A.M.-L., R.d.H., B.M.-S., D.S.F., E.S.-G., I.L.-C., M.D.P.-D., J.J.S., J.M.R., M.L-G. and A.I.R. All authors have read and agreed to the published version of the manuscript.

Funding: This work was supported by: (i) the Ophthalmological Network OFTARED (RD16/0008/0005, RD16/0008/0022), of the Institute of Health of Carlos III of the Spanish Ministry of Economy; by the PN I+D+i 2008–2011, by the ISCIII-Subdirección General de Redes y Centros de Investigación Cooperativa, and by the European programme FEDER; (ii) Articulo 83 118-2017 (UCM-Pharmactive Biotech); (iii) Santander- Complutense University of Madrid Research Projects (PR 87/19-22579); (iv) Santander- Complutense University of Madrid Research Group (UCM UCM 920105, UCM 951579); (v) José A. Fernández-Albarral is currently supported by a Predoctoral Fellowship (FPU17/01023) from the Spanish Ministry of Science, Innovation, and Universities; (vi) Inés López-Cuenca is currently supported by a Predoctoral Fellowship (CT42/18-CT43/18) from the Complutense University of Madrid.

Institutional Review Board Statement: Experimental designs and procedures were approved by the ethical committees of Complutense University and the regulatory institution ((approval ID number: ES280790000086, 1 April 2016) in accordance with the European Commission regulations (2010/63/EU) for the use of laboratory animals, and the Spanish Royal Decree 53/2013, of 1 February, which sets out the basic rules to protect animals used in experiments and for other scientific purposes, including teaching.

Data Availability Statement: The data supporting the findings of this study are available from the corresponding author upon request.

Acknowledgments: The authors would like to thank Desireé Contreras for technical assistance and the members of the UCM Research Group 951579 (Pathophysiology of multiorgan failure: Therapeutic approaches) for their helpful assistance during the whole study; and to Pharmactive Biotech Products for providing the samples of saffron used in the experiments.

Conflicts of Interest: The authors declare no conflict of interest. The funders had no role in the design of the study; in the collection, analyses, or interpretation of data; in the writing of the manuscript; or in the decision to publish the results.

References

1. Tham, Y.C.; Li, X.; Wong, T.Y.; Quigley, H.A.; Aung, T.; Cheng, C.Y. Global Prevalence of Glaucoma and Projections of Glaucoma Burden through 2040: A Systematic Review and Meta-Analysis. *Ophthalmology* **2014**, *121*, 2081–2090. [CrossRef]
2. Qu, J.; Wang, D.; Grosskreutz, C.L. Mechanisms of retinal ganglion cell injury and defense in glaucoma. *Exp. Eye Res.* **2010**, *91*, 48–53. [CrossRef]
3. Baltmr, A.; Duggan, J.; Nizari, S.; Salt, T.E.; Cordeiro, M.F. Neuroprotection in glaucoma–Is there a future role? *Exp. Eye Res.* **2010**, *91*, 554–566. [CrossRef]
4. Tezel, G.; Ben-Hur, T.; Gibson, G.E.; Stevens, B.; Streit, W.J.; Wekerle, H.; Bhattacharya, S.K.; Borras, T.; Burgoyne, C.F.; Caspi, R.R.; et al. The role of glia, mitochondria, and the immune system in glaucoma. *Investig. Ophthalmol. Vis. Sci.* **2009**, *50*, 1001–1012. [CrossRef] [PubMed]
5. Ramirez, A.I.; de Hoz, R.; Salobrar-Garcia, E.; Salazar, J.J.; Rojas, B.; Ajoy, D.; López-Cuenca, I.; Rojas, P.; Triviño, A.; Ramírez, J.M. The Role of Microglia in Retinal Neurodegeneration: Alzheimer's Disease, Parkinson, and Glaucoma. *Front. Aging Neurosci.* **2017**, *9*, 214. [CrossRef] [PubMed]

6. de Hoz, R.; Rojas, B.; Ramirez, A.I.; Salazar, J.J.; Gallego, B.I.; Trivino, A.; Ramirez, J.M. Retinal Macroglial Responses in Health and Disease. *Biomed. Res. Int.* **2016**, *2016*, 2954721. [CrossRef] [PubMed]

7. Ramírez, A.I.; Rojas, B.; de Hoz, R.; Salazar, J.J.; Gallego, B.; Triviño, A.; Ramírez, J.M. Microglia, inflammation, and glaucoma. In *Glaucoma*; SM Group Open Access eBooks: Dover, DE, USA, 2015; pp. 1–16.

8. Russo, R.; Varano, G.P.; Adornetto, A.; Nucci, C.; Corasaniti, M.T.; Bagetta, G.; Morrone, L.A. Retinal ganglion cell death in glaucoma: Exploring the role of neuroinflammation. *Eur. J. Pharmacol.* **2016**, *787*, 134–142. [CrossRef] [PubMed]

9. Salobrar-García, E.; Hoyas, I.; Leal, M.; de Hoz, R.; Rojas, B.; Ramirez, A.I.; Salazar, J.J.; Yubero, R.; Gil, P.; Triviño, A.; et al. Analysis of Retinal Peripapillary Segmentation in Early Alzheimer's Disease Patients. *Biomed. Res. Int.* **2015**, *2015*, 636548. [CrossRef] [PubMed]

10. Gallego, B.I.; Salazar, J.J.; de Hoz, R.; Rojas, B.; Ramírez, A.I.; Salinas-Navarro, M.; Ortín-Martínez, A.; Valiente-Soriano, F.J.; Avilés-Trigueros, M.; Villegas-Perez, M.P.; et al. IOP induces upregulation of GFAP and MHC-II and microglia reactivity in mice retina contralateral to experimental glaucoma. *J. Neuroinflamm.* **2012**, *9*, 92. [CrossRef] [PubMed]

11. Ramírez, A.I.; de Hoz, R.; Fernández-Albarral, J.A.; Salobrar-García, E.; Rojas, B.; Valiente-Soriano, F.J.; Avilés-Trigueros, M.; Villegas-Pérez, M.P.; Vidal-Sanz, M.; Triviño, A.; et al. Time course of bilateral microglial activation in a mouse model of laser-induced glaucoma. *Sci. Rep.* **2020**, *10*, 4890. [CrossRef] [PubMed]

12. Rojas, B.; Gallego, B.I.; Ramírez, A.I.; Salazar, J.J.; de Hoz, R.; Valiente-Soriano, F.J.; Avilés-Trigueros, M.; Villegas-Perez, M.P.; Vidal-Sanz, M.; Triviño, A.; et al. Microglia in mouse retina contralateral to experimental glaucoma exhibit multiple signs of activation in all retinal layers. *J. Neuroinflamm.* **2014**, *11*, 133. [CrossRef] [PubMed]

13. de Hoz, R.; Gallego, B.I.; Ramírez, A.I.; Rojas, B.; Salazar, J.J.; Valiente-Soriano, F.J.; Avilés-Trigueros, M.; Villegas-Perez, M.P.; Vidal-Sanz, M.; Triviño, A.; et al. Rod-like microglia are restricted to eyes with laser-induced ocular hypertension but absent from the microglial changes in the contralateral untreated eye. *PLoS ONE* **2013**, *8*, e83733. [CrossRef]

14. Fernández-Albarral, J.A.; Salazar, J.J.; de Hoz, R.; Marco, E.M.; Martín-Sánchez, B.; Flores-Salguero, E.; Salobrar-García, E.; López-Cuenca, I.; Barrios-Sabador, V.; Avilés-Trigueros, M.; et al. Retinal Molecular Changes Are Associated with Neuroinflammation and Loss of RGCs in an Experimental Model of Glaucoma. *Int. J. Mol. Sci.* **2021**, *22*, 2066. [CrossRef] [PubMed]

15. Haynes, S.E.; Hollopeter, G.; Yang, G.; Kurpius, D.; Dailey, M.E.; Gan, W.-B.; Julius, D. The P2Y12 receptor regulates microglial activation by extracellular nucleotides. *Nat. Neurosci.* **2006**, *9*, 1512–1519. [CrossRef]

16. Salinas-Navarro, M.; Alarcón-Martínez, L.; Valiente-Soriano, F.J.; Ortín-Martínez, A.; Jiménez-López, M.; Avilés-Trigueros, M.; Villegas-Pérez, M.P.; de la Villa, P.; Vidal-Sanz, M. Functional and morphological effects of laser-induced ocular hypertension in retinas of adult albino Swiss mice. *Mol. Vis.* **2009**, *15*, 2578–2598.

17. Poma, A.; Fontecchio, G.; Carlucci, G.; Chichiriccò, G.; Chichiricco, G. Anti-inflammatory properties of drugs from saffron crocus. *Antiinflamm. Antiallergy. Agents Med. Chem.* **2012**, *11*, 37–51. [CrossRef] [PubMed]

18. Yamauchi, M.; Tsuruma, K.; Imai, S.; Nakanishi, T.; Umigai, N.; Shimazawa, M.; Hara, H. Crocetin prevents retinal degeneration induced by oxidative and endoplasmic reticulum stresses via inhibition of caspase activity. *Eur. J. Pharmacol.* **2011**, *650*, 110–119. [CrossRef]

19. Ohno, Y.; Nakanishi, T.; Umigai, N.; Tsuruma, K.; Shimazawa, M.; Hara, H. Oral administration of crocetin prevents inner retinal damage induced by N-methyl-D-aspartate in mice. *Eur. J. Pharmacol.* **2012**, *690*, 84–89. [CrossRef]

20. Hosseinzadeh, H.; Younesi, H.M. Antinociceptive and anti-inflammatory effects of Crocus sativus L. stigma and petal extracts in mice. *BMC Pharmacol.* **2002**, *2*, 7. [CrossRef]

21. Bathaie, S.Z.; Farajzade, A.; Hoshyar, R. A review of the chemistry and uses of crocins and crocetin, the carotenoid natural dyes in saffron, with particular emphasis on applications as colorants including their use as biological stains. *Biotech. Histochem.* **2014**, *89*, 401–411. [CrossRef]

22. Rameshrad, M.; Razavi, B.M.; Hosseinzadeh, H. Saffron and its derivatives, crocin, crocetin and safranal: A patent review. *Expert Opin. Ther. Pat.* **2018**, *28*, 147–165. [CrossRef] [PubMed]

23. Hashemi, M.; Hosseinzadeh, H. A comprehensive review on biological activities and toxicology of crocetin. *Food Chem. Toxicol.* **2019**, *130*, 44–60. [CrossRef]

24. Fernández-Albarral, J.A.; Hoz, R.; de Ramírez, A.I.; López-Cuenca, I.; Salobrar-García, E.; Pinazo-Durán, M.D.; Ramírez, J.M.; Salazar, J.J. Beneficial effects of saffron (Crocus sativus L.) in ocular pathologies, particularly neurodegenerative retinal diseases. *Neural Regen. Res.* **2020**, *15*, 1408. [CrossRef]

25. Falsini, B.; Piccardi, M.; Minnella, A.; Savastano, M.C.; Capoluongo, E.; Fadda, A.; Balestrazzi, E.; Maccarone, R.; Bisti, S. Influence of Saffron Supplementation on Retinal Flicker Sensitivity in Early Age-Related Macular Degeneration. *Investig. Opthalmology Vis. Sci.* **2010**, *51*, 6118–6124. [CrossRef]

26. Korani, S.; Korani, M.; Sathyapalan, T.; Sahebkar, A. Therapeutic effects of Crocin in autoimmune diseases: A review. *BioFactors* **2019**, *45*, 835–843. [CrossRef] [PubMed]

27. Nam, K.N.; Park, Y.M.; Jung, H.J.; Lee, J.Y.; Min, B.D.; Park, S.U.; Jung, W.S.; Cho, K.H.; Park, J.H.; Kang, I.; et al. Anti-inflammatory effects of crocin and crocetin in rat brain microglial cells. *Eur. J. Pharmacol.* **2010**, *648*, 110–116. [CrossRef]

28. Natoli, R.; Zhu, Y.; Valter, K.; Bisti, S.; Eells, J.; Stone, J. Gene and noncoding RNA regulation underlying photoreceptor protection: Microarray study of dietary antioxidant saffron and photobiomodulation in rat retina. *Mol. Vis.* **2010**, *16*, 1801–1822.

29. Soeda, S.; Ochiai, T.; Paopong, L.; Tanaka, H.; Shoyama, Y.; Shimeno, H. Crocin suppresses tumor necrosis factor-α-induced cell death of neuronally differentiated PC-12 cells. *Life Sci.* **2001**, *69*, 2887–2898. [CrossRef]

30. Wang, K.; Zhang, L.; Rao, W.; Su, N.; Hui, H.; Wang, L.; Peng, C.; Tu, Y.; Zhang, S.; Fei, Z. Neuroprotective effects of crocin against traumatic brain injury in mice: Involvement of notch signaling pathway. *Neurosci. Lett.* **2015**, *591*, 53–58. [CrossRef]

31. Zeinali, M.; Zirak, M.R.; Rezaee, S.A.; Karimi, G.; Hosseinzadeh, H. Immunoregulatory and anti-inflammatory properties of Crocus sativus (Saffron) and its main active constituents: A review. *Iran. J. Basic Med. Sci.* **2019**, *22*, 334–344. [CrossRef] [PubMed]

32. Bukhari, S.I.; Manzoor, M.; Dhar, M.K. A comprehensive review of the pharmacological potential of Crocus sativus and its bioactive apocarotenoids. *Biomed. Pharmacother.* **2018**, *98*, 733–745. [CrossRef]

33. Cerdá-Bernad, D.; Valero-Cases, E.; Pastor, J.-J.; Frutos, M.J. Saffron bioactives crocin, crocetin and safranal: Effect on oxidative stress and mechanisms of action. *Crit. Rev. Food Sci. Nutr.* **2020**, 1–18. [CrossRef]

34. Assimopoulou, A.N.; Sinakos, Z.; Papageorgiou, V.P. Radical scavenging activity of Crocus sativus L. extract and its bioactive constituents. *Phyther. Res.* **2005**, *19*, 997–1000. [CrossRef]

35. Urbani, E.; Blasi, F.; Simonetti, M.S.; Chiesi, C.; Cossignani, L. Investigation on secondary metabolite content and antioxidant activity of commercial saffron powder. *Eur. Food Res. Technol.* **2016**, *242*, 987–993. [CrossRef]

36. Fernández-Albarral, J.A.; Ramírez, A.I.; de Hoz, R.; López-Villarín, N.; Salobrar-García, E.; López-Cuenca, I.; Licastro, E.; Inarejos-García, A.M.; Almodóvar, P.; Pinazo-Durán, M.D.; et al. Neuroprotective and anti-inflammatory effects of a hydrophilic saffron extract in a model of glaucoma. *Int. J. Mol. Sci.* **2019**, *20*, 4110. [CrossRef] [PubMed]

37. Almodóvar, P.; Prodanov, M.; Arruñada, O.; Inarejos-García, A.M. affron®, a natural extract of saffron (*Crocus sativus* L.) with colorant properties as novel replacer of saffron stigmas in culinary and food applications. *Int. J. Gastron. Food Sci.* **2018**, *12*, 1–5. [CrossRef]

38. Kell, G.; Rao, A.; Beccaria, G.; Clayton, P.; Inarejos-García, A.M.; Prodanov, M. affron®a novel saffron extract (*Crocus sativus* L.) improves mood in healthy adults over 4 weeks in a double-blind, parallel, randomized, placebo-controlled clinical trial. *Complement. Ther. Med.* **2017**, *33*, 58–64. [CrossRef]

39. Cuenca, N.; Pinilla, I.; Fernández-Sánchez, L.; Salinas-Navarro, M.; Alarcón-Martínez, L.; Avilés-Trigueros, M.; de la Villa, P.; Miralles de Imperial, J.; Villegas-Pérez, M.P.; Vidal-Sanz, M. Changes in the inner and outer retinal layers after acute increase of the intraocular pressure in adult albino Swiss mice. *Exp. Eye Res.* **2010**, *91*, 273–285. [CrossRef]

40. Salinas-Navarro, M.; Alarcón-Martínez, L.; Valiente-Soriano, F.J.; Jiménez-López, M.; Mayor-Torroglosa, S.; Avilés-Trigueros, M.; Villegas-Pérez, M.P.; Vidal-Sanz, M. Ocular hypertension impairs optic nerve axonal transport leading to progressive retinal ganglion cell degeneration. *Exp. Eye Res.* **2010**, *90*, 168–183. [CrossRef]

41. Naskar, R.; Wissing, M.; Thanos, S. Detection of early neuron degeneration and accompanying microglial responses in the retina of a rat model of glaucoma. *Investig. Ophthalmol. Vis. Sci.* **2002**, *43*, 2962–2968.

42. Quigley, H.A.; Hohman, R.M. Laser energy levels for trabecular meshwork damage in the primate eye. *Investig. Ophthalmol. Vis. Sci.* **1983**, *24*, 1305–1307.

43. Neufeld, A.H. Microglia in the optic nerve head and the region of parapapillary chorioretinal atrophy in glaucoma. *Arch. Ophthalmol.* **1999**, *117*, 1050–1056. [CrossRef]

44. Ding, H.; Chen, J.; Su, M.; Lin, Z.; Zhan, H.; Yang, F.; Li, W.; Xie, J.; Huang, Y.; Liu, X.; et al. BDNF promotes activation of astrocytes and microglia contributing to neuroinflammation and mechanical allodynia in cyclophosphamide-induced cystitis. *J. Neuroinflammation* **2020**, *17*, 19. [CrossRef]

45. Guo, X.; Wang, X.; Dong, J.; Lv, W.; Zhao, S.; Jin, L.; Guo, J.; Wang, M.; Cai, C.; Sun, J.; et al. Effects of Ginkgo biloba on Early Decompression after Spinal Cord Injury. *Evid. Based Complement. Altern. Med.* **2020**, *2020*, 6958246. [CrossRef]

46. Sun, L.; Zhang, H.; Wang, W.; Chen, Z.; Wang, S.; Li, J.; Li, G.; Gao, C.; Sun, X. Astragaloside IV Exerts Cognitive Benefits and Promotes Hippocampal Neurogenesis in Stroke Mice by Downregulating Interleukin-17 Expression via Wnt Pathway. *Front. Pharmacol.* **2020**, *11*, 421. [CrossRef]

47. Johnson, S.; Duncan, J.; Hussain, S.A.; Chen, G.; Luo, J.; Mclaurin, C.; May, W.; Rajkowska, G.; Ou, X.M.; Stockmeier, C.A.; et al. The IFNγ-PKR pathway in the prefrontal cortex reactions to chronic excessive alcohol use. *Alcohol. Clin. Exp. Res.* **2015**, *39*, 476–484. [CrossRef] [PubMed]

48. Vaquié, A.; Sauvain, A.; Duman, M.; Nocera, G.; Egger, B.; Meyenhofer, F.; Falquet, L.; Bartesaghi, L.; Chrast, R.; Lamy, C.M.; et al. Injured Axons Instruct Schwann Cells to Build Constricting Actin Spheres to Accelerate Axonal Disintegration. *Cell Rep.* **2019**, *27*, 3152–3166.e7. [CrossRef]

49. Chen, G.; Zhou, Z.; Sha, W.; Wang, L.; Yan, F.; Yang, X.; Qin, X.; Wu, M.; Li, D.; Tian, S.; et al. A novel CX3CR1 inhibitor AZD8797 facilitates early recovery of rat acute spinal cord injury by inhibiting inflammation and apoptosis. *Int. J. Mol. Med.* **2020**, *45*, 1373–1384. [CrossRef] [PubMed]

50. Zhang, S.Z.; Wang, Q.Q.; Yang, Q.Q.; Gu, H.Y.; Yin, Y.Q.; Li, Y.D.; Hou, J.C.; Chen, R.; Sun, Q.Q.; Sun, Y.F.; et al. NG2 glia regulate brain innate immunity via TGF-β2/TGFBR2 axis. *BMC Med.* **2019**, *17*, 204. [CrossRef]

51. Honjoh, K.; Nakajima, H.; Hirai, T.; Watanabe, S.; Matsumine, A. Relationship of Inflammatory Cytokines from M1-Type Microglia/Macrophages at the Injured Site and Lumbar Enlargement with Neuropathic Pain After Spinal Cord Injury in the CCL21 Knockout (plt) Mouse. *Front. Cell. Neurosci.* **2019**, *13*, 525. [CrossRef] [PubMed]

52. Li, B.; Liu, J.; Gu, G.; Han, X.; Zhang, Q.; Zhang, W. Impact of neural stem cell-derived extracellular vesicles on mitochondrial dysfunction, sirtuin 1 level, and synaptic deficits in Alzheimer's disease. *J. Neurochem.* **2020**, *154*, 502–518. [CrossRef]

53. Yamamoto, M.; Kim, M.; Imai, H.; Itakura, Y.; Ohtsuki, G. Microglia-Triggered Plasticity of Intrinsic Excitability Modulates Psychomotor Behaviors in Acute Cerebellar Inflammation. *Cell Rep.* **2019**, *28*, 2923–2938.e8. [CrossRef]

54. Niesman, I.R.; Schilling, J.M.; Shapiro, L.A.; Kellerhals, S.E.; Bonds, J.A.; Kleschevnikov, A.M.; Cui, W.; Voong, A.; Krajewski, S.; Ali, S.S.; et al. Traumatic brain injury enhances neuroinflammation and lesion volume in caveolin deficient mice. *J. Neuroinflammation* **2014**, *11*, 39. [CrossRef]

55. Bocquet, A.; Berges, R.; Frank, R.; Robert, P.; Peterson, A.C.; Eyer, J. Neurofilaments bind tubulin and modulate its polymerization. *J. Neurosci.* **2009**, *29*, 11043–11054. [CrossRef] [PubMed]

56. Hoaglin, D.C.; Iglewicz, B. Fine-tuning some resistant rules for outlier labeling. *J. Am. Stat. Assoc.* **1987**, *82*, 1147–1149. [CrossRef]

57. Wilson, G.N.; Inman, D.M.; Denger-Crish, C.M.; Smith, M.A.; Crish, S.D. Early pro-inflammatory cytokine elevations in the DBA/2J mouse model of glaucoma. *J. Neuroinflammation* **2015**, *12*, 1–13. [CrossRef] [PubMed]

58. Yang, F.; Wu, L.; Guo, X.; Wang, D.; Li, Y. Improved retinal ganglion cell survival through retinal microglia suppression by a chinese herb extract, triptolide, in the dba/2j mouse model of glaucoma. *Ocul. Immunol. Inflamm.* **2013**, *21*, 378–389. [CrossRef] [PubMed]

59. Mohammadzadeh, L.; Abnous, K.; Razavi, B.M.; Hosseinzadeh, H. Crocin-protected malathion-induced spatial memory deficits by inhibiting TAU protein hyperphosphorylation and antiapoptotic effects. *Nutr. Neurosci.* **2020**, *23*, 221–236. [CrossRef]

60. Mozaffari, S.; Yasuj, S.R.; Motaghinejad, M.; Motevalian, M.; Kheiri, R. Crocin acting as a neuroprotective agent against methamphetamine-induced neurodegeneration via CREB-BDNF signaling pathway. *Iran. J. Pharm. Res.* **2019**, *18*, 745–758. [CrossRef]

61. Sadoughi, D. The effect of crocin on apoptotic, inflammatory, BDNF, Pt, and Aβ40 indicators and neuronal density of CA1, CA2, and CA3 regions of hippocampus in the model of Alzheimer suffering rats induced with trimethyltin chloride. *Comp. Clin. Path.* **2019**, *28*, 1403–1413. [CrossRef]

62. Lv, B.; Huo, F.; Zhu, Z.; Xu, Z.; Dang, X.; Chen, T.; Zhang, T.; Yang, X. Crocin Upregulates CX3CR1 Expression by Suppressing NF-κB/YY1 Signaling and Inhibiting Lipopolysaccharide-Induced Microglial Activation. *Neurochem. Res.* **2016**, *41*, 1949–1957. [CrossRef] [PubMed]

63. Fernández-Sánchez, L.; Lax, P.; Esquiva, G.; Martín-Nieto, J.; Pinilla, I.; Cuenca, N. Safranal, a saffron constituent, attenuates retinal degeneration in P23H rats. *PLoS ONE* **2012**, *7*, e43074. [CrossRef] [PubMed]

64. Xie, Y.; He, Q.; Chen, H.; Lin, Z.; Xu, Y.; Yang, C. Crocin ameliorates chronic obstructive pulmonary disease-induced depression via PI3K/Akt mediated suppression of inflammation. *Eur. J. Pharmacol.* **2019**, *862*, 172640. [CrossRef]

65. Du, J.; Chi, Y.; Song, Z.; Di, Q.; Mai, Z.; Shi, J.; Li, M. Crocin reduces Aspergillus fumigatus-induced airway inflammation and NF-κB signal activation. *J. Cell. Biochem.* **2018**, *119*, 1746–1754. [CrossRef]

66. Rezaee-Khorasany, A.; Razavi, B.M.; Taghiabadi, E.; Yazdi, A.T.; Hosseinzadeh, H. Effect of crocin, an active saffron constituent, on ethanol toxicity in the rat: Histopathological and biochemical studies. *Iran. J. Basic Med. Sci.* **2020**, *23*, 51–62. [CrossRef]

67. Kalantar, M.; Kalantari, H.; Goudarzi, M.; Khorsandi, L.; Bakhit, S.; Kalantar, H. Crocin ameliorates methotrexate-induced liver injury via inhibition of oxidative stress and inflammation in rats. *Pharmacol. Rep.* **2019**, *71*, 746–752. [CrossRef]

68. Elsherbiny, N.M.; Salama, M.F.; Said, E.; El-Sherbiny, M.; Al-Gayyar, M.M.H. Crocin protects against doxorubicin-induced myocardial toxicity in rats through down-regulation of inflammatory and apoptic pathways. *Chem. Biol. Interact.* **2016**, *247*, 39–48. [CrossRef]

69. Baradaran Rahim, V.; Khammar, M.T.; Rakhshandeh, H.; Samzadeh-Kermani, A.; Hosseini, A.; Askari, V.R. Crocin protects cardiomyocytes against LPS-Induced inflammation. *Pharmacol. Rep.* **2019**, *71*, 1228–1234. [CrossRef]

70. Adali, F.; Gonul, Y.; Aldemir, M.; Hazman, O.; Ahsen, A.; Bozkurt, M.F.; Sen, O.G.; Keles, I.; Keles, H. Investigation of the effect of crocin pretreatment on renal injury induced by infrarenal aortic occlusion. *J. Surg. Res.* **2016**, *203*, 145–153. [CrossRef] [PubMed]

71. Liu, Y.; Qin, X.; Lu, X. Crocin improves endometriosis by inhibiting cell proliferation and the release of inflammatory factors. *Biomed. Pharmacother.* **2018**, *106*, 1678–1685. [CrossRef] [PubMed]

72. Chidlow, G.; Wood, J.P.M.; Ebneter, A.; Casson, R.J. Interleukin-6 is an efficacious marker of axonal transport disruption during experimental glaucoma and stimulates neuritogenesis in cultured retinal ganglion cells. *Neurobiol. Dis.* **2012**, *48*, 568–581. [CrossRef]

73. Koeberle, P.D.; Gauldie, J.; Ball, A.K. Effects of adenoviral-mediated gene transfer of interleukin-10, interleukin-4, and transforming growth factor-β on the survival of axotomized retinal ganglion cells. *Neuroscience* **2004**, *125*, 903–920. [CrossRef]

74. Echevarria, F.D.; Formichella, C.R.; Sappington, R.M. Interleukin-6 deficiency attenuates retinal ganglion cell axonopathy and glaucoma-related vision loss. *Front. Neurosci.* **2017**, *11*, 318. [CrossRef] [PubMed]

75. Sappington, R.M.; Chan, M.; Calkins, D.J. Interleukin-6 protects retinal ganglion cells from pressure-induced death. *Investig. Ophthalmol. Vis. Sci.* **2006**, *47*, 2932–2942. [CrossRef] [PubMed]

76. Nakagawa, Y.; Chiba, K. Role of microglial M1/M2 polarization in relapse and remission of psychiatric disorders and diseases. *Pharmaceuticals* **2014**, *7*, 1028–1048. [CrossRef]

77. Gaffen, S.L. Structure and signalling in the IL-17 receptor family. *Nat. Rev. Immunol.* **2009**, *9*, 556–567. [CrossRef]

78. Valiente-Soriano, F.J.; Nadal-Nicolás, F.M.; Salinas-Navarro, M.; Jiménez-López, M.; Bernal-Garro, J.M.; Villegas-Pérez, M.P.; Agudo-Barriuso, M.; Vidal-Sanz, M. BDNF rescues RGCs but not intrinsically photosensitive RGCs in ocular hypertensive albino rat retinas. *Investig. Ophthalmol. Vis. Sci.* **2015**, *56*, 1924–1936. [CrossRef] [PubMed]

79. Barleon, B.; Sozzani, S.; Zhou, D.; Weich, H.A.; Mantovani, A.; Marmé, D. Migration of human monocytes in response to vascular endothelial growth factor (VEGF) is mediated via the VEGF receptor flt-1. *Blood* **1996**, *87*, 3336–3343. [CrossRef]

80. Luna, J.D.; Chan, C.-C.; Derevjanik, N.L.; Mahlow, J.; Chiu, C.; Peng, B.; Tobe, T.; Campochiaro, P.A.; Vinores, S.A. Blood-Retinal Barrier (BRB) Breakdown in Experimental Autoimmune Uveoretinitis: Comparison with Vascular Endothelial Growth Factor, Tumor Necrosis Factor a, and Interleukin-1b-Mediated Breakdown. *J. Neurosci. Res.* **1997**, *49*, 268–280. [CrossRef]
81. Hatori, K.; Nagai, A.; Heisel, R.; Ryu, J.K.; Kim, S.U. Fractalkine and fractalkine receptors in human neurons and glial cells. *J. Neurosci. Res.* **2002**, *69*, 418–426. [CrossRef]
82. Zujovic, V.; Benavides, J.; Vigé, X.; Carter, C.; Taupin, V. Fractalkine modulates TNF-α secretion and neurotoxicity induced by microglial activation. *Glia* **2000**, *29*, 305–315. [CrossRef]
83. Sokolowski, J.D.; Chabanon-Hicks, C.N.; Han, C.Z.; Heffron, D.S.; Mandell, J.W. Fractalkine is a "find-me" signal released by neurons undergoing ethanol-induced apoptosis. *Front. Cell. Neurosci.* **2014**, *8*, 360. [CrossRef] [PubMed]
84. Lawrence, T. The nuclear factor NF-kappaB pathway in inflammation. *Cold Spring Harb. Perspect. Biol.* **2009**, *1*, a001651. [CrossRef] [PubMed]
85. Kawabata, K.; Tung, N.H.; Shoyama, Y.; Sugie, S.; Mori, T.; Tanaka, T. Dietary crocin inhibits colitis and colitis-associated colorectal carcinogenesis in male ICR mice. *Evid. Based Complement. Altern. Med.* **2012**, *2012*, 820415. [CrossRef]
86. Li, K.; Li, Y.; Ma, Z.; Zhao, J. Crocin exerts anti-inflammatory and anti-catabolic effects on rat intervertebral discs by suppressing the activation of JNK. *Int. J. Mol. Med.* **2015**, *36*, 1291–1299. [CrossRef]
87. Dong, N.; Dong, Z.; Chen, Y.; Gu, X. Crocetin Alleviates Inflammation in MPTP-Induced Parkinson's Disease Models through Improving Mitochondrial Functions. *Parkinsons. Dis.* **2020**, *2020*, 9864370. [CrossRef] [PubMed]

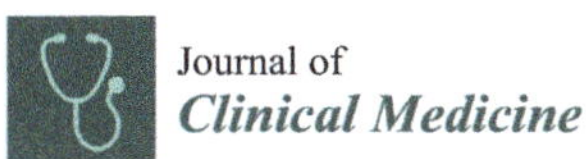

Journal of
Clinical Medicine

Article

Do Age and Sex Play a Role in the Intraocular Pressure Changes after Acrobatic Gymnastics?

Javier Gene-Morales [1,2], Andrés Gené-Sampedro [2,3,*], Alba Martín-Portugués [3] and Inmaculada Bueno-Gimeno [3,*]

[1] Research Group Prevention and Health in Exercise and Sport (PHES), University of Valencia, St. Gascó Oliag 3, 46010 Valencia, Spain; javier.gene@uv.es

[2] Research Institute on Traffic and Road Safety (INTRAS), University of Valencia, St. Serpis 29, 46022 Valencia, Spain

[3] Department of Optics, Optometry & Vision Science, University of Valencia, St. Dr Moliner 50, 46100 Burjassot, Spain; alba.mv17@hotmail.com

* Correspondence: andres.gene@uv.es (A.G.-S.); inmaculada.bueno@uv.es (I.B.-G.)

Abstract: To evaluate the effects of an acrobatic gymnastics (AG) training session on intraocular pressure (IOP), a familiarization session was employed to confirm the participant's suitability for the study. Forty-nine gymnasts (63.27% females, 18–40 years old) voluntarily agreed to participate. As age, sex, baseline IOP, and central corneal thickness (CCT) were considered as potential predictors of the IOP variations, in the second session measurements of the above parameters were taken before and after 90 min of AG. A mixed-factorial analysis of variance evaluated differences. Linear regression was conducted to potentially predict the IOP variation with the exercise. After the scheduled exercise, highly significant ($p < 0.001$, effect size: 0.73) reductions in IOP, but no significant changes in CCT ($p = 0.229$), were observed. IOP was significantly modified in males, older than 25 years, and subjects with baseline IOP > 14 mmHg ($p \leq 0.001$, effect sizes: 0.57–1.02). In contrast, the IOP of females, younger participants, and subjects with baseline IOP $\leq$ 14 mmHg was not significantly modified ($p = 0.114$). With the regression analyses, we concluded that both sex and baseline IOP levels were significant predictors of the IOP fluctuation with AG. These findings could be of interest for gymnasts, coaches, ophthalmologists, and/or optometrists in the prevention and control of risk factors associated with glaucoma.

Keywords: physical exercise; sport; acrobatic gymnastics; baseline intraocular pressure; central corneal thickness; ocular health; tumbling skills; hand balance

Citation: Gene-Morales, J.; Gené-Sampedro, A.; Martín-Portugués, A.; Bueno-Gimeno, I. Do Age and Sex Play a Role in the Intraocular Pressure Changes after Acrobatic Gymnastics? *J. Clin. Med.* **2021**, *10*, 4700. https://doi.org/10.3390/jcm10204700

Academic Editors: Jose Javier Garcia-Medina and Maria Dolores Pinazo-Duran

Received: 26 August 2021
Accepted: 11 October 2021
Published: 13 October 2021

Publisher's Note: MDPI stays neutral with regard to jurisdictional claims in published maps and institutional affiliations.

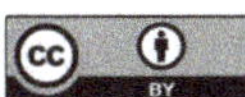

1. Introduction

Intraocular pressure (IOP) and its fluctuations are still recognized as the main modifiable factor in the control, management, and prevention of glaucoma [1–3]. IOP can fluctuate due to different internal and external factors. Among them, age and sex are acknowledged factors that condition IOP [4,5]. Additionally, corneal thickness [6] and baseline IOP levels [2,7] have been identified to play a role in the short-term IOP fluctuations. As far as we know, no previous research has analyzed the potential effects of baseline IOP levels and corneal thickness (CCT) on the IOP fluctuations caused by acrobatic gymnastics (AG) exercise.

Exercise is a key external factor that modifies intraocular pressure [3–5,8,9] and cardiovascular parameters [10]. More specifically, aerobic, continuous exercise such as running or cycling at low to moderate intensities has proven to acutely reduce IOP [8,11–13]. Regarding resistance exercises involving muscular strength such as weightlifting, controversial results appear in the scientific literature, with many studies ensuring IOP elevations [14–20] and other studies reporting IOP reductions due to the exercise effect [21–30]. As shown in previous expert literature, recovery of pre-exercise IOP values could take from several minutes after resistance exercises to up to one hour after aerobic exercise [4,8]. In addition to the exercise methodology itself, certain positions during the activity such as head-down positions could increase IOP [3,5,8]. Considering the above concerns, it remains necessary to study sport disciplines that in their practice combine the aerobic and muscular systems and changes of position, such as AG. Nevertheless, knowledge on AG remains incomplete [31], especially in terms of ocular adaptations. No previous studies dealing with IOP variations after AG were found.

AG is growing in popularity among different age groups [31,32]. AG is a combined activity that can be performed in pairs or groups and includes static elements such as balances and figure holds (hand balances, bridges, splits, human pyramids) and dynamic elements such as partner lifts, throws with complex somersaults and twists, and tumbling skills [33–35]. This motor and social sport requires high levels of strength, flexibility, balance, agility, coordination, speed, and cardiovascular performance [36]. Due to the aforementioned topics, it is scientifically necessary to evaluate the IOP acute adaptations that could occur after an AG session, to obtain a better understanding of the effects of this activity that could not be reached within a laboratory environment. Furthermore, the question arises as to whether sociodemographic and ocular variables such as sex, age, baseline IOP, and baseline CCT could play a role in the IOP variations.

The main aim was to evaluate IOP and CCT variations after an AG session. Additionally, a set of demographics (age and sex) and ocular parameters (baseline IOP and CCT) were considered as potential predictors of the IOP variation due to the exercise effect (difference between post-exercise and pre-exercise intraocular pressure values).

We hypothesized that exercise would reduce the IOP and CCT would remain unchanged. We also expected to find that the independent variables (age, sex, baseline IOP, and CCT) would affect the IOP variations.

2. Materials and Methods

An observational, prospective, longitudinal study was conducted to compare the IOP and CCT of gymnasts pre- and post-exercise. Additionally, the prediction potential of age, sex, baseline IOP, and CCT on the variation of IOP was addressed. We conducted the study in conformity with the Code of Ethics of the World Medical Association (Declaration of Helsinki [37]), and ethical approval was provided by the Research Ethics Committee on human research of the University of Valencia (H1499867368458). The study was also approved by the Club Dynamic Gym of Manises (Valencia, Spain). The subjects were informed of the study characteristics and protocols, and signed, informed consent was obtained from all the participants at the beginning of the procedures. Participants were free to withdraw from the study at any time. Data were confidential and participation was anonymous, implying no potential risks for the integrity of the subjects apart from those derived from the physical activity.

2.1. Participants

The sample size was determined by a priori power analyses, assuming an α of 0.05, power levels (1-ß) of between 0.80 and 0.95, a non-sphericity correction of $\varepsilon = 1$, and an effect size of f(V) = 0.45 for ANOVA tests and $f^2 = 0.24$ for the regression analyses. Thus, 49 participants were recruited for this study. Main inclusion criteria were: (1) older than 18 and younger than 40 years old, (2) experience with acrobatic gymnastics of at least 6 months and performing at least 2 days per week, (3) no musculoskeletal issues, (4) baseline IOP between 10.00 and 21.00 mmHg, (5) normal anterior chamber depth, (6) no history of ophthalmic laser procedures, ocular surgery, traumatism, or use of topic/systemic medications potentially affecting the IOP. Subjects with a family history of glaucoma and/or contact lens wearers were excluded from this study.

At the beginning of the study, 51 athletes were recruited, but only 49 met the criteria (18 male and 31 female). All these subjects voluntarily agreed to participate in the study. Participants were classified into two groups according to their age: (1) adults (>25 years old) and (2) young adults (≤25 years old) [38]. Additionally, three more groups were formed regarding the baseline IOP levels (low, medium, and high). For such purpose, baseline IOP was divided into terciles (with limits at 14 and 17 mmHg) as previously reported [2,7]. Further characteristics of the sample, including demographics and spherocylindrical refraction values, are reflected in Table 1. The spherocylindrical refraction values were converted to power vector notation (M, J0, and J45). Refractive error was determined in terms of (1) the spherical equivalent (M component) and (2) a pair of Jackson Crossed Cylinder lenses oriented at $0°/90°$ (J0 component) and $45°/135°$ (J45 component) for determination of astigmatism. Refractive error was measured to characterize the sample considering its potential influences on IOP [39].

Table 1. Characteristics of the general sample ($n = 49$).

Variable	Mean	Standard Deviation	95% Confidence Interval	
			Lower	Upper
Age (years)	27.67	7.10	25.66	29.69
M (D)	−0.86	1.62	−1.32	−0.41
J0 (D)	−0.01	0.31	−0.09	0.08
J45 (D)	−0.03	0.15	−0.07	0.02

M: spherical equivalent; J0 and J45: Jackson crossed cylinder lenses, representing the three components of refractive error in power vector notation; D: diopters.

All participants were instructed to avoid alcohol/tobacco consumption and to not perform vigorous exercise 24 h before any programmed session. They were asked to sleep for at least 8 h, to not consume stimulants, to not drink more than 1 L of liquids [4], and to not perform prolonged near-viewing activities within the 3 h before the trials [40].

2.2. Procedures

All procedures were conducted in the same gymnastic facilities by the same researchers (one optometrist (in charge of the measurements) and one sports scientist (responsible for the gymnastics session)). All data were collected in a thermoneutral environment ($\sim$22 °C and $\sim$60% humidity), under the same lighting, and at the same period (between 7:20 p.m. and 9:10 p.m.) to reduce the effects of circadian rhythm variations in the eyes [41]. Measurement tools were installed in a room next to the training facilities to improve access and performance of techniques. Two sessions separated by 1 week were scheduled: one for assessment of sociodemographic data, participants' characteristics, and systematized ophthalmological examination at baseline, and a second session to carry out all experimental procedures to evaluate the dependent variables before and after the AG session.

In the first session, an ocular examination was performed to ensure the validity of participants, including measurements of best-corrected visual acuity, subjective refraction, IOP (Auto Kerato-Refracto-Tonometer TRK-2P; Topcon®, Tokyo, Japan), stereopsis, motility, and biomicroscopic anterior eye segment examination (Slit Lamp SL-D4, Topcon Europe Medical BV, The Netherlands). Objective refraction was measured with the Auto Kerato-Refracto Tonometer (TRK-2P, Topcon®, Tokyo, Japan) and was followed by a subjective refinement.

In the second session, pre-exercise eye parameters were measured 5 to 10 min before starting the exercise. All subjects underwent the same 90-min acrobatic gymnastics training session (as reflected in the previous section, for further information on the specific characteristics of this type of sport). IOP and CCT were measured again 5 to 10 min after finishing the exercise.

Intraocular Pressure and Central Corneal Thickness

As above reflected, IOP and CCT were measured in mmHg and microns, respectively, with the Auto Kerato-Refracto-Tonometer TRK-2P (Topcon®, Tokyo, Japan). This non-contact instrument is composed of Rotary Prism Technology and provides unmatched accuracy and reliability as well as permitting accurate and reliable measurements with a pupil as small as 2 mm in diameter. The device uses optical pachymetry to determine CCT, which involves using a tangential slit of light directed onto the cornea at a known angle. The illuminated slit is measured, and corneal thickness is calculated using trigonometry. All parameters, including horizontal and vertical alignment and vertex distance, were determined by the instrument. Additionally, TRK-2P allows adjusting the value of pneumotonometry with pachymetry, so that it automatically adjusts the IOP value based on corneal thickness [42]. The measurements were taken using the full screening mode, which includes intraocular pressure, keratometry, autorefraction, and pachymetry values. Three readings for each patient were obtained, averaged, and recorded.

Measurements were taken in both eyes in this study. Right eye measurements were used since no significant difference ($p = 0.112$) was observed between the eyes.

2.3. Statistical Analysis

First, a basic data curation was performed, and descriptive statistics of the sample features were calculated. Variation of IOP was calculated as post-exercise IOP minus pre-exercise IOP, which, in turn, was converted to a percentage ($\Delta\%$). Normality of data distribution and homoscedasticity was assessed through the Shapiro–Wilk and Levene tests, respectively. Data showed a normal-Gaussian distribution with homogeneous variances.

At this point, a mixed factorial analysis of variance (ANOVA), with the exercise (baseline and post-exercise measurements) as the within-subject factor, and sex (male, female), age (young adult, adult), and baseline IOP levels (low, medium, high) as the between-subject factors, was used to evaluate the effects of the exercise as well as to assess differences in the study-dependent variables. Effect size was evaluated with eta partial squared (ηp^2), where $0.01 < \eta p^2 < 0.06$ constitutes a small effect, $0.06 \leq \eta p^2 \leq 0.14$ constitutes a medium effect, and $\eta p^2 > 0.14$ constitutes a large effect. Pairwise post hoc comparisons were evaluated using Bonferroni correction. The effect size for post hoc comparisons was calculated as Cohen's d with Hedges' corrections to avoid biases due to sample size or standard deviation differences [43]. This corrected value is reported as unbiased Cohen's d (d_{unb}) [44], with $d_{unb} < 0.50$ constituting a small effect, $0.50 \leq d_{unb} \leq 0.79$ a moderate effect, and $d_{unb} \geq 0.80$ a large effect [45].

Afterward, Multiple Linear Regression analyses (MLR–method: enter) were carried out for the variation of intraocular pressure (difference between post-exercise and pre-exercise IOP values). Two models' fit were tested as potential predictors of the IOP variation, one including socio-demographic (age and sex) and one including ocular variables (baseline levels of IOP and CCT).

All the statistical analyses were carried out using the software IBM SPSS Statistics for Macintosh (Version 26.0; IBM Corp., Armonk, NY, USA), while statistical power analyses were carried out with the software G*Power (Version 3.1.9.6; [46]). The level of statistical significance was set at $p < 0.05$, and tendencies were identified from $0.05 \leq p \leq 0.13$.

3. Results

The ANOVA performed on IOP revealed a significant effect of the exercise ($F[1, 43] = 33.77$, $p < 0.001$, $\eta p^2 = 0.46$), the interaction exercise*sex ($F[1, 43] = 6.53$, $p = 0.015$, $\eta p^2 = 0.14$), and exercise*age ($F[1, 43] = 7.76$, $p = 0.008$, $\eta p^2 = 0.17$). The interaction exercise*baseline IOP levels resulted non-significant, although with medium effect size ($F[2, 43] = 1.70$, $p = 0.196$, $\eta p^2 = 0.08$). All the rest of the interactions analyzed were not significant ($p > 0.05$). Regarding the CCT, the ANOVA revealed a non-significant effect of exercise ($F[1, 43] = 3.97$, $p = 0.05$, $\eta p^2 = 0.09$), or for any of the interactions analyzed (exercise*sex: $F[1, 43] = 3.62$, $p = 0.064$, $\eta p^2 = 0.09$; exercise*age: $F[1, 43] = 0.70$, $p = 0.407$, $\eta p^2 = 0.02$; exercise*baseline IOP levels ($F[2, 43] = 0.24$, $p = 0.788$, $\eta p^2 = 0.01$). Table 2 presents the general results of the sample. It is worth highlighting that, while IOP was significantly modified ($p < 0.001$), as a consequence of the exercise, with a moderate-large effect size (d_{unb} = 0.73), CCT showed non-significant differences from pre- to post-exercise experimental points (p = 0.229).

Table 2. Data comparison between the pre- and post-exercise intraocular pressure values in the study participants (n = 49).

	Pre-Exercise	Post-Exercise	Δ%	p-Value	Cohen's d_{unb}
IOP (mmHg)	15.28 ± 0.95 [14.78–15.83]	14.30 ± 1.61 [13.93–14.97]	−6.27	<0.001	0.73
CCT (microns)	557.34 ± 35.51 [544.78–566.05]	557.91 ± 35.23 [545.98–566.94]	0.19	0.229	0.03

Post hoc tests' outcomes with Bonferroni adjustments are presented for intraocular pressure (IOP) and central corneal thickness (CCT). Results are displayed as mean ± standard deviation [95% confidence interval] and percentage of change (Δ%). Cohen's d represents the effect size of the pre- and post- differences, being d_{unb} < 0.50 a small effect, 0.50 ≤ d_{unb} ≤ 0.79 a moderate effect, and d_{unb} ≥ 0.80 a large effect.

3.1. Between-Group Comparisons

Bonferroni's post hoc comparisons for the IOP and CCT results are presented in Table 3 (sex), Table 4 (age), and Table 5 (baseline IOP levels grouping). First, regarding between-sexes comparisons, significant differences were found in pre- (p = 0.01, d_{unb} = 0.59) and post-exercise intraocular pressure (p = 0.04, d_{unb} = 0.45), but not in the CCT (pre-exercise, p = 0.097; post-exercise, p = 0.071). Highly significant differences were detected between sexes in the value of the variation of IOP (Δ%), with a significantly higher reduction found in males (mean difference (m.d.) 1.60 mmHg, 95% CI [1.11–2.13], p < 0.001, d_{unb} = 1.50). Concerning the pre- and post- comparison (within-group comparison), on the one hand, male athletes obtained a significant decrease in IOP with a large effect size (d_{unb} = 1.02). On the other hand, the variation of this variable was non-significant in females (p = 0.312). It is also remarkable that CCT was significantly modified (p = 0.007) from pre- to post-exercise in females, with the effect size being negligible (d_{unb} = 0.03).

The post hoc analyses performed for age showed significant between-group differences in the post-exercise IOP values (m.d. 1.17 mmHg, 95% CI [1.12–1.22], p = 0.016, d_{unb} = 0.50), but not in the pre-exercise values (m.d. 0.02 mmHg, 95% CI [0.01–0.05], p > 0.05). Additionally, both age groups showed a statistical tendency of significantly different IOP variation (Δ%) with moderate effect size (m.d. 0.75 mmHg, 95% CI [0.09–0.98], p = 0.07, d_{unb} = 0.50). Only the subjects over 25 years old presented significant (p < 0.001) IOP fluctuations from pre- to post-exercise with a moderate-large effect size (d_{unb} = 0.78). The young adults did not show significant fluctuations with the exercise (p = 0.154). No significant changes were observed for either of the groups in terms of the CCT (young adults: p = 0.605; adults: p = 0.243).

Table 3. Data comparison between the pre- and post-exercise intraocular pressure values, according to the sex of the participants (males, n = 18; females, n = 31).

	Group	Pre-Exercise	Post-Exercise	Δ%	p-Value	Cohen's d_{unb}
IOP (mmHg)	Male	15.60 ± 1.31 * [15.28–16.04]	13.82 ± 2.29 * [13.06–14.38]	−11.41 **	<0.001	1.02
	Female	14.91 ± 1.04 [15.11–15.71]	14.73 ± 1.81 [14.66–15.70]	−1.20	0.312	0.15
CCT (microns)	Male	546.94 ± 57.95 [526.11–559.51]	546.66 ± 57.13 [526.93–559.85]	0.09	0.395	0.01
	Female	568.02 ± 45.73 [554.84–581.20]	569.53 ± 45.09 [556.54–582.52]	0.27	0.007	0.03

Post hoc tests' outcomes with Bonferroni adjustments are presented for intraocular pressure (IOP) and central corneal thickness (CCT). Results are displayed as mean ± standard deviation [95% confidence interval] and percentage of change (Δ%). * and ** characterize statistically significant and highly statistically significant differences between sexes, respectively. Cohen's d represents the effect size of the pre- and post- differences, with d_{unb} < 0.50 being a small effect, 0.50 ≤ d_{unb} ≤ 0.79 a moderate effect, and d_{unb} ≥ 0.80 a large effect.

Table 4. Data comparison between the pre- and post-exercise intraocular pressure values, according to the age of the participants (young adults [minor or equal to 25 years], $n = 21$; adults [older than 25 years], $n = 28$).

	Group	Pre-Exercise	Post-Exercise	Δ%	*p*-Value	Cohen's d_{unb}
IOP (mmHg)	Young adults	15.27 ± 1.30 [14.89–15.64]	14.88 ± 2.21 * [14.25–15.52]	−2.55	0.154	0.21
	Adults	15.25 ± 1.39 [14.84–15.65]	13.71 ± 2.37 [13.03–14.40]	−10.10	<0.001	0.78
CCT (microns)	Young adults	564.62 ± 58.28 [547.78–581.46]	564.95 ± 57.74 [548.27–581.64]	0.06	0.605	0.00
	Adults	550.05 ± 62.57 [531.97–569.13]	550.87 ± 62.00 [532.95–568.78]	0.15	0.243	0.01

Post hoc tests' outcomes with Bonferroni adjustments are presented for intraocular pressure (IOP) and central corneal thickness (CCT). Results are displayed as mean ± standard deviation [95% confidence interval] and percentage of change (Δ%). * characterize statistically significant differences between age groups. Cohen's d represents the effect size of the pre- and post- differences, with $d_{unb} < 0.50$ being a small effect, $0.50 \leq d_{unb} \leq 0.79$ a moderate effect, and $d_{unb} \geq 0.80$ a large effect.

Table 5. Data comparison between the pre- and post- exercise intraocular pressure values, according to the baseline IOP of the participants (lowest [$\leq$14.00 mmHg], $n = 18$; medium [14.01 to 16.99 mmHg], $n = 17$; highest [$\geq$17.00 mmHg], $n = 14$).

	Group	Pre-Exercise	Post-Exercise	Δ%	*p*-Value	Cohen's d_{unb}
IOP (mmHg)	Low	13.42 ± 1.43 ** [13.00–13.83]	12.91 ± 2.50 ** [12.19–13.63]	−3.80 [3]	0.114	0.25
	Medium	15.75 ± 1.44 ** [15.33–16.17]	14.56 ± 2.53 * [13.83–15.29]	−7.56	0.001	0.57
	High	17.44 ± 1.46 [17.02–17.86]	15.88 ± 2.56 [15.14–16.61]	−8.95	<0.001	0.74
CCT (microns)	Low	551.58 ± 63.13 [533.39–569.77]	552.70 ± 62.24 [534.77–570.63]	0.20	0.136	0.02
	Medium	552.03 ± 63.86 [533.63–570.42]	553.24 ± 62.97 [535.10–571.38]	0.22	0.111	0.02
	High	562.65 ± 64.79 [543.98–581.31]	563.44 ± 63.88 [545.03–581.84]	0.14	0.303	0.01

Post hoc tests' outcomes with Bonferroni adjustments are presented for intraocular pressure (IOP) and central corneal thickness (CCT). Results are displayed as mean ± standard deviation [95% confidence interval] and percentage of change (Δ%). * and ** characterize statistically significant and highly statistically significant differences with the rest of the groups, respectively. [3]: significant differences with Group 3 (high baseline IOP). Cohen's d represents the effect size of the pre- and post-differences, with $d_{unb} < 0.50$ being a small effect, $0.50 \leq d_{unb} \leq 0.79$ a moderate effect, and $d_{unb} \geq 0.80$ a large effect.

Regarding the baseline IOP, significant differences were found in the post-exercise IOP values, as shown in Table 5. In fact, IOP variation (Δ%) showed significantly lower values in the participants with lower baseline IOP ($\leq$14.00 mmHg) than those with higher IOP at baseline ($\geq$17.00 mmHg; m.d. 1.60 mmHg, 95% CI [0.37–2.83], $p = 0.008$, $d_{unb} = 0.96$). The IOP variation (Δ%) in subjects with medium baseline IOP and those with higher IOP did not reflect statistical differences (m.d. 0.37 mmHg, 95% CI [0.28–1.87], $p = 0.420$, $d_{unb} = 0.18$). Furthermore, while subjects with moderate (between 14.01 and 16.99 mmHg) and higher baseline IOP displayed significant ($p \leq 0.001$) IOP decreases with moderate effect sizes (d_{unb} from 0.57 to 0.74), subjects with lower baseline IOP did not show statistically significant differences ($p = 0.114$) with a small effect size ($d_{unb} = 0.25$).

Differences in IOP variation (post-exercise minus pre-exercise) of each of the three groups of participants that were subdivided by IOP values can be found in Figure 1. It is worth mentioning that some subjects of the Lower-Tercile Group (baseline IOP under 14.00 mmHg) and a few of the Upper-Tercile group (baseline IOP over 17.00 mmHg) had their IOP increased due to the exercise effect, as can see in the boxplots on the left and right. Significant differences were encountered between the Lower- and Upper-Tercile Groups ($p = 0.008$, $d_{unb} = 0.96$).

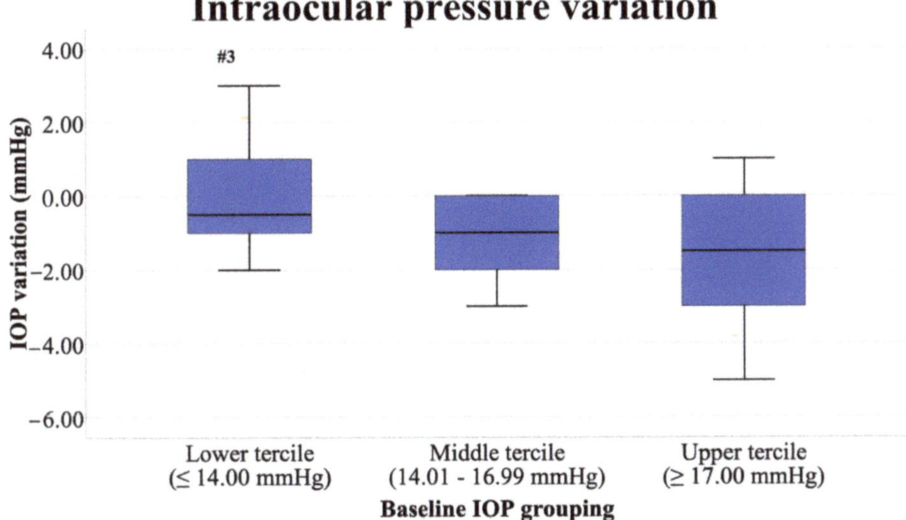

Figure 1. Intraocular pressure variation (post-exercise IOP minus pre-exercise IOP) of each of the three groups formed considering the baseline IOP levels (lower: n = 18; middle: n = 17; upper: n = 14). Values of the vertical axis (IOP variation) are presented in mmHg. The symbol "#3" highlights significant differences with the Upper-Tercile Group (p = 0.008, d_{unb} = 0.96).

3.2. Regression Analyses

Multiple linear regression was calculated to potentially predict the IOP variation based on different features of the sample (age, gender, levels of baseline IOP, and levels of baseline CCT). A significant regression equation was found (F[3, 45] = 10.159, p < 0.001, with an adjusted R^2 of 0.433). Baseline CCT and age were discarded from the equation due to non-significant results. The predicted variation of IOP was equal to 1.430 (sex)–0.270 (baseline IOP), where age is measured in years and the baseline IOP in mmHg. Regression analyses' models are displayed in Table 6, where the significant model and its coefficients are described. Model 2 was retained, as it was the one with the greatest prediction potential. This model predicted 43.3% of the variance in IOP. Sex and baseline IOP levels were significant (p = 0.001, and p = 0.007, respectively) predictors of the test outcomes. As shown in Table 6, while the baseline IOP levels were negatively correlated with the IOP variation, sex showed a positive correlation.

Table 6. Regression analyses.

Model	Predictor	Unstandardized Coefficients		Standardized Coefficients	t	Sig.	Adj. R^2	$\triangle R^2$	Durbin-Watson
		B	S.E.	β					
1	(Constant)	−2.799	1.035		−2.704	0.010			
	Age	−0.036	0.026	−0.164	−1.392	0.171	0.358	0.284	
	Sex	1.800	0.372	0.569	4.835	0.000			
2 *	(Constant)	−0.606	3.059		−0.198	0.844			
	Age	−0.035	0.024	−0.158	−1.429	0.160			
	Sex	1.430	0.383	0.452	3.730	0.001	0.433	0.096	1.975
	Baseline IOP	−0.270	0.096	−0.322	−2.817	0.007			
	Baseline CCT	0.005	0.005	0.104	0.892	0.377			

IOP: Intraocular pressure; CCT: Central corneal thickness; * Retained model; B = Unstandardized effect coefficient; S.E. = Standard Error; β = Standardized effect coefficient (Beta can be interpreted as controlling for the effects of other variables); t = Value of the Student's *t*-test; Sig = *p*-value of the test; Adj. R^2 = Adjusted R-square; $\triangle R^2$ = Changes in R-square.

4. Discussion

To the best of our knowledge, this is the first study aimed at evaluating the effect of an AG session on IOP. Additionally, a set of variables were selected to potentially predict the variation of IOP. The most notable findings were that a session of AG significantly reduced the IOP values, but did not significantly modify CCT (see Table 2), which is consistent with most previous studies on the effects of dynamic exercise on IOP [4,5,8] and confirms our first hypothesis. The small changes observed in CCT, such as those detected in females, could be due to physiological diurnal variations [47]. Additionally, it is worth highlighting that sex and baseline IOP levels were significant predictors of the fluctuation on IOP due to the exercise (see Table 6), which only partially confirms the second hypothesis. Accordingly, male gender and lower baseline IOP demonstrated in a previous study a possible association with visual field progression [48].

Bearing the aforementioned results in mind, it is worth discussing the outputs of this research under the light of other empirical evidence that addressed the influence of the independent variables selected in this study (sex, age, baseline IOP) on intraocular pressure. However, caution should be applied when comparing different methodologies of exercise and it should be borne in mind that the results presented in this study concern specifically acrobatic gymnastics.

First, sex could be a potential factor conditioning intraocular pressure due to sex hormones and genetic variants [49–51]. However, the findings encountered in the scientific literature are not consistent. Our results suggest that significant differences exist in both the baseline and post-exercise IOP values (see Table 3). Furthermore, while males had their IOP significantly modified due to the exercise effect, the intraocular pressure of females did not significantly change. This is in contrast with authors who encountered non-significant differences between sexes in the IOP changes due to treadmill running and isometric efforts [52,53]. On the other hand, the results presented concerning the sex of the participants are consistent with previous research that encountered differences between sexes [54–58] or identify sex as a confounding variable in the relationship between exercise and glaucoma [59]. More specifically, Vera et al. [60] detected further IOP fluctuations in males compared with women after isometric squats. Further research needs to be done in this regard eliminating confounding variables to elucidate if there is an actual difference in the IOP response to exercise between sexes and the origin of these differences.

Age has been widely studied as a conditioning factor of the IOP with significant positive correlations [6,52,55,61]: Only one study was found reporting non-significant correlations between age and IOP [62]. The age of 40 is recognized by the American Academy of Ophthalmology as the cutoff criterion to start comprehensive medical eye evaluation screening [63]. Due to this, only subjects under 40 years old were selected for the study. Although age was excluded from the prediction equation and was not correlated with IOP variations, significantly different behaviors were observed in the IOP of young adults under 25 years old and adults over 25. The fact of not finding a significant correlation with age in the present study could be due to the age of the sample being limited to subjects under 40 years, with studies reporting that the significant increase in baseline values occurs after the age of 40 [64]. This is interesting and coincides with the information presented in Table 4. While the baseline IOP of both groups (under 40 years old) was not significantly different, the after-exercise IOP showed significant between-group differences with a moderate effect size ($d_{unb} = 0.50$). These results suggest that once finished with the effort, the young adults under 25 years old return faster to pre-exercise values than adults over 25 years old. This could be due to the compensatory mechanisms in charge of maintaining tissue stability [2], which may function better in younger subjects, as demonstrated in rats [65].

As for the third independent variable included in this study, it is worth highlighting that IOP followed different behaviors in subjects with medium and high baseline IOP compared to subjects with lower baseline IOP (see Table 5). This is consistent with previous research that encountered larger fluctuations in subjects with higher baseline IOP and less pronounced fluctuations in subjects with lower baseline IOP [2,7,66]. More specifically, larger post-exercise decreases in subjects with higher pre-test values are reported by the expert literature [54,67–69]. In contrast, one study encountered a negative significant correlation between baseline IOP and its change (elevation) after an incremental running test [70] and other non-significant correlations [71]. The results presented are to be considered of relevance, bearing in mind that subjects with lower IOP are more susceptible to optical nerve damage with fluctuations [7,48]. It could be stated that the baseline level of IOP influences the post-exercise IOP and, therefore, this should be a factor to consider in the management of subjects with glaucoma risk factors.

Finally, the analysis and comparison with animal studies could shed some light on the behavior of IOP with exercise. For instance, Castro et al. [72] found positive results in the IOP of rats on a high-fructose diet with treadmill exercise at low intensity. These authors proposed as potential underlying mechanisms improved insulin sensitivity, reduced arterial pressure, and diminished peripheral sympathetic modulation [72]. Additionally, one study reported that swimming can reverse the negative impact of aging on the optic nerve function of rats [73]. As reported by previous expert literature, exercise-related IOP diminishments could be related to lower norepinephrine concentrations, increased colloid osmotic pressure, co-action of nitric oxide and endothelin after exercise, and the association with a β2-adrenergic receptor gene polymorphism [74–76]. Future studies should evaluate the specific mechanisms that led to lower post-exercise IOP with AG.

Limitations and Future Directions

Although all the procedures carried out in this study were carefully designed and supervised, several limitations should be listed. Validated non-contact air-puff tonometry was chosen as it is easy to use and does not require the use of anesthesia [77,78]. However, one should bear in mind that the values presented in this study only reflect pre- and post-exercise values. In this regard, continuous monitoring devices [79] would provide the scientific literature with relevant information on what exactly happens during the practice. Additionally in this concern, future studies should address the time needed for IOP to return to pre-exercise values with similar exercise procedures. As per the results on the different IOP behaviors depending on the age of subjects, it could be interesting to include adults over 40 years in a similar study design. Finally, and as presented in the introduction, the importance of field-based studies like this is unnegotiable; however, it could be of great scientific interest to continuously monitor IOP while performing somersaults and/or tumbling skills in a controlled laboratory environment.

5. Conclusions

In summary, IOP significantly decreased and CCT remained unchanged from pre- to post-exercise. The IOP of males was lowered from baseline to the end of the study. On the other hand, females did not reflect IOP changes. Similarly, the IOP of adults was further reduced compared to young adults. Finally, subjects with higher IOP at baseline (middle and upper terciles) had more pronounced decreases than the participants with lower IOP. Sex and baseline intraocular pressure were obtained as significant predictors of IOP variation.

Taken together, the analyses presented in this article shed some light on the behavior of specific ocular parameters after exercise. The combination of findings presented herein could be of interest for the programming of physical exercise for gymnastics coaches and ophthalmologists or optometrists in the prevention, management, and control of risk factors associated with IOP and glaucoma.

Author Contributions: Conceptualization, I.B.-G. and A.G.-S.; methodology, I.B.-G. and A.M.-P.; software, A.G.-S. and J.G.-M.; validation, I.B.-G., A.G.-S. and J.G.-M.; formal analysis, J.G.-M.; investigation, I.B.-G. and A.M.-P.; resources, I.B.-G.; data curation, I.B.-G. and J.G.-M.; writing—original draft preparation, I.B.-G., A.G.-S. and J.G.-M.; writing—review and editing, I.B.-G., A.G.-S. and J.G.-M.; visualization, I.B.-G. and A.G.-S.; supervision, I.B.-G. and A.G.-S.; project administration, I.B.-G. All authors have read and agreed to the published version of the manuscript.

Funding: This research received no external funding.

Institutional Review Board Statement: The study was conducted in conformity with the Code of Ethics of the World Medical Association (Declaration of Helsinki [37]), and ethical approval was provided by the Research Ethics Committee on human research of the University of Valencia (H1499867368458 approved on 15 September 2017).

Informed Consent Statement: Informed consent was obtained from all subjects involved in the study.

Data Availability Statement: The data presented in this study are available on request from the corresponding author.

Acknowledgments: The authors would like to acknowledge all the participants and the research staff members supporting the data collection. Finally, a special mention to the Club Dynamic Gym (Manises, Spain) for facilitating the investigation.

Conflicts of Interest: The authors declare no conflict of interest.

References

1. Guo, Z.-Z.; Chang, K.; Wei, X. Intraocular Pressure Fluctuation and the Risk of Glaucomatous Damage Deterioration: A Meta-Analysis. *Int. J. Ophthalmol.* **2019**, *12*, 123–128. [CrossRef] [PubMed]
2. Kim, J.H.; Caprioli, J. Intraocular Pressure Fluctuation: Is It Important? *J. Ophthalmic Vis. Res.* **2018**, *13*, 170–174. [CrossRef] [PubMed]
3. Kim, Y.W.; Park, K.H. Exogenous Influences on Intraocular Pressure. *Br. J. Ophthalmol.* **2019**, *103*, 1209–1216. [CrossRef]
4. McMonnies, C.W. Intraocular Pressure and Glaucoma: Is Physical Exercise Beneficial or a Risk? *J. Optom.* **2016**, *9*, 139–147. [CrossRef]
5. Wylęgała, A. The Effects of Physical Exercises on Ocular Physiology: A Review. *J. Glaucoma* **2016**, *25*, e843–e849. [CrossRef]
6. Wong, T.T.; Wong, T.Y.; Foster, P.J.; Crowston, J.G.; Fong, C.-W.; Aung, T. The Relationship of Intraocular Pressure with Age, Systolic Blood Pressure, and Central Corneal Thickness in an Asian Population. *Investig. Ophthalmol. Vis. Sci.* **2009**, *50*, 4097–4102. [CrossRef]
7. Caprioli, J.; Coleman, A.L. Intraocular Pressure Fluctuation: A Risk Factor for Visual Field Progression at Low Intraocular Pressures in the Advanced Glaucoma Intervention Study. *Ophthalmology* **2008**, *115*, 1123–1129. [CrossRef]
8. Zhu, M.M.; Lai, J.S.M.; Choy, B.N.K.; Shum, J.W.H.; Lo, A.C.Y.; Ng, A.L.K.; Chan, J.C.H.; So, K.F. Physical Exercise and Glaucoma: A Review on the Roles of Physical Exercise on Intraocular Pressure Control, Ocular Blood Flow Regulation, Neuroprotection and Glaucoma-Related Mental Health. *Acta Ophthalmol.* **2018**, *96*, e676–e691. [CrossRef]
9. Tribble, J.R.; Hui, F.; Jöe, M.; Bell, K.; Chrysostomou, V.; Crowston, J.G.; Williams, P.A. Targeting Diet and Exercise for Neuroprotection and Neurorecovery in Glaucoma. *Cells* **2021**, *10*, 295. [CrossRef]
10. Gene-Morales, J.; Gené-Sampedro, A.; Salvador, R.; Colado, J.C. Adding the Load Just above the Sticking Point Using Elastic Bands Optimizes Squat Performance, Perceived Effort Rate, and Cardiovascular Responses. *J. Sports Sci. Med.* **2020**, *19*, 735–744.
11. Roddy, G.; Curnier, D.; Ellemberg, D. Reductions in Intraocular Pressure after Acute Aerobic Exercise: A Meta-Analysis. *Clin. J. Sport Med.* **2014**, *24*, 364–372. [CrossRef]
12. Yuan, Y.; Lin, T.P.H.; Gao, K.; Zhou, R.; Radke, N.V.; Lam, D.S.C.; Zhang, X. Aerobic Exercise Reduces Intraocular Pressure and Expands Schlemm's Canal Dimensions in Healthy and Primary Open-Angle Glaucoma Eyes. *Indian J. Ophthalmol.* **2021**, *69*, 1127–1134. [CrossRef]
13. Vera, J.; Jiménez, R.; Redondo, B.; Perez-Castilla, A.; García-Ramos, A. Effects of Wearing the Elevation Training Mask during Low-Intensity Cycling Exercise on Intraocular Pressure. *J. Glaucoma* **2021**, *30*, e193–e197. [CrossRef]
14. Rüfer, F.; Schiller, J.; Klettner, A.; Lanzl, I.; Roider, J.; Weisser, B. Comparison of the Influence of Aerobic and Resistance Exercise of the Upper and Lower Limb on Intraocular Pressure. *Acta Ophthalmol.* **2014**, *92*, 249–252. [CrossRef] [PubMed]
15. Song, H.-Y.; Jeoung, S.-M.; Im, J.-S.; Lee, E.; Kwon, J.-D. The effect of positional changes during heavy weight lifting on intraocular pressure. *J. Korean Ophthalmol. Soc.* **2009**, *50*, 1831–1839. [CrossRef]
16. Vera, J.; Jiménez, R.; Redondo, B.; Torrejón, A.; De Moraes, C.G.V.; García-Ramos, A. Effect of the Level of Effort during Resistance Training on Intraocular Pressure. *Eur. J. Sport Sci.* **2018**, *19*, 394–401. [CrossRef] [PubMed]
17. Vera, J.; Jiménez, R.; Redondo, B.; Torrejón, A.; De Moraes, C.G.V.; García-Ramos, A. Impact of Resistance Training Sets Performed until Muscular Failure with Different Loads on Intraocular Pressure and Ocular Perfusion Pressure. *Eur. J. Ophthalmol.* **2019**, *30*, 1342–1348. [CrossRef]

18. Vera, J.; García-Ramos, A.; Jiménez, R.; Cárdenas, D. The Acute Effect of Strength Exercises at Different Intensities on Intraocular Pressure. *Graefes Arch. Clin. Exp. Ophthalmol.* **2017**, *255*, 2211–2217. [CrossRef]

19. Vieira, G.M.; Oliveira, H.B.; de Andrade, D.T.; Bottaro, M.; Ritch, R. Intraocular Pressure Variation during Weight Lifting. *Arch. Ophthalmol.* **2006**, *124*, 1251–1254. [CrossRef] [PubMed]

20. Vaghefi, E.; Shon, C.; Reading, S.; Sutherland, T.; Borges, V.; Phillips, G.; Niederer, R.L.; Danesh-Meyer, H. Intraocular Pressure Fluctuation during Resistance Exercise. *BMJ Open Ophthalmol.* **2021**, *6*, e000723. [CrossRef] [PubMed]

21. Avunduk, A.M.; Yilmaz, B.; Şahin, N.; Kapicioglu, Z.; Dayanır, V. The Comparison of Intraocular Pressure Reductions after Isometric and Isokinetic Exercises in Normal Individuals. *Ophthalmologica* **1999**, *213*, 290–294. [CrossRef]

22. Chromiak, J.A.; Abadie, B.R.; Braswell, R.A.; Koh, Y.S.; Chilek, D.R. Resistance Training Exercises Acutely Reduce Intraocular Pressure in Physically Active Men and Women. *J. Strength Cond. Res.* **2003**, *17*, 715–720. [PubMed]

23. Conte, M.; Scarpi, M.J.; Rossin, R.A.; Beteli, H.R.; Lopes, R.G.; Marcos, H.L. Intraocular pressure variation after submaximal strength test in resistance training. *Arq. Bras. Oftalmol.* **2009**, *72*, 351–354. [CrossRef]

24. Conte, M.; Ciolac, E.G.; Rosa, M.R.R.; Cozza, H.; Baldin, A.D. Efeito agudo do exercicio resistido, aerobico continuo e intervalado na pressao intraocular de individuos fisicamente ativos. *Ens. Ciênc* **2012**, *16*, 27–37.

25. Conte, M.; Scarpi, M.J. A Comparison of the Intraocular Pressure Response between Two Different Intensities and Volumes of Resistance Training. *Rev. Bras. Oftalmol.* **2014**, *73*, 23–27. [CrossRef]

26. Soares, A.S.; Caldara, A.A.; Storti, L.R.; Teixeira, L.F.M.; Terzariol, J.G.T.; Conte, M. Variation of Intraocular Pressure in Resistance Exercise Performed in Two Different Positions. *Rev. Bras. Oftalmol.* **2015**, *74*, 160–163. [CrossRef]

27. Tamura, S.D.; Caldara, A.A.; Soares, A.S.; Storti, L.R.; Teixeira, L.F.M.; Conte, M. Association between Plasma Lactate Concentrations after Resistance Exercise with Intraocular Pressure. *Perspect. Med.* **2013**, *24*, 5–10. [CrossRef]

28. Teixeira, L.F.M.; Tamura, S.D.; Possebom, H.M.; Conte, M. Effect of Resistance Training Session on Intraocular Pressure in Patients with Open Angle Glaucoma. *Med. Sci. Sports Exerc.* **2019**, *51*, 988. [CrossRef]

29. Vieira, G.M.; Penna, E.P.; Marques, M.B.; Bezerra, R.F. The Accute Effects of Resistance Exercise on Intraocular Pressure. *Arq. Bras. Oftalmol.* **2003**, *66*, 431–435. [CrossRef]

30. Gene-Morales, J.; Gené-Sampedro, A.; Salvador, R.; Colado, J.C. Effects of Squatting with Elastic Bands or Conventional Resistance-Training Equipment at Different Effort Levels in the Post-Exercise Intraocular Pressure of Healthy Men. *Biol. Sport.* **2022**, *39*, in press.

31. Taboada-Iglesias, Y.; Santana, M.V.; Gutiérrez-Sánchez, Á. Anthropometric Profile in Different Event Categories of Acrobatic Gymnastics. *J. Hum. Kinet.* **2017**, *57*, 169–179. [CrossRef] [PubMed]

32. Taboada-Iglesias, Y.; Gutiérrez-Sánchez, Á.; Vernetta Santana, M. Anthropometric Profile of Elite Acrobatic Gymnasts and Prediction of Role Performance. *J. Sports Med. Phys. Fitness* **2016**, *56*, 433–442. [PubMed]

33. Fédération Internationale de Gymnastique World Age Group Competition Rules. Acrobatic Gymnastics. 2017–2020. 2016. Available online: https://www.gymnastics.sport/publicdir/rules/files/en_ACRO%20WAGC%20Rules%202017-2020%20(with%20videos).pdf (accessed on 26 July 2021).

34. Fédération Internationale de Gymnastique Technical Regulations 2020. Section 1 General Regulations. 2020. Available online: https://www.gymnastics.sport/publicdir/rules/files/en_Technical%20Regulations%202021%20with%20changes.pdf (accessed on 26 July 2021).

35. Fédération Internationale de Gymnastique Acrobatic Gymnastics. Available online: https://www.gymnastics.sport/site/pages/disciplines/pres-acro.php (accessed on 5 October 2021).

36. Höög, S.; Andersson, E.P. Sex and Age-Group Differences in Strength, Jump, Speed, Flexibility, and Endurance Performances of Swedish Elite Gymnasts Competing in TeamGym. *Front. Sports Act. Living* **2021**, *3*, 653503. [CrossRef]

37. Hutchinson, D. *World Medical Association Declaration of Helsinki, Edinburgh 2000*; Canary Publications: Guildford, UK, 2002.

38. Bonnie, R.J.; Stroud, C.; Breiner, H.; Committee on Improving the Health, Safety, and Well-Being of Young Adults; Board on Children, Youth, and Families; Institute of Medicine; National Research Council. *Investing in the Health and Well-Being of Young Adults*; National Academies Press (US): Washington, DC, USA, 2015.

39. Wong, T.Y.; Klein, B.E.K.; Klein, R.; Knudtson, M.; Lee, K.E. Refractive Errors, Intraocular Pressure, and Glaucoma in a White Population. *Ophthalmology* **2003**, *110*, 211–217. [CrossRef]

40. Vera, J.; Jiménez, R.; García, J.A.; Cárdenas, D. Intraocular Pressure Is Sensitive to Cumulative and Instantaneous Mental Workload. *Appl. Ergon.* **2017**, *60*, 313–319. [CrossRef] [PubMed]

41. Lau, W.; Pye, D.C. Associations between Diurnal Changes in Goldmann Tonometry, Corneal Geometry, and Ocular Response Analyzer Parameters. *Cornea* **2012**, *31*, 639–644. [CrossRef] [PubMed]

42. Kocamis, O.; Kilic, R. Repeatability, Reproducibility and Agreement of Central Corneal Thickness Measurements by Two Noncontact Pachymetry Devices. *Med. Hypothesis Discov. Innov. Ophthalmol.* **2019**, *8*, 34–39.

43. Lakens, D. Calculating and Reporting Effect Sizes to Facilitate Cumulative Science: A Practical Primer for t-Tests and ANOVAs. *Front. Psychol.* **2013**, *4*, 863. [CrossRef]

44. Cumming, G. The New Statistics: Why and How. *Psychol. Sci.* **2014**, *25*, 7–29. [CrossRef]

45. Cohen, J. *Statistical Power Analysis for the Behavioral Sciences*, 2nd ed.; L. Erlbaum Associates: Hillsdale, NJ, USA, 1988; ISBN 978-0-8058-0283-2.

46. Faul, F.; Erdfelder, E.; Lang, A.-G.; Buchel, A. G*Power 3: A Flexible Statistical Power Analysis Program for the Social, Behavioral, and Biomedical Sciences. *Behav. Res. Methods* **2007**, *39*, 175–191. [CrossRef]

47. Ariza-Gracia, M.A.; Piñero, D.P.; Rodriguez, J.F.; Pérez-Cambrodí, R.J.; Calvo, B. Interaction between Diurnal Variations of Intraocular Pressure, Pachymetry, and Corneal Response to an Air Puff: Preliminary Evidence. *JCRS Online Case Rep.* **2015**, *3*, 12–15. [CrossRef]

48. Nouri-Mahdavi, K.; Hoffman, D.; Coleman, A.L.; Liu, G.; Li, G.; Gaasterland, D.; Caprioli, J. Predictive Factors for Glaucomatous Visual Field Progression in the Advanced Glaucoma Intervention Study. *Ophthalmology* **2004**, *111*, 1627–1635. [CrossRef]

49. Dane, Ş.; Aslankurt, M.; Yazici, A.T.; Gümüştekin, K. Sex-Related Difference in Intraocular Pressure in Healthy Young Subjects. *Percept. Mot. Skills* **2003**, *96*, 1314–1316. [CrossRef]

50. Simcoe, M.J.; Khawaja, A.P.; Mahroo, O.A.; Hammond, C.J.; Hysi, P.G. The Role of Chromosome X in Intraocular Pressure Variation and Sex-Specific Effects. *Investig. Ophthalmol. Vis. Sci.* **2020**, *61*, 20. [CrossRef]

51. Vajaranant, T.S.; Nayak, S.; Wilensky, J.T.; Joslin, C.E. Gender and Glaucoma: What We Know and What We Need to Know. *Curr. Opin. Ophthalmol.* **2010**, *21*, 91–99. [CrossRef]

52. Esfahani, M.A.; Gharipour, M.; Fesharakinia, H. Changes in Intraocular Pressure after Exercise Test. *Oman J. Ophthalmol.* **2017**, *10*, 17–20. [CrossRef]

53. Vera, J.; Raimundo, J.; García-Durán, B.; Pérez-Castilla, A.; Redondo, B.; Delgado, G.; Koulieris, G.-A.; García-Ramos, A. Acute Intraocular Pressure Changes during Isometric Exercise and Recovery: The Influence of Exercise Type and Intensity, and Participant's Sex. *J. Sports Sci.* **2019**, *37*, 2213–2219. [CrossRef] [PubMed]

54. Era, P.; Pärssinen, O.; Kallinen, M.; Suominen, H. Effect of Bicycle Ergometer Test on Intraocular Pressure in Elderly Athletes and Controls. *Acta Ophthalmol.* **1993**, *71*, 301–307. [CrossRef] [PubMed]

55. Jeelani, M.; Taklikar, R.; Taklikar, A.; Itagi, V.; Bennal, A. Variation of Intraocular Pressure with Age and Gender. *Natl. J. Physiol. Pharm. Pharmacol.* **2014**, *4*, 57. [CrossRef]

56. Mori, K.; Ando, F.; Nomura, H.; Sato, Y.; Shimokata, H. Relationship between Intraocular Pressure and Obesity in Japan. *Int. J. Epidemiol.* **2000**, *29*, 661–666. [CrossRef] [PubMed]

57. Qureshi, I.A. Intraocular Pressure: A Comparative Analysis in Two Sexes. *Clin. Physiol.* **1997**, *17*, 247–255. [CrossRef] [PubMed]

58. Son, J.; Koh, H.; Son, J. The Association between Intraocular Pressure and Different Combination of Metabolic Syndrome Components. *BMC Ophthalmol.* **2016**, *16*, 76. [CrossRef] [PubMed]

59. Lin, S.-C.; Wang, S.Y.; Pasquale, L.R.; Singh, K.; Lin, S.C. The Relation between Exercise and Glaucoma in a South Korean Population-Based Sample. *PLoS ONE* **2017**, *12*, e0171441. [CrossRef] [PubMed]

60. Vera, J.; Jiménez, R.; Redondo, B.; Torrejón, A.; Koulieris, G.-A.; De Moraes, C.G.V.; García-Ramos, A. Investigating the Immediate and Cumulative Effects of Isometric Squat Exercise for Different Weight Loads on Intraocular Pressure: A Pilot Study. *Sports Health* **2019**, *11*, 247–253. [CrossRef] [PubMed]

61. Baek, S.U.; Kee, C.; Suh, W. Longitudinal Analysis of Age-Related Changes in Intraocular Pressure in South Korea. *Eye* **2015**, *29*, 625–629. [CrossRef]

62. Rochtchina, E.; Mitchell, P.; Wang, J.J. Relationship between Age and Intraocular Pressure: The Blue Mountains Eye Study. *Clin. Exp. Ophthalmol.* **2002**, *30*, 173–175. [CrossRef] [PubMed]

63. Machiele, R.; Motlagh, M.; Patel, B.C. Intraocular Pressure. In *StatPearls*; StatPearls Publishing: Treasure Island, FL, USA, 2021.

64. Qureshi, I.A. Age and Intraocular Pressure: How Are They Correlated? *J. Pak. Med. Assoc.* **1995**, *45*, 150–152.

65. Jiang, X.; Johnson, E.; Cepurna, W.; Lozano, D.; Men, S.; Wang, R.K.; Morrison, J. The Effect of Age on the Response of Retinal Capillary Filling to Changes in Intraocular Pressure Measured by Optical Coherence Tomography Angiography. *Microvasc. Res.* **2018**, *115*, 12–19. [CrossRef]

66. Tojo, N.; Abe, S.; Miyakoshi, M.; Hayashi, A. Correlation between Short-Term and Long-Term Intraocular Pressure Fluctuation in Glaucoma Patients. *Clin. Ophthalmol.* **2016**, *10*, 1713–1717. [CrossRef]

67. Ashkenazi, I.; Melamed, S.; Blumenthal, M. The Effect of Continuous Strenuous Exercise on Intraocular Pressure. *Investig. Ophthalmol. Vis. Sci.* **1992**, *33*, 2874–2877.

68. Leighton, D.A.; Phillips, C.I. Effect of Moderate Exercise on the Ocular Tension. *Br. J. Ophthalmol.* **1970**, *54*, 599–605. [CrossRef]

69. Najmanova, E.; Pluhacek, F.; Botek, M. Intraocular Pressure Response to Moderate Exercise during 30-Min Recovery. *Optom. Vis. Sci.* **2016**, *93*, 281–285. [CrossRef]

70. Najmanova, E.; Pluhacek, F.; Botek, M. Intraocular Pressure Response to Maximal Exercise Test during Recovery. *Optom. Vis. Sci.* **2018**, *95*, 136–142. [CrossRef]

71. Price, E.L.; Gray, L.S.; Humphries, L.; Zweig, C.; Button, N.F. Effect of Exercise on Intraocular Pressure and Pulsatile Ocular Blood Flow in a Young Normal Population. *Optom. Vis. Sci.* **2003**, *80*, 460–466. [CrossRef] [PubMed]

72. Castro, E.F.S.; Mostarda, C.T.; Rodrigues, B.; Moraes-Silva, I.C.; Feriani, D.J.; De Angelis, K.; Irigoyen, M.C. Exercise Training Prevents Increased Intraocular Pressure and Sympathetic Vascular Modulation in an Experimental Model of Metabolic Syndrome. *Braz. J. Med. Biol. Res.* **2015**, *48*, 332–338. [CrossRef]

73. Chrysostomou, V.; Kezic, J.M.; Trounce, I.A.; Crowston, J.G. Forced Exercise Protects the Aged Optic Nerve against Intraocular Pressure Injury. *Neurobiol. Aging* **2014**, *35*, 1722–1725. [CrossRef]

74. Risner, D.; Ehrlich, R.; Kheradiya, N.S.; Siesky, B.; McCranor, L.; Harris, A. Effects of Exercise on Intraocular Pressure and Ocular Blood Flow: A Review. *J. Glaucoma* **2009**, *18*, 429–436. [CrossRef] [PubMed]

75. Gale, J.; Wells, A.P.; Wilson, G. Effects of Exercise on Ocular Physiology and Disease. *Surv. Ophthalmol.* **2009**, *54*, 349–355. [CrossRef] [PubMed]
76. Martin, B.; Harris, A.; Hammel, T.; Malinovsky, V. Mechanism of Exercise-Induced Ocular Hypotension. *Investig. Ophthalmol. Vis. Sci.* **1999**, *40*, 1011–1015.
77. Kato, Y.; Nakakura, S.; Matsuo, N.; Yoshitomi, K.; Handa, M.; Tabuchi, H.; Kiuchi, Y. Agreement among Goldmann Applanation Tonometer, ICare, and Icare PRO Rebound Tonometers; Non-Contact Tonometer; and Tonopen XL in Healthy Elderly Subjects. *Int. Ophthalmol.* **2018**, *38*, 687–696. [CrossRef]
78. Radhakrishnan, B.; Hemapriya, S.; Ghouse, N.F.; Rajagopalan, A. Comparison of Intraocular Pressure Measurement with Non-Contact Tonometry and Applanation Tonometry among Various Central Corneal Thickness Groups. *J. Evid. Based Med. Healthc.* **2018**, *5*, 531–536. [CrossRef]
79. Kim, Y.W.; Kim, M.J.; Park, K.H.; Jeoung, J.W.; Kim, S.H.; Jang, C.I.; Lee, S.H.; Kim, J.H.; Lee, S.; Kang, J.Y. Preliminary Study on Implantable Inductive-Type Sensor for Continuous Monitoring of Intraocular Pressure. *Clin. Exp. Ophthalmol.* **2015**, *43*, 830–837. [CrossRef] [PubMed]

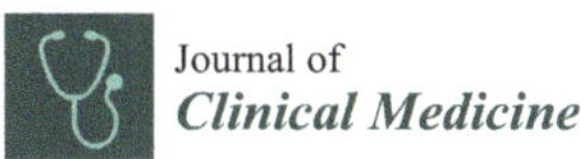

Journal of
Clinical Medicine

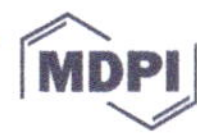

Article

Is Obesity a Risk or Protective Factor for Open-Angle Glaucoma in Adults? A Two-Database, Asian, Matched-Cohort Study

Wei-Dar Chen [1,2], Li-Ju Lai [1,2], Kang-Lung Lee [3,4], Tzeng-Ji Chen [4,5], Chia-Yen Liu [6] and Yao-Hsu Yang [6,7,8,*]

1   Department of Ophthalmology, Chang Gung Memorial Hospital, Chiayi 33305, Taiwan; weidar1023@gmail.com (W.-D.C.); lynnlai@cgmh.org.tw (L.-J.L.)
2   College of Medicine, Chang Gung University, Taoyuan 33302, Taiwan
3   Department of Radiology, Taipei Veterans General Hospital, Taipei 11217, Taiwan; miguelkllee@gmail.com
4   School of Medicine, National Yang Ming Chiao Tung University, Taipei 11221, Taiwan; tjchen@vghtpe.gov.tw
5   Department of Family Medicine, Taipei Veterans General Hospital, Taipei 11217, Taiwan
6   Health Information and Epidemiology Laboratory, Chang Gung Memorial Hospital, Chiayi 33305, Taiwan; qchiayen@gmail.com
7   Department of Traditional Chinese Medicine, Chang Gung Memorial Hospital, Chiayi 33305, Taiwan
8   School of Traditional Chinese Medicine, College of Medicine, Chang Gung University, Taoyuan 33302, Taiwan
*   Correspondence: r95841012@ntu.edu.tw; Tel.: +886-5-3621000 (ext. 3613)

Citation: Chen, W.-D.; Lai, L.-J.; Lee, K.-L.; Chen, T.-J.; Liu, C.-Y.; Yang, Y.-H. Is Obesity a Risk or Protective Factor for Open-Angle Glaucoma in Adults? A Two-Database, Asian, Matched-Cohort Study. *J. Clin. Med.* **2021**, *10*, 4021. https://doi.org/10.3390/jcm10174021

Academic Editors: Jose Javier Garcia-Medina and Maria Dolores Pinazo-Duran

Received: 7 August 2021
Accepted: 2 September 2021
Published: 6 September 2021

Publisher's Note: MDPI stays neutral with regard to jurisdictional claims in published maps and institutional affiliations.

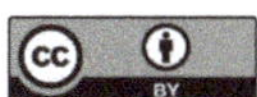

Abstract: Obesity contributes to multiple systemic disorders; however, extensive discussion regarding obesity and open-angle glaucoma (OAG) remains limited, and conclusions in the existing literature diverge. This study aims to analyze the risk of OAG among obese adults in Taiwan. In this study, adults (aged ≥18 years) with a diagnostic code of obesity or morbid obesity registered in the Longitudinal Health Insurance Database (LHID) 2000 and LHID2005 from 1 January 2001 to 31 December 2010 were included. All adults were traced until the diagnosis of OAG, the occurrence of death, or 31 December 2013. Risk of OAG was significantly higher in obese adults than in non-obese adults after multivariable adjustment (adjusted hazard ratio (aHR): 1.43 (95% confidence interval (CI) 1.11–1.84)/aHR: 1.54 (95% CI 1.23–1.94) in the LHID2000/LHID2005). Both databases demonstrated that young obese adults (aged ≤40 years) had a remarkably increased risk of OAG compared with young non-obese adults (aHR 3.08 (95% CI 1.82–5.21)/aHR 3.81 (95% CI 2.26–6.42) in the LHID2000/LHID2005). This two-database matched-cohort study suggests that obese adults have an increased risk of OAG. In young adults, in particular, obesity could be a potential risk factor of OAG.

Keywords: obesity; open-angle glaucoma; risk factor; young adults

1. Introduction

Obesity represents one of the biggest health emergency issues worldwide. According to the World Health Organization, the prevalence of obesity (body mass index (BMI) $\geq$ 30 kg/m^2) in the United States was 36.2% in 2016 [1]; this figure was projected to soar to 50.7% by 2030 [2]. Similarly, the prevalence of obesity in Europe and Asia has increased exponentially over the past decade. Obesity has a multifactorial association with the environment, dietary habits, sedentary lifestyles, and genetics [3]. Obesity-derived metabolic dysregulation, inflammatory stress, and neural degeneration lead to a series of pathophysiological processes [4]. Numerous studies have indicated that obesity has a strong connection with diabetes mellitus, hypertension, ischemic heart disease, stroke, and Alzheimer's disease [5,6].

Although discussing the association between obesity and sight-threatening disorders has recently intensified [7], the relationship between obesity and open-angle glaucoma (OAG) remains controversial. OAG, the most prevalent subtype of glaucoma globally, is characterized by progressive damage of retinal ganglion cells (RGCs), enlarged optic disc cupping, and irreversible deterioration of the visual field. Lowering intraocular pressure

(IOP) is considered to be the most effective strategy in preventing disease progression, although the etiology of OAG has been not completely elucidated.

To date, several studies have reported that obesity has a positive correlation with increased IOP [8–10]. Nevertheless, whether obesity is a risk factor for OAG remains inconclusive [11,12]. In the Rotterdam study, there was no significant association between BMI and OAG after multivariable adjustment [13]. However, Newman-Casey showed that obese patients had a 14% increased risk of OAG in the univariable analysis, and obese women had a 6% increased hazard for OAG after multivariable adjustment [14]. Conversely, Pasquale reported that increased BMI was associated with a 6% lower risk of OAG in Caucasian women [15]. Additionally, Kim et al. showed that overweight status is a protective factor of OAG [16]. Prompted by inconsistent reports of the association between obesity and OAG, the present 13-year matched-cohort study aimed to analyze the risk of OAG among obese individuals using data from two Taiwanese population-based longitudinal databases.

2. Materials and Methods

2.1. Databases

In this study, participant data were collected from the Longitudinal Health Insurance Database (LHID) 2000 and LHID2005, which belong to the National Health Insurance research database (NHIRD) in Taiwan. The National Health Insurance program is a universal and compulsory health insurance program benefiting >99.6% of the Taiwanese population to date, and data of the NHIRD, including registration files and original claim data, have been used in many studies with high academic value. The LHID2000 contains 1,000,000 de-identified insurance claim data randomly retrieved from the year 2000 Registry of Beneficiaries of the NHIRD (23.75 million) during the period of 1 January 2000 to 31 December 2000 by Oracle's internal random number generator. Likewise, the LHID2005 encompasses 1,000,000 insurance claim data drawn from the year 2005 Registry of Beneficiaries of the NHIRD (25.68 million) during the period of 1 January 2005 to 31 December 2005 following the same method. Through statistic validation, there was no selection bias on age, sex, or insurance premiums between the LHID and the NHIRD. Both the LHID2000 and LHID2005 adopted the 2001 Edition of International Classification of Diseases, Ninth Revision, Clinical Modification (ICD-9-CM). This study was approved by the Institutional Review Board (IRB) of Chang Gung Medical Foundation, and adhered to the tenets of the Declaration of Helsinki. Given the retrospective nature of this study and the use of de-identified patient data in the LHID, the IRB of the Chang Gung Medical foundation approved that the requirements of informed consent were waived.

2.2. Study Design

A flowchart of enrollment of obese and non-obese groups is presented in Figure 1. The LHID2000 and LHID2005 were separately reviewed in this matched-cohort study. There were 17,256 and 17,474 individuals aged ≥18 years included from the LHID2000 and LHID2005. The obese individuals were qualified with the coding of obesity or morbid obesity (ICD-9-CM codes 278.0, 278.00, 278.01) between 1 January 1997 and 31 December 2013. We washed out the initial 4-year period to eliminate individuals with incomplete data and those diagnosed with obesity before 2001 (LHID2000/LHID2005: 1889/1880 individuals). Simultaneously, individuals with a new diagnosis of obesity after 2010 were excluded to confirm that individuals can be traced for at least 3 years (LHID2000/LHID2005: 3365/3397 individuals). Further, individuals diagnosed with OAG before a coding of obesity were also excluded (LHID2000/LHID2005: 60/74 individuals). Final numbers of 11,939 and 12,118 individuals with a new diagnosis of obesity between 2001 and 2010 were recruited in obese groups of the LHID2000 and LHID2005. Individuals without a diagnosis of overweight or obesity (ICD-9-CM codes: 278.0, 278.00, 278.01, 278.02, and 278.1) were included in the non-obese group. The obese individuals were matched with the non-obese individuals at a 1:4 ratio by sex, age, urbanized level, and income. The stratification of urbanization level and income followed the criteria reported in a previous LHID study [17]. All individuals were traced from the index date to the diagnosis of OAG, occurrence of death, or 31 December 2013.

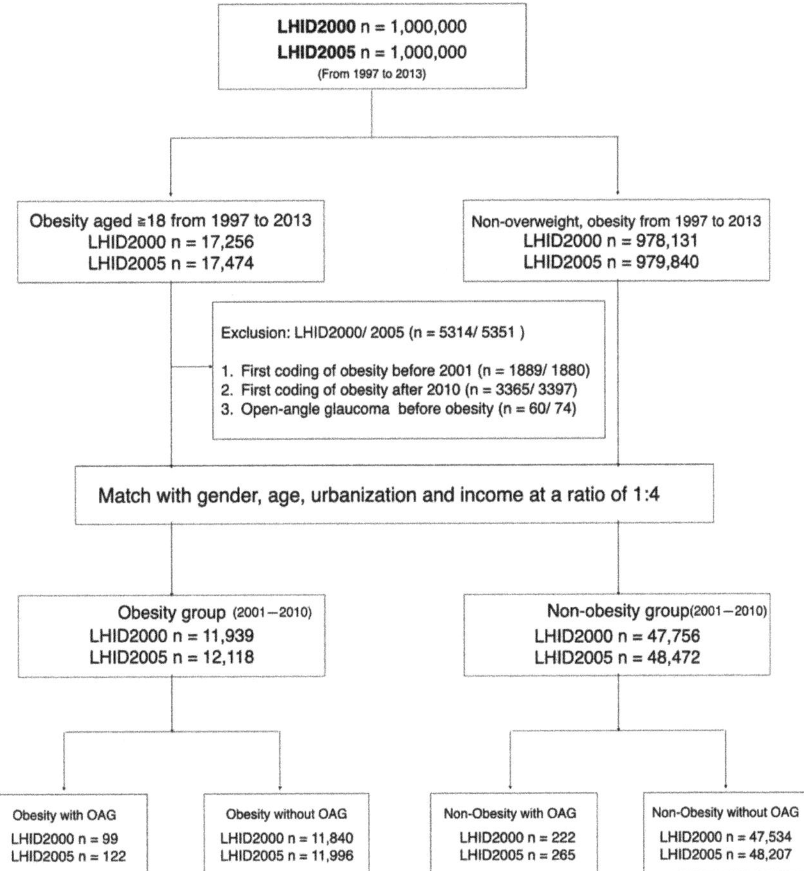

Figure 1. Flowchart of enrollment and allocation of adults with obesity and non-obesity in a two-database matched-cohort study. Obese adults aged ≥18 years in the LHID2000 and LHID2005 between 1 January 1997 and 31 December 2013 were included. Adults first diagnosed with obesity before 2001, adults first diagnosed with obesity after 2010, and adults diagnosed with OAG before obesity were excluded in this study. Obese adults were matched with non-obese adults at a 1:4 ratio by sex, age, urbanization level, and income. All adults were traced until the death, occurrence of OAG, or 31 December 2013. LHID = longitudinal health insurance database; OAG = open-angle glaucoma.

To increase the validation of OAG, outcomes were rigorously defined as the coding of OAG (ICD-9-CM codes 365.1, 365.10, 365.11, 365.12), with a treatment involving anti-glaucoma drugs or surgeries ≥2 times, adjudicated by an ophthalmologist(s) over one year. Multiple covariates were collected for adjustment of the risk of OAG: diabetes mellitus (ICD-9-CM codes 250x), hypertension (ICD-9-CM codes 401x–405x), hyperlipidemia (ICD-9-CM codes 272x), ischemic heart disease (IHD) (ICD-9-CM codes 410x–414x), chronic kidney disease (CKD) (ICD-9-CM codes 585x and 586x), myopia (ICD-9-CM codes 367.1), migraine (ICD-9-CM codes 346x), hypothyroidism (ICD-9-CM code 244.9), obstructive sleep apnea (OSA) (ICD-9-CM codes 327.23, 780.51, 780.53, and 780.57), and hypotension (ICD-9-

CM codes 458x). The inclusion criteria for covariates were diagnostic coding ≥ 1 time in admission or ≥ 3 times in ambulatory visits.

2.3. Statistical Analyses

All statistical data in this study were processed and analyzed using SAS version 9.4 (SAS Inc., Cary, NC, USA). For baseline characteristics, a chi-squared test and Student's *t* test were used to analyze categorical and continuous variables, respectively. The cumulative incidence of OAG was calculated using the Kaplan–Meier method and a log-rank test. A multivariable Cox proportional regression was applied to estimate the adjusted hazard ratio (aHR) and 95% confidence interval (CI) for risk of OAG. The main model for adjustment consisted of demographic variables: sex, age, urbanization level, and income, and five cardinal covariates associated with risk of OAG: diabetes mellitus, hypertension, hyperlipidemia, ischemic heart disease, and chronic kidney disease. Another five potential covariates of OAG—myopia, hypothyroidism, migraine, obstructive sleep apnea, and hypotension—were added one by one into the main model for testing the stability of the sensitivity analysis. Ultimately, sex, age, and covariates were tested for risk of OAG in multivariable stratified analysis. Statistical significance was defined as a two-sided $p < 0.05$.

3. Results

In the LHID2000, OAG occurrence was 99 in 11,939 obese individuals, and the incidence rate of OAG was 1.0 and 0.6 per 1000 person-years in the obese and non-obese groups (incidence rate ratio (IRR) 1.79), respectively. In the LHID2005, OAG occurrence was 122 in 12,118 obese individuals, and the incidence rate of OAG was 1.3 and 0.7 per 1000 person-years in the obese and non-obese groups (IRR 1.85), respectively. The average follow-up was $7.91 \pm 2.93/7.93 \pm 2.93$ years in the obese/non-obese groups of the LHID2000, respectively, and $7.88 \pm 2.92/7.89 \pm 2.92$ years in the obese/non-obese groups of LHID2005, respectively. The ratio of females to males was 2:1 in both databases. For age distribution, the ratio of obese individuals aged ≤ 40 and >40 years was approximately 1:1 in both databases. Obese adults had a higher rate and frequency of ophthalmology visits than non-obese adults. Additionally, obese adults had higher rates of diabetes mellitus, hypertension, hyperlipidemia, ischemic heart disease, chronic kidney disease, myopia, obstructive sleep apnea, migraine, and hypothyroidism than non-obese adults in both databases (Table 1).

Table 1. Baseline characteristics with incidence of open-angle glaucoma in obese and non-obese adults.

	LHID2000			LHID2005		
	Obesity	Non-Obesity		Obesity	Non-Obesity	
Variables	*n* (%)	*n* (%)	*p*-value	*n* (%)	*n* (%)	*p*-value
Total	11,939	47,756		12,118	48,472	
Gender			1.00			1.00
Female	7718 (64.6)	30,872 (64.6)		7815 (64.5)	31,260 (64.5)	
Male	4221 (35.4)	16,884 (35.4)		4303 (35.5)	17,212 (35.5)	
Age			1.00			1.00
18–30	3135 (26.3)	12,540 (26.3)		3098 (25.6)	12,392 (25.6)	
31–40	2858 (23.9)	11,432 (23.9)		2961 (24.4)	11,844 (24.4)	
41–50	2660 (22.3)	10,640 (22.3)		2645 (21.8)	10,580 (21.8)	
51–60	1992 (16.7)	7968 (16.7)		2054 (17.0)	8216 (17.0)	
61–70	886 (7.4)	3544 (7.4)		944 (7.8)	3776 (7.8)	
>70	408 (3.4)	1632 (3.4)		416 (3.4)	1664 (3.4)	
Urbanization level			1.00			1.00
1(City)	3965 (33.2)	15,860 (33.2)		3765 (31.1)	15,060 (31.1)	
2	5477 (45.9)	21,908 (45.9)		5837 (48.2)	23,348 (48.2)	
3	1673 (14.0)	6692 (14.0)		1746 (14.4)	6984 (14.4)	
4(Villages)	824 (6.9)	3296 (6.9)		770 (6.4)	3080 (6.4)	

Table 1. *Cont.*

	LHID2000			LHID2005		
	Obesity	Non-Obesity		Obesity	Non-Obesity	
Income			1.00			1.00
0	3952 (33.1)	15,808 (33.1)		2447 (20.2)	9788 (20.2)	
1–15,840	1883 (15.8)	7532 (15.8)		1811 (14.9)	7244 (14.9)	
15,841–25,000	3990 (33.4)	15,960 (33.4)		3742 (30.9)	14,968 (30.9)	
≥25,001	2114 (17.7)	8456 (17.7)		4118 (34.0)	16,472 (34.0)	
OPH visit	3856 (32.3)	12,082 (25.3)	<0.001	3995 (33.0)	12,731 (26.3)	<0.001
Frequency of OPH visit			<0.001			<0.001
0	8083 (67.7)	35,674 (74.7)		8123 (67.0)	35,741 (73.7)	
1–2	2458 (20.6)	8061 (16.9)		2564 (21.2)	8470 (17.5)	
>2	1398 (11.7)	4021 (8.4)		1431 (11.8)	4261 (8.8)	
Comorbidity						
Diabetes mellitus	3494 (29.3)	5419 (11.4)	<0.001	3642 (30.1)	5810 (12.0)	<0.001
Hypertension	5576 (46.7)	10,818 (22.7)	<0.001	5571 (46.0)	11,434 (23.6)	<0.001
Hyperlipidemia	5202 (43.6)	8326 (17.4)	<0.001	5353 (44.2)	8939 (18.4)	<0.001
IHD	2275 (19.1)	4510 (9.4)	<0.001	2306 (19.0)	4867 (10.0)	<0.001
CKD	381 (3.2)	969 (2.0)	<0.001	372 (3.1)	1027 (2.1)	<0.001
Myopia	1169 (9.8)	3422 (7.2)	<0.001	1207 (10.0)	3562 (7.4)	<0.001
Migraine	697 (5.8)	1618 (3.4)	<0.001	730 (6.0)	1815 (3.7)	<0.001
Hypothyroidism	269 (2.3)	354 (0.7)	<0.001	266 (2.2)	404 (0.8)	<0.001
OSA	463 (3.9)	319 (0.7)	<0.001	428 (3.5)	313 (0.7)	<0.001
Hypotension	72 (0.6)	225 (0.5)	0.067	71 (0.6)	234 (0.5)	0.151
No. of OAG	99	222		122	265	
Incidence %	1.0	0.6	<0.001	1.3	0.7	<0.001
IRR (95% CI)	1.79 (1.41–2.27)			1.85 (1.49–2.29)		

CI = confidence interval; CKD = chronic kidney disease; IHD = ischemic heart disease; LHID = Longitudinal Health Insurance Database OAG = open-angle glaucoma; OSA = obstructive sleep apnea; OPH = ophthalmology IRR = incidence rate ratio.

Kaplan–Meier curve analysis revealed that the obese group had a significantly higher cumulative incidence of OAG than the non-obese group in both databases ($p < 0.001$) (Figure 2A,B). In the age-stratified analysis, both the young and older obese groups still showed an increased accumulation of OAG compared with the young and older non-obese groups, and the young obese group displayed a remarkable accumulation of OAG in both databases (Figure 2C,D).

The risk of OAG in the multivariable Cox proportional hazard regression are summarized in Table 2. The risk of OAG occurrence was significantly higher in the obese group than in the non-obese group after adjusting for the main model (aHR 1.43 in the LHID2000; aHR 1.54 in the LHID2005). Men appeared to have a higher risk of OAG than women; however, the difference did not reach statistical significance. Older adults (aged >40 years) had an increased risk of OAG compared with young adults (aged ≤40 years). Among covariates, diabetes mellitus was a prominent risk factor for OAG in both databases.

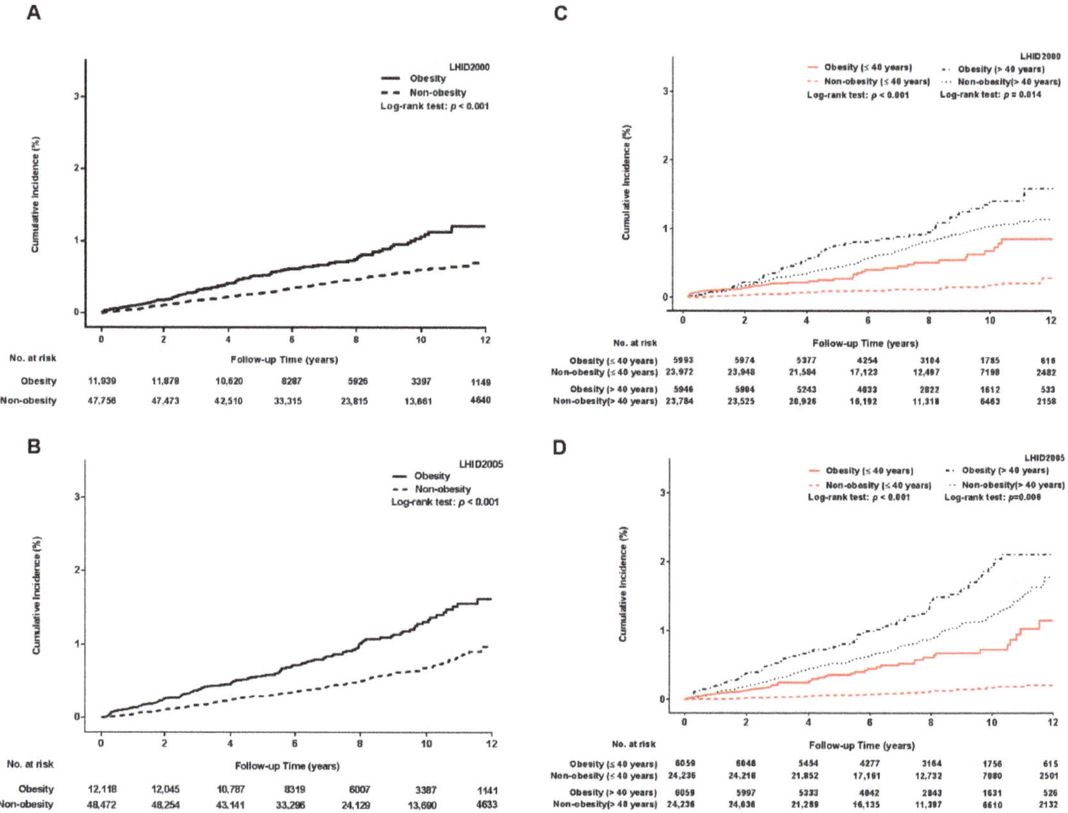

Figure 2. Cumulative incidence of open-angle glaucoma in obese and non-obese adults. (**A**) Cumulative incidence of OAG in the LHID2000; (**B**) cumulative incidence of OAG in the LHID2005; (**C**) age-stratified analysis for the cumulative incidence of OAG in the LHID2000; (**D**) age-stratified analysis for the cumulative incidence of OAG in the LHID2005. Both the LHID2000 and LHID2005 demonstrated that the cumulative incidence of OAG was higher in obese adults than non-obese adults (Log-rank test *p* < 0.001). In the age-stratified analysis, young obese adults (red line) displayed a remarkable cumulative incidence of OAG compared with young non-obese adults (red dotted line) (Log-rank test *p* < 0.001) although both the young and older obese adults had a significantly higher cumulative incidence of OAG. LHID = longitudinal health insurance database; OAG = open-angle glaucoma.

Table 2. Multivariable cox proportional hazard regression of the association between open-angle glaucoma and potential risk factors.

Variables	LHID2000				LHID2005			
	Crude HR (95% CI)	*p*-Value	aHR (95% CI)	*p*-Value	Crude HR (95% CI)	*p*-Value	aHR (95% CI)	*p*-Value
Exposure								
Non-obesity	1 (Reference)		1 (Reference)		1 (Reference)		1 (Reference)	
Obesity	1.79 (1.41–2.27)	<0.001	1.43 (1.11–1.84)	0.006	1.85 (1.49–2.29)	122	1.54 (1.23–1.94)	<0.001
Gender								
Female	1 (Reference)		1 (Reference)		1 (Reference)		1 (Reference)	
Male	1.23 (0.98–1.54)	0.076	1.21 (0.95–1.52)	0.120	1.16 (0.95–1.43)	0.153	1.19 (0.96–1.47)	0.109

Table 2. *Cont.*

Variables	LHID2000				LHID2005			
	Crude HR (95% CI)	*p*-Value	aHR (95% CI)	*p*-Value	Crude HR (95% CI)	*p*-Value	aHR (95% CI)	*p*-Value
Age ≤ 40	1 (Reference)		1 (Reference)		1 (Reference)		1 (Reference)	
Age > 40	3.83 (2.94–5.00)	<0.001	3.09 (2.26–4.25)	<0.001	4.75 (3.66–6.15)	<0.001	3.52 (2.64–4.70)	<0.001
Comorbidity								
Diabetes								
No	1 (Reference)		1 (Reference)		1 (Reference)		1 (Reference)	
Yes	2.91 (2.31–3.66)	<0.001	1.55 (1.18–2.04)	0.002	3.04 (2.47–3.73)	<0.001	1.61 (1.26–2.06)	<0.001
Hypertension								
No	1 (Reference)		1 (Reference)		1 (Reference)		1 (Reference)	
Yes	2.68 (2.16–3.34)	<0.001	1.22 (0.92–1.61)	0.170	3.00 (2.46–3.67)	<0.001	1.38 (1.07–1.77)	0.012
Hyperlipidemia								
No	1 (Reference)		1 (Reference)		1 (Reference)		1 (Reference)	
Yes	2.51 (2.01–3.12)	<0.001	1.14 (0.87–1.50)	0.347	2.27 (1.86–2.78)	<0.001	0.90 (0.71–1.15)	0.412
IHD								
No	1 (Reference)		1 (Reference)		1 (Reference)		1 (Reference)	
Yes	2.66 (2.08–3.42)	<0.001	1.27 (0.95–1.68)	0.106	2.60 (2.07–3.25)	<0.001	(1.170.91–1.50)	0.231
CKD								
No	1 (Reference)		1 (Reference)		1 (Reference)		1 (Reference)	
Yes	2.17 (1.29–3.64)	0.003	1.02 (0.60–1.74)	0.934	2.05 (1.28–3.30)	0.003	0.93 (0.57–1.51)	0.764

CKD = chronic kidney disease; IHD = ischemic heart disease; IRR = incidence rate ratio; LHID = Longitudinal Health Insurance Database OAG = open-angle glaucoma.

In sensitivity analysis of the risk of OAG (Figure 3), after adjustment for full model or potential covariates, the aHR of OAG occurrence in obesity remained steady, from 1.32 to 1.43 in the LHID2000, and from 1.46 to 1.58 in the LHID2005.

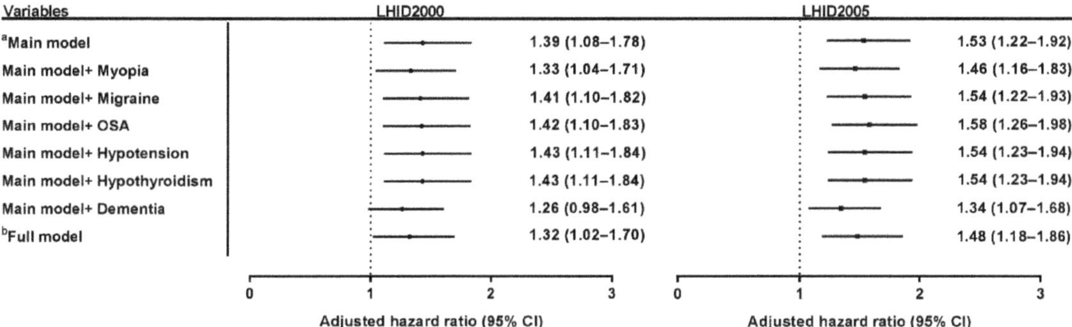

Figure 3. Sensitivity analysis of the risk of open-angle glaucoma in obesity. Sensitivity analysis in both the LHID2000 and LHID2005 showed that the adjusted hazard ratio of OAG remained stable after being adjusted according to the full model and main model with each potential covariate (myopia, migraine, OSA, hypotension, and hypothyroidism). The adjusted hazard ratio of OAG was 1.32 to 1.43 in the LHID2000, and 1.49 to 1.58 in the LHID2005. [a] Main model adjusted for age, gender, income, urbanization, diabetes mellitus, hypertension, hyperlipidemia, ischemic heart disease, and chronic kidney disease [b] Full model adjusted for the main model, myopia, hypothyroidism, migraine, OSA, and hypotension. OAG = open-angle glaucoma; OSA = obstructive sleep apnea.

The multivariable stratified analysis is presented in Figure 4. In the age-stratified analysis, there was a demonstrably higher risk in young obese adults than in young non-obese adults, but there was no statistical significance of OAG risk in older adults. In the sex-stratified analysis, obese men had a higher risk of OAG compared with the non-obese men in both databases; however, obese women had an unremarkable (LHID2000) and borderline (LHID2005) risk of OAG. Moreover, adults with at least one ophthalmology visit were analyzed, and the result showed that obese adults still had a higher risk of OAG than non-obese adults in both databases. In the covariate-stratified analysis, the results revealed that in the LHID2005, obese adults without each covariate had a significantly higher risk of OAG than non-obese adults without each covariate, but obese adults with each covariate had a nonsignificant hazard for OAG compared with non-obese adults with each covariate. There was a similar tendency in most analyses of covariates in the LHID2000, although the analysis of hypertension and hyperlipidemia was discordant between the LHID2000 and LHID2005.

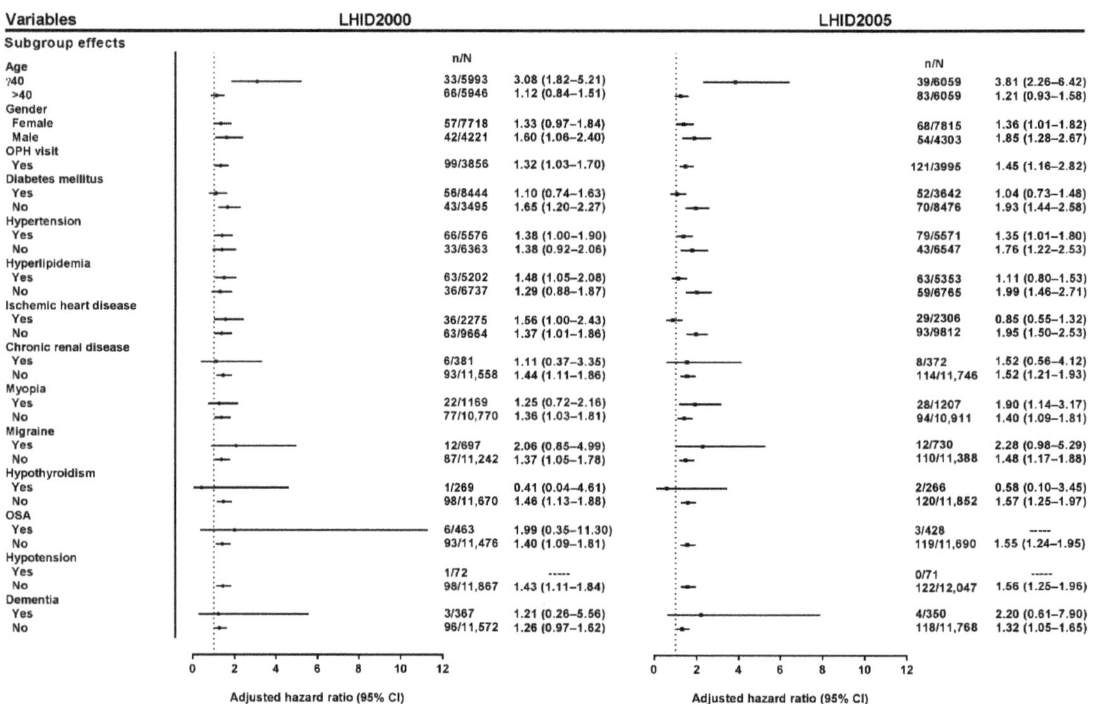

Figure 4. Multivariable stratified hazard analysis of the association between obesity and open-angle glaucoma. All adjusted hazard ratios in the multivariable stratified analysis were adjusted by the main model. The results in both the LHID2000 and LHID2005 displayed that obesity was a remarkable hazard of OAG in young (aged ≤40 years) obese adults compared with young non-obese adults. In gender stratification, the risk of OAG was more significant in obese men than non-obese men. As for the stratified analysis of covariates, in the LHID2005, the obese group without each covariate had an increased risk of OAG compared with the non-obese group without each covariate; however, the obese group with each covariate had a nonsignificant risk of OAG compared with the non-obese group with each covariate. There was a similar tendency in most of the stratified analyses of covariates in the LHID2000, but the analyses of hypertension and hyperlipidemia were inconsistent between the LHID2000 and LHID2005. There was no adjusted hazard ratio in a few subgroups (obesity with OSA in the LHID2005, and obesity with hypotension in both the LHID2000 and LHID2005). LHID = longitudinal health insurance database; OAG = open-angle glaucoma; OSA = obstructive sleep apnea; OPH = ophthalmology.

4. Discussion

In this two-database, matched-cohort study, obese adults had a higher cumulative incidence of OAG at the 13-year follow-up. Overall, obesity was a significant hazard of OAG after adjustment for multivariable covariates. Moreover, young obese adults had a remarkably higher risk of OAG than young non-obese adults.

The cardinal pathogenesis of OAG is the progressive degeneration of RGCs. Several mechanisms could be considered as to how obesity contributes to the damage of RGCs in OAG. Hormonal disequilibrium in obesity plays an integral role in the progressive impairment of RGCs. Decreased adiponectin and increased leptin resistance in obesity result in insulin resistance, dysfunctional lipid metabolism, atherosclerosis, and the activation of proinflammatory cytokines and oxidative stress, which lead to vascular hypo-perfusion and chronic inflammation of RGCs [18–20]. OAG is firmly associated with neurodegenerative pathogeneses such as dysregulation of the brain-derived neurotrophic factor (BDNF), phosphorylation of the tau protein, and overexpression of the apolipoprotein E (APOE) gene [21–23]. These neurodegenerative pathways have crucial connections with obesity. BDNF is a potential neuroprotective molecule that prevents neuron damage and synaptic disturbances. Recent studies have demonstrated that decreased BDNF has a profound effect on neurodegenerative diseases in the obese population [24]. Furthermore, leptin resistance in obesity plays a critical role in the formation of tau phosphorylation, which may have a detrimental effect on the impairment of RGCs [25]. Meanwhile, the fat-mass and obesity-associated (FTO) gene, strongly related to obesity, was found to be associated with risk of Alzheimer's disease through interaction with the APOE gene [26], and modulates cholesterol metabolism in the central neural network [23]. It is possible that obesity orchestrates a similar genetic vulnerability in the pathogenesis of OAG.

This was an Asian population-based study used to substantiate the association between obesity and OAG, and the results suggest that obesity is a potential risk factor for OAG, especially in young obese adults. This result, however, contradicts those of some previous population-based studies, in which the increase of BMI was associated with a lower risk of OAG. There are several possible explanations for this divergence. First, we only included truly obese adults, because physicians in Taiwan coded obesity or morbid obesity as patients with a BMI ≥ 30 kg/m^2 who intended to seek medical assistance (e.g., including dietary consultation, enrollment in a weight-loss program, the use of anti-obesity drugs, or evaluation for bariatric surgery) [27]. Likewise, Newman-Casey's study, in which the result showed obesity is a risk factor of OAG, also included obese patients as the study population [14]. By contrast, the study by Pasquale and Ramdas included patients with a wide range of BMI values, which were not thoroughly specific for an obese population [15]. In Kim's study, they adopted the overweight status (BMI > 25 kg/m^2) to evaluate the risk of OAG instead of the obese status [16]. Body fat is the critical factor that induces a series of physical dysfunctions in obesity. However, increase in BMI cannot truly reflect the increased mass of body fat, especially in adults with who are overweight or have a normal weight [28]. Further, obesity contributes to more severe morbidities and mortality than overweight [29]. Several studies have even reported that overweight is related to lower mortality rates than normal weight [30,31]. This is why our results showed that obesity is a significant hazard of OAG, because this study recruited truly obese adults who were in need of medical assistance.

Second, previous studies have included study populations aged >40 years, whereas our study recruited study populations aged ≥ 18 years. In Table 2, the risk of OAG was significantly higher in older adults than in young adults (aged ≤ 40 years), which is compatible with the concept that OAG is a strong age-related neurodegenerative disease. In the age-stratified analysis, obesity was a nonsignificant hazard for OAG in older adults (aged >40 years) although there was an increased risk of OAG in obese adults. This result is similar to most of the previous studies in that obesity was a nonsignificant risk factor for OAG in adults aged >40 years. This outcome could partially determine age as the most conspicuous risk factor for OAG, and show that age-related neurodegenerative effects result in a more profound risk for OAG than obesity-related neurodegenerative effects. Meanwhile, the degeneration of optic neurons is susceptible to long-term chronic diseases such as hypertension and diabetes, and metabolic diseases among older obese adults. These multiple factors would make the impact of obesity inconspicuous when assessing risk of OAG.

On the other hand, our data indicated that obesity is a remarkable contributor to OAG in young adults (aged ≤40 years) regardless of accumulative incidence or age-stratified analysis. This result may have suggested that without the influence of aging and long-term chronic diseases, obesity would be a decisive factor for accelerating the damage of neurons, and that obesity-related neurodegenerative effects have a crucial impact on OAG occurrence among young adults [32]. Moreover, obesity may be correlated with the pathogenesis of juvenile OAG, such as mutation of the CYP1B1 gene or the glaucoma-associated olfactomedin domain of myocilin [33,34]. With obesity trending among younger populations, it is important to raise the awareness that obesity could be a potential risk factor for OAG in young adults.

In this study, obese adults had a higher rate and frequency of ophthalmology visits than non-obese adults, which is reasonable because obese adults with diabetes, hypertension, or metabolic diseases are often asked for the ophthalmic survey of cataract, retinopathy, or macular degeneration. This may have increased the incidental diagnosis of OAG that resulted in a selection bias of higher OAG risk in obese adults. In order to reduce the effect of higher rates of ophthalmology visits among obese adults, we analyzed the risk of OAG in adults with at least one ophthalmology visit, and the data showed that obesity is still a significant risk factor for OAG after multivariable adjustment. In addition, this study showed that the obese populations skewed towards female and young adults. It is assumed that female and young adults may be more concerned with their physical stature and health than male or older adults, so that these two populations are more active in seeking medical assistance to control weight. To reduce sex and age biases, a complete matching strategy was adopted in this study to mitigate the bias of these factors.

The analysis of both databases demonstrated that men exhibit a higher risk for OAG than women, although the HR did not reach statistical significance. This phenomenon could be explained by the fact that estrogen can protect RGCs in women [35]. In the sex-stratified analysis, obese men had a significantly higher HR of OAG than non-obese men. One reason may be that there are decreased adiponectin levels and an increased insulin resistance among obese men compared with non-obese men [36]. On the other hand, the risk of OAG was relatively indistinct between obese and non-obese women, which could imply that elevated circulating estrogen in obese menopausal women may reduce the risk of OAG [37].

In the multivariable analysis, diabetes mellitus showed a strong association with risk of OAG. Probable pathophysiological mechanisms include insulin resistance, vascular dysregulation, and reduction of neurotrophic factors [38]. In the covariate-stratified analysis, obesity without each covariate was shown to be a significant OAG hazard, but obesity with each covariate revealed a nonsignificant risk of OAG in the LHID2005. Most stratified analyses of covariates had a similar tendency in the LHID2000. These results indicated that even in adults without these covariates, obesity would be a prominent risk factor for OAG. Nevertheless, in adults with these covariates, mutual interaction between obesity and covariates may weaken the impact of obesity on OAG occurrence, and obesity could become a relatively inconspicuous risk factor for OAG. Another reason for the nonsignificant hazard of OAG in obese adults with covariates could be due to the small number of cases because the analysis revealed a wide confidence interval. Further, the stratified analysis of hypertension and hyperlipidemia were inconsistent between the LHID2000 and LHID2005, and a larger study population is required to elucidate their role on the association between obesity and OAG in advanced studies.

This study had several limitations. First, the data of BMI were not collected in the LHID, and the dynamic changes of weight could not be traced. Additionally, the obese population may have been underestimated, as most physicians code obesity only if the obese patient wants to seek out medical assistance. On the other hand, the coding of obesity is rather reliable in Taiwan, because physicians are required to code patients with obesity for medical intervention, otherwise they will face the risk of an audit and heavy penalties under the monthly review of the Bureau of National Health Insurance. In addition, the incidence rate of OAG may have been underestimated. In clinical experience, obese adults often experience a long period of obesity before coding; however, we excluded all adults diagnosed with OAG before the coding of obesity could curtail the incidence of OAG in obese adults. Second, IOP is a critical risk factor for OAG, and most studies have already reported that obesity is highly associated with elevated IOP. However, the data of IOP was not collected in the LHID, so the mutual interaction among obesity, IOP, and OAG could not be evaluated without IOP data. Third, the definition of OAG depends on the coding system of the ICD-9. To validate the accuracy of OAG, we strictly defined the outcome as (at least) a coding of OAG with a treatment involving anti-glaucoma drugs or surgeries ≥ 2 times, adjudicated by an ophthalmologist(s) over one year. Moreover, two independent databases were used to confirm the consistency of the results. Finally, there is no personal history collected in the NHIRD, so the effect of smoking was not taken into account.

To summarize, in a Taiwanese-based population, the results of this two-database matched-cohort study suggested that obese adults have an increased hazard of OAG. In age stratification, obesity could be a potential risk factor of OAG in young adults, but obesity poses a nonsignificant risk for OAG in older adults. In this era of obesity trending among young adults, more attention should be paid to the impact of obesity on OAG occurrence, and a recommendation of ophthalmic survey should be considered in young obese adults, not only for those with metabolic diseases. A comprehensive understanding of the association between obesity and OAG could have a far-reaching influence on the lives of young obese adults. Obesity-related hormonal disequilibrium, neurologic disturbance, and genetic dysregulation are possible pathogenic mechanisms of OAG. Advanced clinical and laboratory research will be essential for elucidating the relationship between obesity and OAG.

Author Contributions: Conceptualization, W.-D.C. and Y.-H.Y.; methodology, W.-D.C., K.-L.L., C.-Y.L. and Y.-H.Y.; software, C.-Y.L. and Y.-H.Y.; validation, L.-J.L., T.-J.C. and Y.-H.Y.; formal analysis, C.-Y.L. and Y.-H.Y.; investigation, W.-D.C., L.-J.L., K.-L.L., T.-J.C., C.-Y.L. and Y.-H.Y.; resources, T.-J.C. and Y.-H.Y.; data curation, W.-D.C., C.-Y.L. and Y.-H.Y.; writing—original draft preparation, W.-D.C.; writing—review and editing, L.-J.L. and Y.-H.Y. All authors have read and agreed to the published version of the manuscript.

Funding: This research received no external funding.

Institutional Review Board Statement: This study was approved by the Institutional Review Board of Chang Gung Medical Foundation (Chiayi County, Taiwan; IRB No: 201701230B0), and thoroughly adhered to the tenets of the Declaration of Helsinki.

Informed Consent Statement: Given the retrospective nature of the present study and the use of de-identified patient data in the LHID, the Institutional Review Board of Chang Gung Medical foundation approved that the requirement of informed consent was waived.

Data Availability Statement: The data presented in this study are available on request from the corresponding author. The data are not publicly available due to privacy and ethical reasons.

Acknowledgments: The authors would like to thank Health Information and Epidemiology Laboratory for the comprehensive comments and assistance in data analysis. Besides, we also would like to thank Chao-Yung Wang, the physician of the department of cardiology at Linkou Chang Gung Memorial Hospital, for the consultation of the information and epidemiology of the obese population in Taiwan.

Conflicts of Interest: The authors declare no conflict of interest.

References

1. Hruby, A.; Hu, F.B. The Epidemiology of Obesity: A Big Picture. *Pharmacoeconomics* **2015**, *33*, 673–689. [CrossRef]
2. Finkelstein, E.A.; Khavjou, O.A.; Thompson, H.; Trogdon, J.G.; Pan, L.; Sherry, B.; Dietz, W. Obesity and severe obesity forecasts through 2030. *Am. J. Prev. Med.* **2012**, *42*, 563–570. [CrossRef]
3. Qi, L.; Cho, Y.A. Gene-environment interaction and obesity. *Nutr. Rev.* **2008**, *66*, 684–694. [CrossRef] [PubMed]
4. Heymsfield, S.B.; Wadden, T.A. Mechanisms, Pathophysiology, and Management of Obesity. *N. Engl. J. Med.* **2017**, *376*, 254–266. [CrossRef] [PubMed]
5. Pi-Sunyer, X. The medical risks of obesity. *Postgrad Med.* **2009**, *121*, 21–33. [CrossRef] [PubMed]
6. Alford, S.; Patel, D.; Perakakis, N.; Mantzoros, C.S. Obesity as a risk factor for Alzheimer's disease: Weighing the evidence. *Obes Rev.* **2018**, *19*, 269–280. [CrossRef] [PubMed]
7. Ling, C.N.Y.; Lim, S.C.; Jonas, J.B.; Sabanayagam, C. Obesity and risk of age-related eye diseases: A systematic review of prospective population-based studies. *Int. J. Obes* **2021**, *45*, 1863–1885. [CrossRef]
8. Cohen, E.; Kramer, M.; Shochat, T.; Goldberg, E.; Garty, M.; Krause, I. Relationship Between Body Mass Index and Intraocular Pressure in Men and Women: A Population-based Study. *J. Glaucoma* **2016**, *25*, e509–e513. [CrossRef]
9. Mori, K.; Ando, F.; Nomura, H.; Sato, Y.; Shimokata, H. Relationship between intraocular pressure and obesity in Japan. *Int. J. Epidemiol.* **2000**, *29*, 661–666. [CrossRef]
10. Tham, Y.C.; Cheng, C.Y. Associations between chronic systemic diseases and primary open angle glaucoma: An epidemiological perspective. *Clin. Exp. Ophthalmol.* **2017**, *45*, 24–32. [CrossRef]
11. Cheung, N.; Wong, T.Y. Obesity and eye diseases. *Surv. Ophthalmol.* **2007**, *52*, 180–195. [CrossRef] [PubMed]
12. Liu, W.; Ling, J.; Chen, Y.; Wu, Y.; Lu, P. The Association between Adiposity and the Risk of Glaucoma: A Meta-Analysis. *J. Ophthalmol.* **2017**, *2017*, 9787450. [CrossRef]
13. Springelkamp, H.; Wolfs, R.C.; Ramdas, W.D.; Hofman, A.; Vingerling, J.R.; Klaver, C.C.; Jansonius, N.M. Incidence of glaucomatous visual field loss after two decades of follow-up: The Rotterdam Study. *Eur. J. Epidemiol.* **2017**, *32*, 691–699. [CrossRef]
14. Newman-Casey, P.A.; Talwar, N.; Nan, B.; Musch, D.C.; Stein, J.D. The relationship between components of metabolic syndrome and open-angle glaucoma. *Ophthalmology* **2011**, *118*, 1318–1326. [CrossRef]
15. Pasquale, L.R.; Willett, W.C.; Rosner, B.A.; Kang, J.H. Anthropometric measures and their relation to incident primary open-angle glaucoma. *Ophthalmology* **2010**, *117*, 1521–1529. [CrossRef]
16. Kim, K.E.; Kim, M.J.; Park, K.H.; Jeoung, J.W.; Kim, S.H.; Kim, C.Y.; Kang, S.W. Epidemiologic Survey Committee of the Korean Ophthalmological, S. Prevalence, Awareness, and Risk Factors of Primary Open-Angle Glaucoma: Korea National Health and Nutrition Examination Survey 2008–2011. *Ophthalmology* **2016**, *123*, 532–541. [CrossRef]
17. Tsai, M.S.; Lee, L.A.; Tsai, Y.T.; Yang, Y.H.; Liu, C.Y.; Lin, M.H.; Hsu, C.M.; Chen, C.K.; Li, H.Y. Sleep apnea and risk of vertigo: A nationwide population-based cohort study. *Laryngoscope* **2018**, *128*, 763–768. [CrossRef] [PubMed]
18. Martin, S.S.; Qasim, A.; Reilly, M.P. Leptin resistance: A possible interface of inflammation and metabolism in obesity-related cardiovascular disease. *J. Am. Coll. Cardiol.* **2008**, *52*, 1201–1210. [CrossRef] [PubMed]
19. McArdle, M.A.; Finucane, O.M.; Connaughton, R.M.; McMorrow, A.M.; Roche, H.M. Mechanisms of obesity-induced inflammation and insulin resistance: Insights into the emerging role of nutritional strategies. *Front. Endocrinol.* **2013**, *4*, 52. [CrossRef]
20. Stewart, R.M.; Clearkin, L.G. Insulin resistance and autoregulatory dysfunction in glaucoma and retinal vein occlusion. *Am. J. Ophthalmol.* **2008**, *145*, 394–396. [CrossRef]
21. Shpak, A.A.; Guekht, A.B.; Druzhkova, T.A.; Kozlova, K.I.; Gulyaeva, N.V. Brain-Derived Neurotrophic Factor in Patients with Primary Open-Angle Glaucoma and Age-related Cataract. *Curr. Eye Res.* **2018**, *43*, 224–231. [CrossRef]
22. Chiasseu, M.; Cueva Vargas, J.L.; Destroismaisons, L.; Vande Velde, C.; Leclerc, N.; Di Polo, A. Tau Accumulation, Altered Phosphorylation, and Missorting Promote Neurodegeneration in Glaucoma. *J. Neurosci.* **2016**, *36*, 5785–5798. [CrossRef]
23. Wang, Y.; Zhou, Y.F.; Zhao, B.Y.; Gu, Z.Y.; Li, S.L. Apolipoprotein E gene epsilon4epsilon4 is associated with elevated risk of primary open angle glaucoma in Asians: A meta-analysis. *BMC Med. Genet.* **2014**, *15*, 60. [CrossRef]
24. Motamedi, S.; Karimi, I.; Jafari, F. The interrelationship of metabolic syndrome and neurodegenerative diseases with focus on brain-derived neurotrophic factor (BDNF): Kill two birds with one stone. *Metab. Brain Dis.* **2017**, *32*, 651–665. [CrossRef] [PubMed]
25. Platt, T.L.; Beckett, T.L.; Kohler, K.; Niedowicz, D.M.; Murphy, M.P. Obesity, diabetes, and leptin resistance promote tau pathology in a mouse model of disease. *Neuroscience* **2016**, *315*, 162–174. [CrossRef]
26. Keller, L.; Xu, W.; Wang, H.X.; Winblad, B.; Fratiglioni, L.; Graff, C. The obesity related gene, FTO, interacts with APOE, and is associated with Alzheimer's disease risk: A prospective cohort study. *J. Alzheimers Dis.* **2011**, *23*, 461–469. [CrossRef] [PubMed]
27. Huang, C.C.; Huang, Y.T.; Chiu, C.C. A population-based analysis of use and outcomes of laparoscopic bariatric surgery across socioeconomic groups in Taiwan. *Int. J. Equity Health* **2015**, *14*, 127. [CrossRef]
28. Nuttall, F.Q. Body Mass Index: Obesity, BMI, and Health: A Critical Review. *Nutr. Today* **2015**, *50*, 117–128. [CrossRef] [PubMed]
29. Zheng, W.; McLerran, D.F.; Rolland, B.; Zhang, X.; Inoue, M.; Matsuo, K.; He, J.; Gupta, P.C.; Ramadas, K.; Tsugane, S.; et al. Association between body-mass index and risk of death in more than 1 million Asians. *N. Engl. J. Med.* **2011**, *364*, 719–729. [CrossRef]
30. Flegal, K.M.; Kit, B.K.; Orpana, H.; Graubard, B.I. Association of all-cause mortality with overweight and obesity using standard body mass index categories: A systematic review and meta-analysis. *JAMA* **2013**, *309*, 71–82. [CrossRef] [PubMed]

31. Orpana, H.M.; Berthelot, J.M.; Kaplan, M.S.; Feeny, D.H.; McFarland, B.; Ross, N.A. BMI and mortality: Results from a national longitudinal study of Canadian adults. *Obes. Silver Spring* **2010**, *18*, 214–218. [CrossRef]

32. Nevalainen, T.; Kananen, L.; Marttila, S.; Jylhava, J.; Mononen, N.; Kahonen, M.; Raitakari, O.T.; Hervonen, A.; Jylha, M.; Lehtimaki, T.; et al. Obesity accelerates epigenetic aging in middle-aged but not in elderly individuals. *Clin. Epigenetics* **2017**, *9*, 20. [CrossRef]

33. Li, F.; Jiang, C.; Larsen, M.C.; Bushkofsky, J.; Krausz, K.W.; Wang, T.; Jefcoate, C.R.; Gonzalez, F.J. Lipidomics reveals a link between CYP1B1 and SCD1 in promoting obesity. *J. Proteome Res.* **2014**, *13*, 2679–2687. [CrossRef]

34. Donegan, R.K.; Hill, S.E.; Freeman, D.M.; Nguyen, E.; Orwig, S.D.; Turnage, K.C.; Lieberman, R.L. Structural basis for misfolding in myocilin-associated glaucoma. *Hum. Mol Genet.* **2015**, *24*, 2111–2124. [CrossRef] [PubMed]

35. Dewundara, S.S.; Wiggs, J.L.; Sullivan, D.A.; Pasquale, L.R. Is Estrogen a Therapeutic Target for Glaucoma? *Semin. Ophthalmol.* **2016**, *31*, 140–146. [CrossRef] [PubMed]

36. Hara, T.; Fujiwara, H.; Shoji, T.; Mimura, T.; Nakao, H.; Fujimoto, S. Decreased plasma adiponectin levels in young obese males. *J. Atheroscler. Thromb.* **2003**, *10*, 234–238. [CrossRef] [PubMed]

37. Cleary, M.P.; Grossmann, M.E. Minireview: Obesity and breast cancer: The estrogen connection. *Endocrinology* **2009**, *150*, 2537–2542. [CrossRef]

38. Song, B.J.; Aiello, L.P.; Pasquale, L.R. Presence and Risk Factors for Glaucoma in Patients with Diabetes. *Curr. Diab. Rep.* **2016**, *16*, 124. [CrossRef]

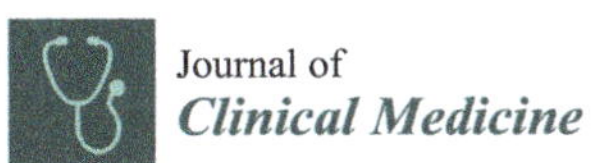

Journal of
Clinical Medicine

Article

Fully Automated Colorimetric Analysis of the Optic Nerve Aided by Deep Learning and Its Association with Perimetry and OCT for the Study of Glaucoma

Marta Gonzalez-Hernandez [1,2], Daniel Gonzalez-Hernandez [1], Daniel Perez-Barbudo [1], Paloma Rodriguez-Esteve [3], Nisamar Betancor-Caro [3] and Manuel Gonzalez de la Rosa [1,3,*]

[1] INSOFT S.L., 25 de Julio, 34, 38004 Santa Cruz de Tenerife, Spain; martaglezhdez@gmail.com (M.G.-H.); management@insoft.es (D.G.-H.); danieltf@gmail.com (D.P.-B.)
[2] Ophthalmology Department, Hospital Universitario de Canarias, Carretera Ofra s/n, 38320 San Cristobal de La Laguna, Spain
[3] Facultad de Ciencias de la Salud, Universidad de La Laguna, C/Sta, María Soledad s/n, 38200 San Cristobal de La Laguna, Spain; paloma.rguezesteve@gmail.com (P.R.-E.); nisamar89@hotmail.com (N.B.-C.)
* Correspondence: mgdelarosa1950@gmail.com

Citation: Gonzalez-Hernandez, M.; Gonzalez-Hernandez, D.; Perez-Barbudo, D.; Rodriguez-Esteve, P.; Betancor-Caro, N.; Gonzalez de la Rosa, M. Fully Automated Colorimetric Analysis of the Optic Nerve Aided by Deep Learning and Its Association with Perimetry and OCT for the Study of Glaucoma. *J. Clin. Med.* **2021**, *10*, 3231. https://doi.org/10.3390/jcm10153231

Academic Editors: Jose Javier Garcia-Medina and Maria Dolores Pinazo-Duran

Received: 6 July 2021
Accepted: 20 July 2021
Published: 22 July 2021

Publisher's Note: MDPI stays neutral with regard to jurisdictional claims in published maps and institutional affiliations.

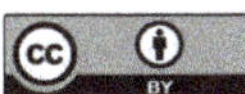

Abstract: Background: Laguna-ONhE is an application for the colorimetric analysis of optic nerve images, which topographically assesses the cup and the presence of haemoglobin. Its latest version has been fully automated with five deep learning models. In this paper, perimetry in combination with Laguna-ONhE or Cirrus-OCT was evaluated. Methods: The morphology and perfusion estimated by Laguna ONhE were compiled into a "Globin Distribution Function" (GDF). Visual field irregularity was measured with the usual pattern standard deviation (PSD) and the threshold coefficient of variation (TCV), which analyses its harmony without taking into account age-corrected values. In total, 477 normal eyes, 235 confirmed, and 98 suspected glaucoma cases were examined with Cirrus-OCT and different fundus cameras and perimeters. Results: The best Receiver Operating Characteristic (ROC) analysis results for confirmed and suspected glaucoma were obtained with the combination of GDF and TCV (AUC: 0.995 and 0.935, respectively. Sensitivities: 94.5% and 45.9%, respectively, for 99% specificity). The best combination of OCT and perimetry was obtained with the vertical cup/disc ratio and PSD (AUC: 0.988 and 0.847, respectively. Sensitivities: 84.7% and 18.4%, respectively, for 99% specificity). Conclusion: Using Laguna ONhE, morphology, perfusion, and function can be mutually enhanced with the methods described for the purpose of glaucoma assessment, providing early sensitivity.

Keywords: glaucoma; deep learning; perimetry; optic nerve

1. Introduction

Glaucoma is a disease with a relatively high incidence, estimated between 2.09% and 5.82% of the adult population [1]. Its diagnosis in early stages is difficult due to its almost asymptomatic onset and controversy of criteria regarding its initial signs.

Intraocular pressure is an important pathogenesis factor; while not the only one, it is currently the only one that can be targeted for treatment. Many other factors seem to have an influence on the disease: genetic, morphological, vasospasm, intracranial pressure, tissue thickness and morphology, sleep apnoea, etc.

For many years, visual field assessment and optic nerve head examination were the main diagnostic procedures. More recently, morphological tests have been proposed, and many authors have argued their greater precocity [2], although, as shown in this paper, this opinion is debatable. Examples are the scanning laser polarimeter (GDx), the Heidelberg retina tomograph (HRT) and the optical coherence tomograph (OCT), which is

J. Clin. Med. **2021**, *10*, 3231. https://doi.org/10.3390/jcm10153231   https://www.mdpi.com/journal/jcm

currently widely used. More recently, OCT angiographies have been introduced to analyse vascularization [3], especially in the retinal areas surrounding the optic nerve.

We developed a simple colorimetric procedure to estimate the presence of haemoglobin and its distribution on the optic disc, which reflects its perfusion and morphology, using conventional colour retinographies (Laguna ONhE) [4]. The method has been shown to have good sensitivity and specificity in previous studies [5–12]. However, deep learning methods for the segmentation of optic nerve edges were later incorporated to facilitate its use and improve its reproducibility [13].

Artificial intelligence, especially convolutional networks, allow the experience of experts to be transferred with great precision to other possible users in different medical specialties, most notably in ophthalmology [14]. Transfer Learning's new procedures simplify the development work, taking advantage of the previous training of networks on generic problems [15].

In a previous experiment [13], we used a deep learning U-Net architecture for semantic segmentation [16]. In this case, 40,000 images were used to segment the optic disc, identifying the inner edge of Elschnig's scleral ring.

The importance of perfusion in glaucoma is well recognised [3]. A recent paper using this same version of the algorithm showed that its results are in the range of an OCT angiography [17]. The aim of this paper was to take advantage of these new automatic procedures based on experience to facilitate the use of the application and to improve its reproducibility, sensitivity, and specificity. In particular, an attempt was made to combine the morphological and perfusion information provided by the method with functional perimetric data representative of visual field homogeneity [18] to assess whether this provided robustness in the diagnostic decision.

2. Materials and Methods

The study protocol of this cross-sectional retrospective study adhered to the principles of the 1975 Declaration of Helsinki revised in 2013, and was approved by the Research Ethics Committee of the Hospital Universitario de Canarias (CHUC_2018_09 (V3)). Consent was obtained from all participants.

2.1. Automation of the Laguna ONhE Method for Estimation of Haemoglobin in the Optic Nerve Head

The presence of haemoglobin in the tissue was estimated by Laguna ONhE with reference to the colour of the vessels. Haemoglobin mainly absorbs green radiation and reflects most of the red. Therefore, the reference colour of the vessels was calculated using the values of the red (R) and green (G) channels of their pixels, to which the formula $(R-G)/R$ is applied. The same equation was used for the pixels of the tissue, and finally, the result was expressed as a percentage. An estimate of cup size and position was also obtained, and the results of the cup, rim sectors, vertical cup/disc ratio (Hb-C/D) and cup/disc area ratio were compared with the percentiles achieved in the normal population [10]. Each fundus camera model was calibrated to achieve an equivalent response.

To achieve full automation of the method, five neural networks were used: one to segment the edges of the optic nerve already described [13], one for vessel segmentation using 4195 optic disc images, one to identify the eye as left or right using 4201 images, one to recognize image quality using 7048 images, and one to identify between normality (using 1518 images) and confirmed or suspected glaucoma (using 1596 images). The technical method is described in detail in the Appendix A "Computing development setup".

The classification results obtained by deep learning were associated with the distribution of haemoglobin and the estimated Cup/Disc ratios to define a new value for the "Globin Distribution Function" (GDF) index, as previously described [4,5]. Once the value of the deep learning classifier was normalized to the mean values and standard deviation in the normal population, it influenced the result of the current GDF index by 45%. In the remaining 55%, the rest of the usual variables that we used in previous studies also intervened with normalized values. An example of the graphic results is shown in Figure 1.

It shows how the method automatically performs the analysis of a retinography (a). Once its quality has been checked, the position of the optic nerve is identified, the inner edge of Elschnig's scleral ring is defined, which is more internal than the apparent clear edge, and the size and shape of the cup is estimated (b). Its veins and arteries are then segmented, the colour of which is used to estimate the relative haemoglobin of the rest of the nerve tissue, shown in a colour code (c). In each sector of the optic disc, cup or rim, their areas are estimated as a percentage of the total disk area and expressed in colour if it corresponds to what is expected in a normal optic nerve (d).

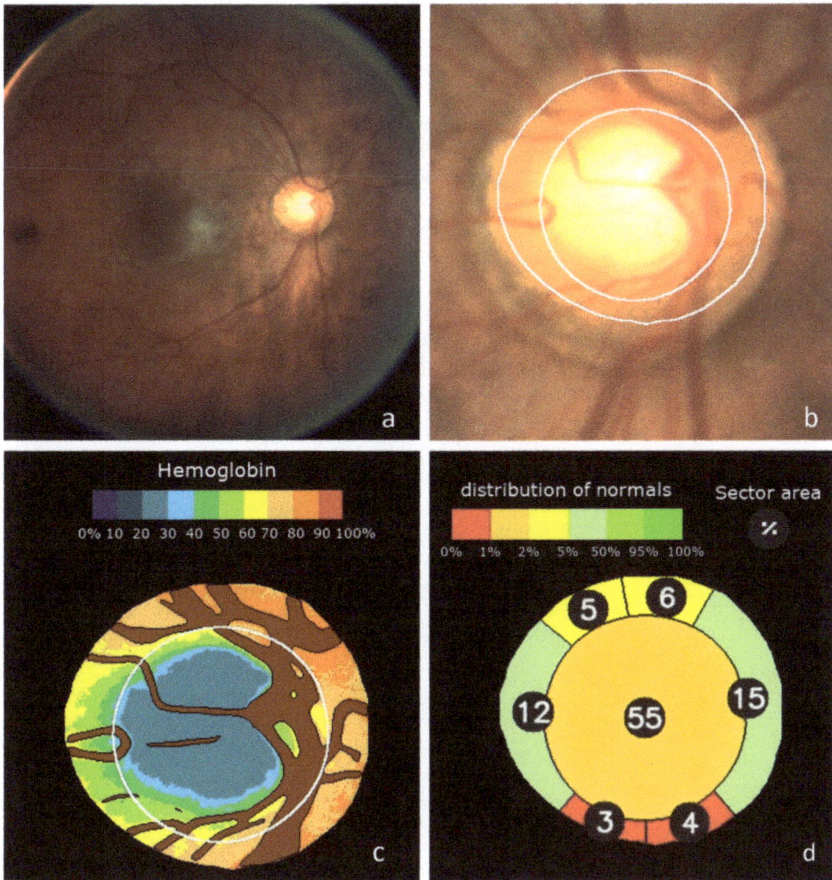

Figure 1. Example of Laguna ONhE analysis: (**a**) Original wide-field eye fundus image. (**b**) Identification of the optic disc and boundaries segmentation. Central cup estimated from the haemoglobin distribution. (**c**) Segmentation of reference vessels and pseudo-colour image of haemoglobin distribution. (**d**) Estimated sector areas as a percentage of the total area, and compared to a normal reference population.

2.2. Combination of Laguna ONhE and Perimetric Indices

The pattern standard deviation (PSD) perimetric index and its equivalent in the Octopus perimeters, the square root of loss variance (sLV), are well known. In essence, the pointwise differences between the patient's sensitivity thresholds and the expected value in a subject of the same age were calculated, and the standard deviation of all values was obtained. In general, these values increase as the disease progresses, but in advanced defects they reduce as the number of points with no detectable sensitivity (0 dB) increases. To achieve a linear response, in advanced glaucoma, a modification was made, as previously described [19], taking into account the mean defect/deviation (MD), using Equation (1).

Equation (1): sLV modification to provide a linear response.

$$\text{If abs(MD)} > 16.33, \text{ then sLV} = \text{sLV} + \frac{\text{abs(MD)} - 16.33}{0.84} \tag{1}$$

The threshold coefficient of variation (TCV) is an index of regularity described by our research group, which represents the harmony of one's own visual field, without comparing it with patterns of normality [18]. A characteristic for normality is stability or harmony, and for pathology, is irregularity or fluctuation. We aimed to analyse them in the subject themself, regardless of whether their thresholds are close or far from the normal average, in the same way that a subject can be harmonious and of short stature or harmonious and tall. This way, TCV is a less complex index than PSD, as it is independent of the age of the subject. In normal subjects and initial and moderate glaucoma, it is calculated by dividing the standard deviation of the thresholds in 16 symmetrical positions of the visual field by their mean value, and multiplying by 100. In advanced glaucoma, where absolute scotomas are present, both values are adjusted to their number.

2.3. Datasets for the Laguna ONhE, OCT and Perimetric Indices

Two groups were included, consisting of 477 healthy eyes from 409 subjects and 333 eyes with confirmed or suspected chronic open-angle glaucoma from 246 subjects. Healthy subjects consisted of hospital staff, patient relatives, or people who needed refraction but did not have eye abnormalities.

All cases had corrected visual acuity of 20/40 or higher, refractive error with spherical equivalent of less than ±5.00 dioptres, astigmatism less than ±2 dioptres, and open anterior chamber angle. Subjects with cataracts reaching the specified visual acuity were not excluded. Previous cataract or glaucoma surgery were also not exclusion criteria. Patients with associated ocular diseases which could interfere with the interpretation of the results, such as optic neuritis, coloboma, and papillary oedema, were not included. All the participants underwent a complete examination, including visual acuity, slit lamp examination, Goldmann tonometry, and fundus examination, within a maximum time interval of one week.

All cases were examined with the Cirrus spectral-domain optical coherence tomograph (OCT; Carl Zeiss Meditec, Jena, Germany), using the optic disc cube 200 × 200 acquisition protocol (software version 5.2). All images were acquired with a quality greater than 6/10.

Three fundus cameras, two perimeters, and two different perimetric strategies were used to verify that the results of the evaluated method did not depend on the instruments used. In total, 213 normal cases and 110 glaucomas were examined with a Nidek AFC-210 non-mydriatic fundus retinograph (Nidek Co., LTD, Aichi, Japan) and a white-on-white Spark strategy in an Easyfield perimeter (Oculus Optikgeräte GmbH, Wetzlar, Germany) [20]. Then, 87 normal cases and 70 glaucomas were examined with a Kowa Wx non-mydriatic fundus retinograph (Kowa Co. Ltd., Tokyo, Japan) and with the Easyfield perimeter using Spark strategy, and 177 normal and 153 glaucomas were examined with a Horus Scope DEC-200 handheld fundus camera (MiiS, Hsinchu, Taiwan) and an Octopus 300 perimeter (Hagg-Streit AG, Bern, Switzerland) using the Tendency Oriented Perimetry (TOP) strategy [21].

All control and glaucoma patients underwent perimetric assessment, having undergone at least two previous examinations. Healthy eyes had intraocular pressure less than 21 mmHg, and no abnormal results in the visual field or on the optic disc. The "glaucoma" group comprised glaucoma and glaucoma-suspected eyes. Not all patients in the "glaucoma" group had defects characteristic of the optic nerve or visual field. In some cases, there were only signs of suspicion, such as intraocular pressure greater than 21 mmHg, associated with a family history of glaucoma, an optic disc with a dubious appearance, or borderline visual fields, such as a mean deviation exceeding −2 dB or points outside normal limits on the defect curve. Subjects with ocular pressures greater than 25 mmHg, or pressures between 21 and 25 mmHg accompanied by a thin cornea (less than 500 μm), were also included.

Two types of analysis were carried out. In the first, no strict boundary was established between confirmed and suspected glaucoma, so as not to introduce an a priori criterion that could alter an objective interpretation of the results [22]. This methodology was widely discussed in a previous paper [23]. Additionally, two groups were analysed separately (confirmed glaucoma and glaucoma suspects): confirmed glaucoma was defined based on the presence of glaucomatous visual field loss in standard automated perimetry (pattern standard deviation or mean deviation of <5%) and signs of glaucomatous neuropathy (Laguna ONhE GDF or OCT-rim area of <5%). Those who did not meet these criteria, but met some of the criteria described in the previous paragraph, were considered as glaucoma suspects.

2.4. Statistical Analysis

Clinical statistical analyses were performed using the Excel 2016 program (Excel, Microsoft Corp., Redmond, WA, USA) and MedCalc (Version 18.9–64 bits; MedCalc software bvba, Mariakerke, Belgium). The statistical comparison between the results of the different AUCs were calculated in MedCalc using the criteria described by DeLonng et al. [24].

For statistical purposes, the sign of MD values of the Octopus Perimeter was inverted, to use the same criterion in both perimeters.

In order to associate different indices, they were previously normalized in relation to the mean value and standard deviation of all normal cases.

3. Results

The reference group was composed of 167 male eyes and 310 female eyes, aged 44.56 ± 13.23 years, with a perimetric MD of 0.18 ± 1.56 dB and PSD-sLV of 1.48 ± 0.52 dB. The rim area of the Cirrus-OCT was 1.42 ± 0.29 mm^2, the retinal nerve fibre layer thickness (RNFLT) was 91.67 ± 9.77 μm, and the vertical cup/disc ratio (OCT-C/D) was 0.45 ± 0.15.

The glaucoma group consisted of 176 male eyes and 157 female eyes, aged 63.63 ± 11.74 years, with a perimetric MD of -8.85 ± 8.45 dB and PSD-sLV of 4.43 ± 2.82 dB. The rim area was 0.77 ± 0.34 mm^2, the RNFLT was 68.75 ± 16.44 μm, and the OCT-C/D was 0.74 ± 0.14. Differences were statistically significant in all cases ($p < 0.0001$). Among them, 235 met the criteria for confirmed glaucoma, and 98 were considered to be suspected glaucoma. Glaucoma suspects had an MD of -0.92 ± 2.71 dB, and confirmed glaucoma had an MD of -12.16 ± 7.81 dB.

3.1. Results of the Indices of the Three Testing Methods on the Total Sample (without Separating Confirmed and Suspected Glaucoma)

The GDF index result in the groups of validation datasets is shown in Table 1. The Laguna ONhE GDF index obtained significantly higher results than all perimetric and Cirrus-OCT indices. The best OCT index was rim area and the best perimetric index TCV, with no significant differences between them.

Figure 2 shows the receiver operating characteristic (ROC) curves obtained for the Laguna ONhE GDF index, the OCT indices, and the perimetric indices. To improve the identification of differences, the upper left part of the curves is enlarged. GDF presented a sensitivity higher than the rim area for 95.0% ($p = 0.0121$) and 99.0% specificities ($p = 0.0131$), which was also higher than the rest of the perimetric indices and OCT ($p < 0.0001$).

Table 1. Performance of Laguna OnhE, OCT, and perimetry indices.

	GDF	RNFLT	Rim Area	OCT-C/D	MD	PSDr	TCV
AUC	0.970	0.875	0.926	0.921	0.897	0.883	0.904
SE	0.0054	0.0135	0.0104	0.0099	0.012	0.013	0.0115
CI	0.956–0.981	0.850–0.897	0.906–0.943	0.901–0.939	0.874–0.917	0.859–0.904	0.881–0.923

	GDF	RNFLT	Rim Area	OCT-C/D	MD	PSD-sLVr
RNFLT	$p < 0.0001$					
Rim Area	$p < 0.0001$	$p < 0.0001$				
OCT-C/D	$p < 0.0001$	$p = 0.0006$	$p = 0.5812$			
MD	$p < 0.0001$	$p = 0.1389$	$p = 0.0422$	$p = 0.0869$		
PSDr	$p < 0.0001$	$p = 0.6013$	$p = 0.0039$	$p = 0.0083$	$p = 0.0692$	
TCV	$p < 0.0001$	$p < 0.0001$	$p = 0.0824$	$p = 0.1731$	$p = 0.5053$	$p = 0.0066$

GDF = Laguna OnhE globin distribution factor; RNFLT = OCT retina nerve fiver layer thickness; OCT-C/D = OCT vertical cup/disc ratio; MD = perimetric mean defect or deviation; PSDr = perimetric pattern standard deviation or square root of loss variance rectified; TCV = perimetric threshold coefficient of variation; AUC = area under the receiver operating characteristic curve; SE = standard error; and CI = 5–95% confidence intervals.

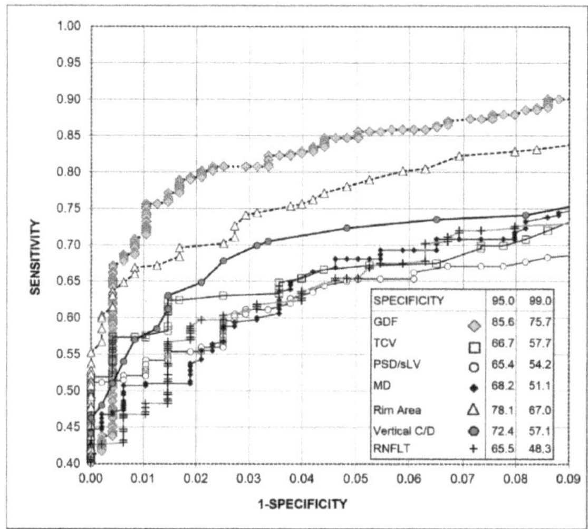

Figure 2. Receiver operating characteristic curve (ROC) obtained with Laguna ONhE (GDF), Cirrus-OCT (rim area, vertical C/D ratio, and RNFLT) and perimetry (MD, TCV, and PSD-sLV) indices, as well as percentage sensitivities for 95% and 99% specificities.

3.2. Combination of Laguna ONhE and Perimetric Indices on the Total Sample (without Separating Confirmed and Suspected Glaucoma)

Table 2 shows the results of the combinations of the two examination methods (Laguna ONhE and OCT) and the perimetric indices of uniformity and harmony. The AUCs did not show significant differences when combining GDF with each of the two perimetric indices, but these two combinations produced significantly larger curves than the combinations of perimetric and OCT indices. The RNFLT and PSDr combination performed better than the other OCT indexes combinations with the perimetric PSDr. The combinations with the perimetric MD performed worse and were thus ignored.

Table 2. Performance of the combination of Laguna ONhE and Cirrus-OCT variables and perimetric variables.

	GDF and TCV	GDF and PSDr	Rim Area and PSDr	OCT-C/D and PSDr	RNFLT and PSDr
AUC	0.978	0.976	0.945	0.947	0.915
SE	0.00459	0.00506	0.00872	0.0079	0.0109
CI	0.965–0.987	0.963–0.986	0.927–0.960	0.929–0.961	0.894–0.933

	GDF and TCV	GDF and PSDr	Rim Area and PSDr	OCT-C/D and PSDr
GDF and PSDr	$p = 0.2974$			
Rim Area and PSDr	$p = 0.0001$	$p = 0.0002$		
OCT-C/D and PSDr	$p < 0.0001$	$p < 0.0001$	$p = 0.8728$	
RNFLT and PSDr	$p < 0.0001$	$p < 0.0001$	$p = 0.0015$	$p = 0.0004$

GDF = Laguna ONhE globin distribution factor; RNFLT = OCT retina nerve fiver layer thickness; OCT-C/D = OCT vertical cup/disc ratio; MD = perimetric mean defect or deviation; PSDr = perimetric pattern standard deviation or square root of loss variance rectified; TCV = perimetric threshold coefficient of variation; AUC = area under the receiver operating characteristic curve; SE = standard error; and CI = 5–95% confidence intervals.

Figure 3 shows the ROC curves obtained for the combinations of the Laguna ONhE and OCT indices with those of perimetry. The combinations of GDF and TCV and GDF and rectified PSD-sLV did not present differences in sensitivity for 95.0% ($p = 0.790$) and 99.0% ($p = 0.674$) specificities. For 95.0% specificity, both combinations had higher sensitivities than the combinations of perimetry and OCT ($p < 0.0005$). For 99.0% specificity, the combination GDF and TCV had higher sensitivity than the rim area and rectified PSD-sLV ($p = 0.011$). GDF and rectified PSD-sLV surpassed this with $p = 0.032$. Both combinations surpassed the combinations used by the other OCT and perimetrics indices ($p < 0.0005$).

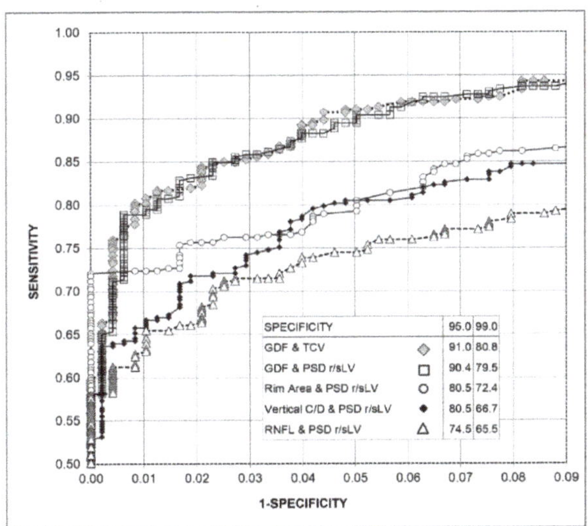

Figure 3. Graph of the receiver operating characteristic curve (ROC) of the combinations of Laguna ONhE and Cirrus-OCT indices with the perimetrics, as well as percentage sensitivities for 95% and 99% specificities.

A linear relationship was observed between perimetric MD and the GDF and TCV combination (Figure 4a), while the relationship was largely curvilinear when comparing MD with the combination of OCT morphological indices and TCV or PSDr (Figure 4b). The correlation between MD and GDF and TCV (r = 0.9132) was significantly higher than that between MD and GDF and PSDr (r = 0.8927) ($p = 0.0252$).

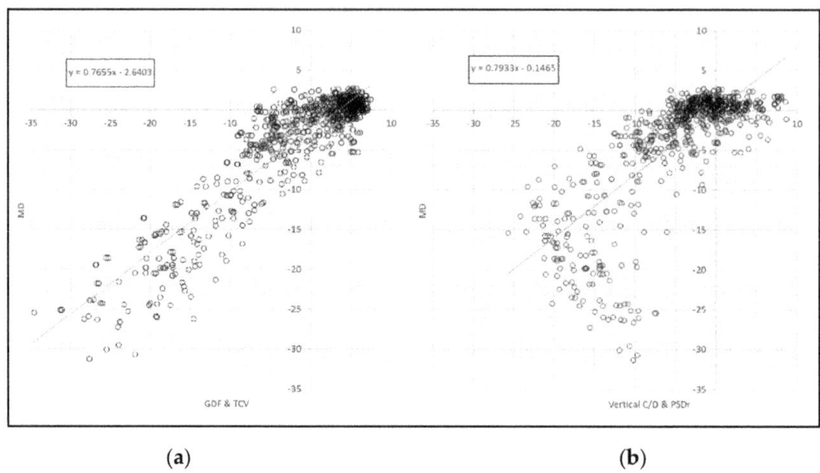

Figure 4. Relationship between the perimetric MD index and (**a**) the combined GDF and TCV and (**b**) the vertical C/D and PSDr (right) indices.

3.3. Results of the Indices of the Three Testing Methods on the Total Sample Compared to Confirmed and to Suspected Glaucoma

Table 3 shows that Laguna ONhE GDF index obtained significantly higher results than all perimetric and Cirrus-OCT indices in suspect glaucomas. It also achieves the highest ROC area in confirmed glaucoma, but without significant differences with several of the other indices.

Table 3. Performance of Laguna ONhE, OCT, and perimetry indices.

	GDF	RNFLT	Rim Area	OCT-C/D	MD	PSDr	TCV
AUC susp.	0.932	0.709	0.827	0.834	0.687	0.651	0.718
AUC conf.	0.986	0.944	0.968	0.958	0.985	0.98	0.981
SE susp.	0.013	0.0303	0.025	0.0223	0.0297	0.0311	0.029
SE conf.	0.00437	0.0107	0.00877	0.00867	0.00316	0.00432	0.00391
CI susp.	0.908–0.951	0.670–0.746	0.794–0.857	0.801–0.864	0.647–0.725	0.611–0.690	0.679–0.754
CI conf.	0.974–0.993	0.925–0.960	0.952–0.979	0.940–0.971	0.973–0.993	0.966–0.989	0.968–0.990

	GDF	RNFLT	Rim Area	OCT-C/D	MD	PSDr
RNFLT susp.	$p < 0.0001$					
RNFLT conf.	$p = 0.0002$					
RimArea susp.	$p < 0.0001$	$p = 0.0002$				
Rim Area conf.	$p = 0.0635$	$p = 0.0490$				
OCT-C/D susp.	$p < 0.0001$	$p = 0.0001$	$p = 0.7755$			
OCT-C/D conf.	$p = 0.0019$	$p = 0.2691$	$p = 0.1642$			
MD susp.	$p < 0.0001$	$p = 0.5917$	$p = 0.0004$	$p = 0.0001$		
MD conf.	$p = 0.8630$	$p = 0.0002$	$p = 0.0636$	$p = 0.0025$		
PSDr susp.	$p < 0.0001$	$p = 0.1429$	$p < 0.0001$	$p < 0.0001$	$p = 0.2399$	
PSDr conf.	$p = 0.2847$	$p = 0.0015$	$p = 0.2264$	$p = 0.0199$	$p = 0.2146$	
TCV susp.	$p < 0.0001$	$p = 0.8057$	$p = 0.0022$	$p = 0.0008$	$p = 0.2796$	$p = 0.0050$
TCV conf.	$p = 0.3720$	$p = 0.0008$	$p = 0.1663$	$p = 0.0106$	$p = 0.2885$	$p = 0.6232$

GDF = Laguna ONhE globin distribution factor; RNFLT = OCT retina nerve fiver layer thickness; OCT-C/D = OCT vertical cup/disc ratio; MD = perimetric mean defect or deviation; PSDr = perimetric pattern standard deviation or square root of loss variance rectified; TCV = perimetric threshold coefficient of variation; AUC = area under the receiver operating characteristic curve; SE = standard error; and CI = 5–95% confidence intervals.

3.4. Performance of Combined Indexes in Normal Subjects as Compared to Confirmed and to Suspected glaucoma

Table 4 shows the results of the best combinations of two non-psychophysical examination methods (Laguna ONhE and OCT), with the perimetric indices of uniformity and harmony in confirmed and suspected glaucoma. Significant differences between the two could be observed in glaucoma suspects. In suspected glaucomas, the combinations of the three OCT indices and the perimetric PSDr did not show significant differences. The combinations with the perimetric MD were worse and thus ignored.

Table 4. Performance of the combination of Laguna ONhE and Cirrus-OCT variables and perimetric variables between reference and confirmed (conf.) and suspect (susp.) glaucoma cases.

	GDF and TCV	GDF and PSDr	Rim Area and PSDr	OCT-C/D and PSDr	RNFLT and PSDr
AUC conf.	0.995	0.995	0.988	0.988	0.987
AUC susp	0.935	0.932	0.843	0.847	0.742
SE conf.	0.0021	0.0021	0.0049	0.0035	0.0033
SE susp.	0.013	0.015	0.024	0.022	0.029
CI conf.	0.987–0.999	0.987–0.999	0.977–0.995	0.977–0.995	0.976–0.994
CI susp	0.912–0.954	0.908–0.951	0.810–0.871	0.815–0.876	0.704–0.77

	GDF and TCV	GDF and PSDr	Rim Area and PSDr	OCT-C/D and PSDr
GDF and PSDr conf.	$p = 0.695$			
GDF and PSDr susp.	$p = 0.323$			
Rim Area and PSDr conf.	$p = 0.187$	$p = 0.195$		
Rim Area and PSDr susp.	$p < 0.0001$	$p = 0.0002$		
OCT-C/D and PSDr conf.	$p = 0.060$	$p = 0.064$	$p = 0.8728$	
OCT-C/D and PSDr susp.	$p < 0.0001$	$p < 0.0001$	$p = 0.839$	
RNFLT and PSDr conf.	$p = 0.036$	$p = 0.037$	$p = 0.852$	$p = 0.859$
RNFLT and PSDr susp.	$p < 0.0001$	$p < 0.0001$	$p = 0.0005$	$p = 0.0001$

GDF = Laguna ONhE globin distribution factor; RNFLT = OCT retina nerve fiver layer thickness; OCT-C/D = OCT vertical cup/disc ratio; MD = perimetric mean defect or deviation; PSDr = perimetric pattern standard deviation or square root of loss variance rectified; TCV = perimetric threshold coefficient of variation; AUC = area under the receiver operating characteristic curve; SE = standard error; and CI = 5–95% confidence intervals.

4. Discussion

Several current papers that apply deep learning to the study of glaucoma exhibit interesting theoretical approaches; however, they are not always based on real-life scenarios, but on samples collected by outside groups. Several review papers [14,25] highlight the results of others that exclude suspected glaucomas from the sample, not fully reflecting the reality of the clinical problem. They often do not clarify the type of sample analysed [26], or they base the reference classification (normal or glaucoma) exclusively on subjective expert opinions on the images [27]. Others include only cases with large cups as glaucomas [28], or do not indicate the specificity achieved [29]. Achieving a good sensitivity is not sufficient in this type of task [15] if the specificity is not high. Our analysis was performed on a real sample, without excluding doubtful or intermediate cases, and trying to avoid biases that may occur when differentiating between confirmed and suspected glaucoma [23], although both groups were analysed separately, according to the most common criteria in the literature.

Selectively analysing the optic nerve and controlling image quality has undoubted advantages over the use of wider eye fundus images [30], although it has been suggested that the sectoral atrophy of fibres could enrich the diagnosis [31].

Attempting to emulate the behaviour of an OCT to obtain its most efficient indices is an interesting approach [32]. However, the classifiers obtained through deep learning produce results that tend to involve the extremes of a dichotomous series (for example: Yes/No glaucoma or Yes/No image of adequate quality) but do not provide a gradual value of the degree of defect. For this reason, in our case, we attempted to combine these results with the estimation of other indices, such as the cup/disc ratio, which is obtained by multiple regression from sectoral haemoglobin estimates [10], and/or with the results of visual field examinations. This type of combination provides new indices with progressive gradation to better assess the level of defect and, likely, its degree of progression.

In general, published procedures require the intervention of experts for pre-processing or assessing if the images are of sufficient quality for analysis. Our procedure reached a degree of full automation in this respect, requiring no human intervention.

It is well known that the relationship between morphology and function estimated by OCT and perimetry is not linear. However, the precocity of detectable morphological damage with respect to functional damage has been questioned by several authors [33,34]. Some aspects can be complementary. Indeed, our study suggests that the association between the Laguna ONhE algorithm and perimetry seems to provide highly promising results. In particular, the linearity between the perimetric mean deviation (MD), the combination of the morphological and perfusion information presented by the Laguna ONhE GDF index, and the functional disharmony assessed by TCV provides a new perspective in the interpretation of these relationships.

It is noteworthy that this combination achieves high sensitivity while retaining high specificity. In a disease of uncertain onset, such as glaucoma, it is advisable to evaluate it with highly specific procedures, in order not to establish unnecessary treatments and to avoid overloading the health systems.

The combination of the indices provided by OCT angiography with perimetric indices should be evaluated in the future, in order to compare their results with those presented in this paper. However, an important factor to take into account in this type of comparison is the cost–benefit ratio for healthcare systems, given the low cost of some current fundus cameras, and the possibility of evaluating their images via telemedicine, without additional equipment. Such an evaluation should also be carried out in the near future.

5. Conclusions

The Laguna ONhE method arose from the observation of differences in RGB frequency histograms of optic disc structures (vessels, rim, and cup) when analysing colour photographs of the optic nerve, as can be seen in Figure 6 of our first publication [4]. The favourable results of a simple, non-invasive test, such as the one we propose for the assessment of glaucoma, were cited in the introduction, and are further evident in this new study, as they are enhanced by functional perimetric results. The application of deep learning facilitates the use of the Laguna ONhE software, taking advantage of expert experience, and improving its reproducibility, sensitivity, and specificity. Morphology, function, and perfusion can be combined for the optimal evaluation of glaucoma. However, these results should be confirmed by other independent studies.

Author Contributions: Conceptualization, M.G.-H., D.G.-H., and M.G.d.l.R.; methodology, M.G.d.l.R., D.G.-H., and M.G.-H.; software, D.G.-H. and D.P.-B.; validation, M.G.d.l.R., D.G.-H., and M.G.-H.; formal analysis, M.G.d.l.R. and M.G.-H.; investigation, M.G.d.l.R., D.G.-H., M.G.-H., P.R.-E., and N.B.-C.; resources, M.G.d.l.R., D.G.-H., and M.G.-H.; data curation, M.G.d.l.R. and D.P.-B.; writing—original draft preparation, M.G.-H. and M.G.d.l.R.; writing—review and editing, M.G.d.l.R., D.G.-H., and M.G.-H.; visualization, M.G.d.l.R.; supervision, M.G.d.l.R.; project administration, M.G.-H.; and funding acquisition, M.G.-H. and D.G.-H. All authors have read and agreed to the published version of the manuscript.

Funding: This study was supported in part by a grant (PI12/02307) from the Instituto de Salud Carlos III with FEDER funds and by Instrumentacion y Oftalmologia (INSOFT SL) company.

Institutional Review Board Statement: The study protocol of this cross-sectional retrospective study adhered to the principles of the 1975 Declaration of Helsinki revised in 2013, and was approved by the Research Ethics Committee of the Hospital Universitario de Canarias (CHUC_2018_09 (V3)).

Informed Consent Statement: Consent was obtained from all participants.

Data Availability Statement: The datasets analysed and generated during the study can be found at the following link: https://cloud.insoft.es/s/sRaFgmjQp7S4sgR.

Acknowledgments: The authors would like to thank RetinaLyze® for their support.

Conflicts of Interest: Daniel Gonzalez-Hernandez, Marta Gonzalez-Hernandez, and Manuel Gonzalez de la Rosa participate in the patent rights of the Laguna ONhE method and partners of INSOFT S.L.; Daniel Perez-Barbudo is employed by INSOFT S.L.; Paloma Rodriguez-Esteve and Nismar Betancor-Caro have no commercial interest.

Appendix A. Computing Development Setup

For the development of the Laguna ONhE program and its neural networks, the Python programming language (ver. 3.7.1, Python Software Foundation, Beaverton, OR, USA) was selected.

Machine learning and deep learning development was carried out using images provided by RetinaLyze®, partner of INSOFT SL. For each neural network, the corresponding image data sets were divided into three subsets. The training process of the neural networks requires two different images and ground-truths subsets (training and validation) to fully pass through them in several cycles in order to complete the training process. Once the network is trained on an independent test subset, which has never been seen by the algorithm, it is used to estimate the method's efficacy.

The libraries used were Keras, with Tensorflow background for the implementation of the architectures; OpenCV, for RGB component analysis, image pre-processing, and post-processing; Numpy, for calculations; Pandas, for data manipulation; and Scikit-learn for splitting the training set between training and validation sets.

A. Optic Disc segmentation: In a previous experiment [13], we used a deep learning U-Net architecture [16] for semantic segmentation. In this case, 40,000 images were used to segment the optic disc, identifying the inner edge of Elschnig's scleral ring. This was achieved by manually identifying by an expert. Elschnig's scleral ring is observed as a thin white ring, immediately adjacent to the margin of the optic disc. An example is shown in Figure 1 of reference [13].

B. Vessel segmentation: 4195 optic disc images were used to train the neural network on vessel segmentation. The vessels were drawn by hand by a single expert on each image, using the GIMP program (Version 2.10.10. http://www.gimp.org, Accessed on 21 July 2019). The data set was then divided into training (3684), validation (921), and test (410) subsets. The training set was used to train the neural network, obtaining information on each pixel belonging to a vessel or to adjacent tissue. The same basic structure of U-Net was used with contracting path filter sizes of 16, 32, 64, 128, 256, and 512 pixels towards a centre filter of 1024 pixels with batch normalization at each convolution block and ReLU activation.

Results: The Sorensen–Dice index of coincidence between the ground truth and the network was 0.932, and its corresponding Jaccard index was 0.877, in the 410 images of the test subset.

C. Eye labelling as right or left: 4201 images of the optic disc and surrounding region were divided into subsets for training (3025), validation (756), and testing (420). The results were compared with two other criteria: the greater presence of vessels in the nasal half of the optic disc and the estimation of a greater presence of haemoglobin in such area. The optic disc position on wide-angle retinographies was not considered, in order to explicitly assess the method's ability to identify it as isolated or centred.

A pre-trained ResNet50-v2 was used, with the top layers cut out. The network was trained in the ImageNet database. The network was fine-tuned with a global average pooling layer and three fully connected layers using stochastic gradient descent (SGD).

Results: 98.5% of the eyes of the test dataset were correctly automatically classified using only the optic nerve image, observing a greater presence of haemoglobin in the nasal sector; 99.3% by the greater presence of vessels in the nasal half; and 95.9% by the neural network. The coincidence of two of these three criteria identified 99.5% of the cases.

D. Image quality: Previous experience in screening systems with multiple users showed us that it is necessary to detect and exclude images of very poor quality, incomplete optic disc, etc. In total, 7048 images were subjectively classified into two groups according to their quality by a single expert (4780 acceptable and 2268 unacceptable quality), and divided into subsets of training (5075), validation (1268), and testing (705).

For this analysis, a ResNet50 network architecture was used with two fully connected layers. A LeakyRelu activation function [35] and an Adam optimizer were used for stochastic optimization [36]. The network was first trained for 50 epochs and a learning rate of 0.0001 and was fine tuned for an extra 20 epochs at a learning rate of 0.00001.

Results: In the test subset, an AUC of 0.958 was obtained, with a 5–95% confidence interval 0.940 to 0.971 ($p < 0.0001$). For a sensitivity of 95.0%, indicating that the image quality was correct, the specificity was 82.8%.

E. Normal vs. glaucoma discrimination: To train the network to distinguish normal cases from glaucoma, the haemoglobin values estimated in the tissue were represented as a pseudo-colour image, preserving the details of its surroundings. Normalization of its colour channels was applied to reduce the differences due to the fundus camera or flash used. In this way, the training was intended to include the atrophies that glaucoma usually produces outside the optic disc.

Then, 3114 such images belonging to subjects verified as normal (1518) and of glaucoma or glaucoma suspects (1596) were divided into subsets of training (2274), validation (529), and testing (311). Transfer learning was used, passing the images to a ResNet50 network [37], with the upper layers cut out, including the pre-trained weights in the ImageNet database [38]. Therefore, independently of the original image size, which was 1956×1934, all images were trimmed around the ONH segmentation and resized to 224×224 in order to fine tune the pretrained ResNet50 network. Random horizontal flip, rotation of up to 25°, and brightness darkening up to a 20% were implemented. A global average pooling layer and three specific layers were then included to classify the case as normal or glaucoma [39]. After each of the first two fully connected layers, a dropout layer with a rate value of 0.5 was included. Additionally, both use a hyperbolic tangent (tanh) activation function. The final one uses a softmax activation function. Categorical cross-entropy was used as a loss function, and accuracy was used as a metric to evaluate the performance of the model. Stochastical gradient decent (SGD) was used as an optimizer with a learning rate of 0.0001 and momentum of 0.9. The classification results obtained by deep learning were associated with the distribution of haemoglobin and the estimated cup/disc ratios to define a new value for the globin distribution function (GDF) index, as previously described [4,5].

Results: In the test subset, an AUC of 0.976 was obtained, with a 5–95% confidence interval of 0.953 to 0.990 ($p < 0.0001$).

In order to assess the model's efficiency [40], the learning curve of the training and validation loss as well as the confusion matrix of the test dataset are shown in Figure A1a,b. These graphical representations are the most commonly accepted methods to determine the model's accuracy and generalization capability [41,42].

These show the capacity of the dataset, and therefore seem to us to be more representative of the effectiveness of the network than other possibilities such as "heat maps", which show examples of how the network focuses on representative details of specific cases, but do not reflect the overall sensitivity of the method [43]. Figure A2 shows four examples of these heat maps.

As can be seen from the learning curve, we achieved an optimal fit, which is the goal of any learning algorithm achieving the minimum generalization gap [44]. Both the training and validation losses decreased to a point of stability. After 1000 epochs, the training was stopped in order to avoid overfitting. Additionally, dropout was activated when training, but deactivated when evaluating the validation data, which makes it reasonable for the validation error to be smaller than training error. The confusion matrix showed that the model had very good accuracy in the test data set. The learning curves show that both the training and validation losses drop rapidly until 100 epochs and then both continue to decrease at a slower pace until both curves meet. Even though the validation error in the graph looks as though it stops lowering from epoch 100 onwards, this is a scale problem. The validation curve does not stop; it continues to descend.

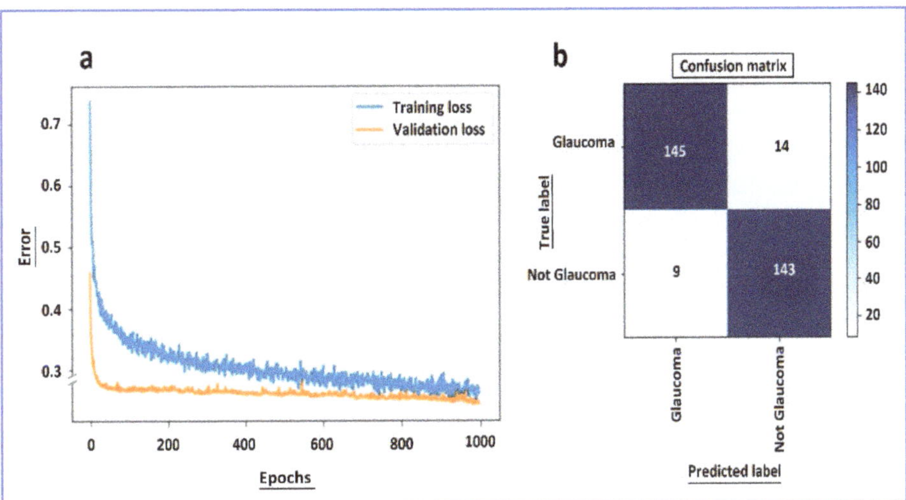

Figure A1. From the normal vs. glaucoma neural network: (**a**) learning curve of the training and validation loss and (**b**) confusion matrix of the test dataset.

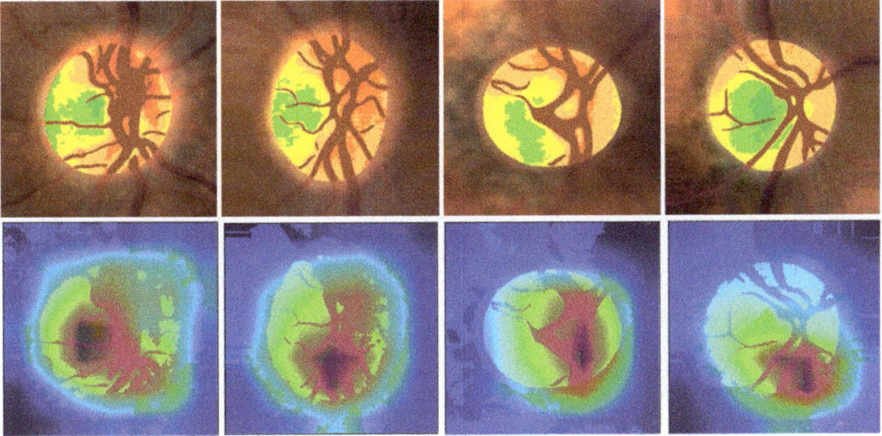

Figure A2. (**Top**): Pseudo-colour images of haemoglobin distribution in two normal optic discs (left) and two glaucomas (right) and the normalised environment, which are used for network training. The eyes are always analysed with the temporal region to the left. (**Below**): The Gradient-weighted Class Activation Maps, known as Grad-CAM saliency map, or heat maps, indicate that the networks seem to be particularly focused on the cup and the upper and lower poles.

References

1. Tham, Y.C.; Li, X.; Wong, T.Y.; Quigley, H.A.; Aung, T.; Cheng, C.Y. Global prevalence of glaucoma and projections of glaucoma burden through 2040: A systematic review and meta-analysis. *Ophthalmology* **2014**, *121*, 2081–2090. [CrossRef] [PubMed]
2. Hoyt, W.F.; Frisén, L.; Newman, N.M. Fundoscopy of nerve fiber layer defects in glaucoma. *Investig. Ophthalmol.* **1973**, *12*, 814–829.
3. Jia, Y.; Morrison, J.C.; Tokayer, J.; Tan, O.; Lombardi, L.; Baumann, B.; Lu, C.D.; Choi, W.; Fujimoto, J.G.; Huang, D. Quantitative OCT angiography of optic nerve head blood flow. *Biomed. Opt. Express* **2012**, *3*, 3127–3137. [CrossRef]
4. de la Rosa, M.G.; Gonzalez-Hernandez, M.; Sigut, J.; Alayon, S.; Radcliffe, N.; Mendez-Hernandez, C.; García-Feijoo, J.; Fuertes-Lazaro, I.; Perez-Olivan, S.; Ferreras, A. Measuring haemoglobin levels in the optic nerve head: Comparisons with other structural and functional parameters of glaucoma. *Investig. Ophthalmol. Vis. Sci.* **2013**, *54*, 482–489. [CrossRef] [PubMed]
5. Pena-Betancor, C.; Gonzalez-Hernandez, M.; Fumero-Batista, F.; Sigut, J.; Medina-Mesa, E.; Alayon, S.; de la Rosa, M.G. Estimation of the relative amount of haemoglobin in the cup and neuroretinal rim using stereoscopic color fundus images. *Investig. Ophthalmol. Vis. Sci.* **2015**, *56*, 1562–1568. [CrossRef] [PubMed]
6. Uña, I.R.; Hernandez, C.M.; Saenz-Frances, F.; Feijóo, J.G. Correlación de la relación excavación/papila óptica medida mediante HRT-III, SD-OCT y el dispositivo de colorimetría fotográfica Laguna On_hE. *Arch. Soc. Esp. Oftalmol.* **2015**, *90*, 212–219.
7. Mendez-Hernandez, C.; Rodriguez-Uña, I.; Rosa, M.G.-d.-l.; Arribas-Pardo, P.; Garcia-Feijoo, J. Glaucoma diagnostic capacity of optic nerve head haemoglobin measures compared with spectral domain OCT and HRT III confocal tomography. *Acta Ophthalmol.* **2016**, *94*, 697–704. [CrossRef]
8. Gonzalez-de-la-Rosa, M.; Gonzalez-Hernandez, M.; Mendez-Hernandez, C.; Garcia-Martin, E.; Fumero-Bautista, F.; Alayon, S.; Sigut, J. Glaucoma imaging: Measuring haemoglobin levels in the optic nerve head for glaucoma management. In *Glaucoma Imaging*; Ferreras, A., Ed.; Springer: Berlin/Heidelberg, Germany, 2016; pp. 265–280.
9. Mendez-Hernandez, C.; Garcia-Feijoo, J.; Arribas-Pardo, P.; Saenz-Frances, F.; Rodriguez-Uña, I.; Fernandez-Perez, C.; de la Rosa, M.G. Reproducibility of optic nerve head haemoglobin measures. *J. Glaucoma* **2016**, *25*, 348–354. [CrossRef]
10. Medina-Mesa, E.; Gonzalez-Hernandez, M.; Sigut, J.; Fumero-Batista, F.; Pena-Betancor, C.; Alayon, S.; de la Rosa, M.G. Estimating the amount of haemoglobin in the neuroretinal rim using color images and OCT. *Curr. Eye Res.* **2016**, *41*, 798–805. [CrossRef]
11. Perucho-González, L.; Méndez-Hernández, C.D.; González-de-la-Rosa, M.; Fernández-Pérez, C.; Sáez-Francés, F.; Andrés-Guerrero, V.; García-Feijóo, J. Preliminary study of the differences in optic nerve head haemoglobin measures between patients with and without childhood glaucoma. *J. Pediatric Ophthalmol. Strabismus* **2017**, *54*, 387–394. [CrossRef]
12. Gonzalez-Hernandez, M.; Sigut Saavedra, J.; de la Rosa, M.G. Relationship between retinal nerve fiber layer thickness and haemoglobin present in the optic nerve head in glaucoma. *J. Ophthalmol.* **2017**, *2017*, 2340236. [CrossRef]
13. Gonzalez-Hernandez, D.; Diaz-Aleman, T.; Perez-Barbudo, D.; Mendez-Hernandez, C.; de la Rosa, M.G. Segmentation of the optic nerve head based on Deep Learning to determine its haemoglobin content in normal and glaucomatous subjects. *J. Clin. Exp. Opthamol.* **2018**, *9*, 1000760. [CrossRef]
14. Kapoor, R.; Walters, S.P.; Al-Aswad, L.A. The current state of artificial intelligence in ophthalmology. *Surv. Ophthalmol.* **2019**, *64*, 233–240. [CrossRef]
15. Shibata, N.; Tanito, M.; Mitsuhashi, K.; Fujino, Y.; Matsuura, M.; Murata, H.; Asaoka, R. Development of a deep residual learning algorithm to screen for glaucoma from fundus photography. *Sci. Rep.* **2018**, *8*, 14665. [CrossRef]
16. Ronneberger, O.; Fischer, P.; Brox, T. U-net: Convolutional networks for biomedical image segmentation. In *Medical Image Computing and Computer-Assisted Intervention—MICCAI 2015, Proceedings of the International Conference on Medical Image Computing and Computer-Assisted Intervention, Munich, Germany, 5–9 October 2015*; Springer: Cham, Switzerland, 2015; pp. 234–241.
17. Mendez-Hernandez, C.; Wang, S.; Arribas-Pardo, P.; Salazar-Quiñones, L.; Güemes-Villahoz, N.; Fernandez-Perez, C.; Garcia-Feijoo, J. Diagnostic validity of optic nerve head colorimetric assessment and optical coherence tomography angiography in patients with glaucoma. *Br. J. Ophthalmol.* **2020**. [CrossRef]
18. Abreu-Gonzalez, R.; Gonzalez-Hernandez, M.; Pena-Betancor, C.; Rodriguez-Esteve, P.; De La Rosa, M.G. New visual field indices of disharmony for early diagnosis of glaucoma, alone or associated with conventional parameters. *Eur. J. Ophthalmol.* **2018**, *28*, 590–597. [CrossRef] [PubMed]
19. De La Rosa, M.G.; Gonzalez-Hernandez, M.; Diaz-Aleman, T. Linear regression analysis of the cumulative defect curve by sectors and other criteria of glaucomatous visual field progression. *Eur. J. Ophthalmol.* **2009**, *19*, 416–424. [CrossRef] [PubMed]
20. de la Rosa, M.G.; Gonzalez-Hernandez, M. A Strategy for averaged estimates of visual field threshold: Spark. *J. Glaucoma* **2013**, *22*, 284–289. [CrossRef] [PubMed]
21. de la Rosa, M.G.; Martinez, A.; Sanchez, M.; Mesa, C.; Cordovés, L.; Losada, M.J. Accuracy of the Tendency Oriented Perimetry (TOP) in the Octopus 1-2-3 Perimeter. In *Perimetry Update 1996/1997*; Wall, M., Wild, J., Eds.; Kugler Publications: Amsterdam, The Netherlands, 1997; pp. 119–123.
22. Ransohoff, D.F.; Feinstein, A.R. Problems of Spectrum and Bias in Evaluating the Efficacy of Diagnostic Tests. *N. Engl. J. Med.* **1978**, *299*, 926–930. [CrossRef] [PubMed]
23. de la Rosa, M.G.; Gonzalez-Hernandez, M. Gold standards may bias clinical test validation. *ARS Clin. Acad.* **2020**, *6*, 5–10.
24. Delong, E.R.; Delong, D.M.; Clarke-Pearson, D.L. Comparing the Areas under Two or More Correlated Receiver Operating Characteristic Curves: A Nonparametric Approach. *Biometrics* **1988**, *44*, 837–845. [CrossRef]
25. Hogarty, D.T.; Mackey, D.A.; Hewitt, A.W. Current state and future prospects of artificial intelligence in ophthalmology: A re-view. *Clin. Exp. Ophthalmol.* **2019**, *47*, 128–139. [CrossRef]

26. Raghavendra, U.; Fujita, H.; Bhandary, S.V.; Gudigar, A.; Tan, J.H.; Acharya, U.R. Deep convolution neural network for accurate diagnosis of glaucoma using digital fundus images. *Inf. Sci.* **2018**, *441*, 41–49. [CrossRef]
27. Liu, H.; Li, L.; Wormstone, I.M.; Qiao, C.; Zhang, C.; Liu, P.; Li, S.; Wang, H.; Mou, D.; Pang, R.; et al. Development and Validation of a Deep Learning System to Detect Glaucomatous Optic Neuropathy Using Fundus Photographs. *JAMA Ophthalmol.* **2019**, *137*, 1353–1360. [CrossRef]
28. Li, Z.; He, Y.; Keel, S.; Meng, W.; Chang, R.T.; He, M. Efficacy of a Deep Learning System for Detecting Glaucomatous Optic Neuropathy Based on Color Fundus Photographs. *Ophthalmology* **2018**, *125*, 1199–1206. [CrossRef]
29. Du, X.-L.; Li, W.-B.; Hu, B.-J. Application of artificial intelligence in ophthalmology. *Int. J. Ophthalmol.* **2018**, *11*, 1555–1561. [CrossRef] [PubMed]
30. Phan, S.; Satoh, S.; Yoda, Y.; Kashiwagi, K.; Oshika, T.; The Japan Ocular Imaging Registry Research Group. Evaluation of deep convolutional neural networks for glaucoma detection. *Jpn. J. Ophthalmol.* **2019**, *63*, 276–283. [CrossRef] [PubMed]
31. Christopher, M.; Belghith, A.; Bowd, C.; Proudfoot, J.A.; Goldbaum, M.H.; Weinreb, R.N.; Girkin, C.A.; Liebmann, J.M.; Zangwill, L.M. Performance of Deep Learning Architectures and Transfer Learning for Detecting Glaucomatous Optic Neuropathy in Fundus Photographs. *Sci. Rep.* **2018**, *8*, 16685. [CrossRef] [PubMed]
32. Thompson, A.C.; Jammal, A.A.; Medeiros, F.A. A Deep Learning Algorithm to Quantify Neuroretinal Rim Loss From Optic Disc Photographs. *Am. J. Ophthalmol.* **2019**, *201*, 9–18. [CrossRef] [PubMed]
33. Gonzalez-Hernandez, M.; Pablo, L.E.; Armas-Dominguez, K.; de La Vega, R.R.; Ferreras, A.; De La Rosa, M.G. Structure-function relationship depends on glaucoma severity. *Br. J. Ophthalmol.* **2009**, *93*, 1195–1199. [CrossRef]
34. Malik, R.; Swanson, W.H.; Garway-Heath, D. Structure–function relationship in glaucoma: Past thinking and current concepts. *Clin. Exp. Ophthalmol.* **2012**, *40*, 369–380. [CrossRef] [PubMed]
35. Zhang, X.; Trmal, J.; Povey, D.; Khudanpur, S. Improving deep neural network acoustic models using generalized maxout networks. In Proceedings of the 2014 IEEE International Conference on Acoustics, Speech and Signal Processing (ICASSP), Florence, Italy, 4–9 May 2014; Institute of Electrical and Electronics Engineers (IEEE): Piscataway, NJ, USA, 2014; pp. 215–219.
36. Kingma, D.P.; Ba, J. Adam: A Method for Stochastic Optimization. In Proceedings of the 3rd International Conference on Learning Representations (ICLR), San Diego, CA, USA, 7–9 May 2015; pp. 1–15.
37. He, K.; Zhang, X.; Ren, S.; Sun, J. Deep Residual Learning for Image Recognition. In Proceedings of the 2016 IEEE Conference on Computer Vision and Pattern Recognition (CVPR), Seattle, WA, USA, 1 June 2016; pp. 770–778.
38. ImageNet Project. Stanford Vision Lab, Stanford University, Princeton University. 2016. Available online: http://www.image-net.org/ (accessed on 9 November 2020).
39. Shin, H.-C.; Roth, H.R.; Gao, M.; Lu, L.; Xu, Z.; Nogues, I.; Yao, J.; Mollura, D.; Summers, R.M. Deep Convolutional Neural Networks for Computer-Aided Detection: CNN Architectures, Dataset Characteristics and Transfer Learning. *IEEE Trans. Med. Imaging* **2016**, *35*, 1285–1298. [CrossRef] [PubMed]
40. Goodfellow, I.; Bengio, Y.; Courville, A. *Deep Learning*; The MIT Press: Cambridge, MA, USA, 2016; pp. 96–161.
41. Anzanello, M.J.; Fogliatto, F.S. Learning curve models and applications: Literature review and research directions. *Int. J. Ind. Ergon.* **2011**, *41*, 573–583. [CrossRef]
42. James, G.; Witten, D.; Hastie, T.; Tibshirani, R. *An Introduction to Statistical Learning: With Applications in R*; Springer-Verlag: New York, NY, USA, 2013; pp. 29–42.
43. Adebayo, J.; Muelly, M.; Liccardi, I.; Kim, B. Debugging Tests for Model Explanations. *arXiv* **2020**, arXiv:2011.05429.
44. Hoffer, E.; Hubara, I.; Soudry, D. Train longer, generalize better: Closing the generalization gap in large batch training of neural networks. In Proceedings of the 31st International Conference on Neural Information Processing Systems, Long Beach, CA, USA, 4 December 2017; pp. 1729–1739.

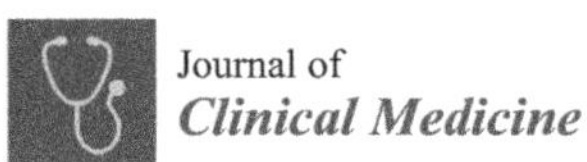

Journal of
Clinical Medicine

Article

Corneal Biomechanical Parameters and Central Corneal Thickness in Glaucoma Patients, Glaucoma Suspects, and a Healthy Population

Mª. Ángeles del Buey-Sayas [1,2,3], Elena Lanchares-Sancho [3,4], Pilar Campins-Falcó [5], María Dolores Pinazo-Durán [6,7] and Cristina Peris-Martínez [7,8,9,*]

[1] Department of Ophthalmology, Hospital Clínico Universitario "Lozano Blesa", Avda. San Juan Bosco 15, 50009 Zaragoza, Spain; madelbuey@gmail.com
[2] Aragón Health Research Institute (IIS Aragon), Avda. San Juan Bosco 13, 50009 Zaragoza, Spain
[3] Aragon Institute of Engineering Research (13A), University of Zaragoza, Mariano Esquillor s/n, 50018 Zaragoza, Spain; elanchar@unizar.es
[4] Centro de Investigación Biomédica en Red en Bioingeniería, Biomateriales y Nanomedicina (CIBER-BBN), 28029 Madrid, Spain
[5] Department of Analytical Chemistry, Faculty of Chemistry, University of Valencia, 46100 Valencia, Spain; pilar.campins@uv.es
[6] Ophthalmic Research Unit "Santiago Grisolía", Foundation for the Promotion of Health and Biomedical Research of Valencia FISABIO, 46017 Valencia, Spain; pinazoduran@yahoo.es
[7] Ophthalmology Department, University of Valencia, 46019 Valencia, Spain
[8] FISABIO Oftalmología Médica (FOM), Foundation for the Promotion of Health and Biomedical Research of Valencia (FISABIO), 46015 Valencia, Spain
[9] Aviñó Peris Eye Clinic, 46001 Valencia, Spain
* Correspondence: Cristina.P.Peris@uv.es

Citation: del Buey-Sayas, Mª.Á.; Lanchares-Sancho, E.; Campins-Falcó, P.; Pinazo-Durán, M.D.; Peris-Martínez, C. Corneal Biomechanical Parameters and Central Corneal Thickness in Glaucoma Patients, Glaucoma Suspects, and a Healthy Population. *J. Clin. Med.* **2021**, *10*, 2637. https://doi.org/10.3390/jcm10122637

Academic Editor: Brent Siesky

Received: 27 April 2021
Accepted: 10 June 2021
Published: 15 June 2021

Publisher's Note: MDPI stays neutral with regard to jurisdictional claims in published maps and institutional affiliations.

Abstract: Purpose: To evaluate and compare corneal hysteresis (CH), corneal resistance factor (CRF), and central corneal thickness (CCT), measurements were taken between a healthy population (controls), patients diagnosed with glaucoma (DG), and glaucoma suspect patients due to ocular hypertension (OHT), family history of glaucoma (FHG), or glaucoma-like optic discs (GLD). Additionally, Goldmann-correlated intraocular pressure (IOPg) and corneal-compensated IOP (IOPcc) were compared between the different groups of patients. Methods: In this prospective analytical-observational study, a total of 1065 patients (one eye of each) were recruited to undergo Ocular Response Analyzer (ORA) testing, ultrasound pachymetry, and clinical examination. Corneal biomechanical parameters (CH, CRF), CCT, IOPg, and IOPcc were measured in the control group ($n = 574$) and the other groups: DG ($n = 147$), FHG ($n = 78$), GLD ($n = 90$), and OHT ($n = 176$). We performed a variance analysis (ANOVA) for all the dependent variables according to the different diagnostic categories with multiple comparisons to identify the differences between the diagnostic categories, deeming $p < 0.05$ as statistically significant. Results: The mean CH in the DG group (9.69 mmHg) was significantly lower compared to controls (10.75 mmHg; mean difference 1.05, $p < 0.001$), FHG (10.70 mmHg; mean difference 1.00, $p < 0.05$), GLD (10.63 mmHg; mean difference 0.93, $p < 0.05$) and OHT (10.54 mmHg; mean difference 0.84, $p < 0.05$). No glaucoma suspects (FHG, GLD, OHT groups) presented significant differences between themselves and the control group ($p = 1.00$). No statistically significant differences were found in the mean CRF between DG (11.18 mmHg) and the control group (10.75 mmHg; mean difference 0.42, $p = 0.40$). The FHG and OHT groups showed significantly higher mean CRF values (12.32 and 12.41 mmHg, respectively) than the DG group (11.18 mmHg), with mean differences of 1.13 ($p < 0.05$) and 1.22 ($p < 0.001$), respectively. No statistically significant differences were found in CCT in the analysis between DG (562 μ) and the other groups (control = 556 μ, FHG = 576 μ, GLD = 569 μ, OHT = 570 μ). The means of IOPg and IOPcc values were higher in the DG patient and suspect groups than in the control group, with statistically significant differences in all groups ($p < 0.001$). Conclusion: This study presents corneal biomechanical values (CH, CRF), CCT, IOPg, and IOPcc for diagnosed glaucoma patients, three suspected glaucoma groups, and a healthy population, using the ORA. Mean CH values were markedly lower in the DG group (diagnosed with glaucoma damage) compared to the other groups. No significant difference was found in CCT

---

between the DG and control groups. Unexpectedly, CRF showed higher values in all groups than in the control group, but the difference was only statistically significant in the suspect groups (FHG, GLD, and OHT), not in the DG group.

Keywords: glaucoma; corneal hysteresis; ocular inflammation; corneal biomechanics; ocular biomarkers

1. Introduction

Corneal biomechanics studies the balance and deformation of the corneal tissue subjected to any external action. This scientific discipline explores the function and the inner structure of the cornea and endeavors to establish some physical-mathematical bases that define it [1]. The possible practical applications range from the diagnosis and assessment of certain pathologies [2–5] to the prediction of response to corneal surgical procedures [6–9].

The Ocular Response Analyzer, ORA (Reichert), was the first device to measure the biomechanical properties of the cornea in vivo. It can determine some parameters of the structure and viscoelastic properties of the cornea, and also intraocular pressure (IOP) [10]. Corneal biomechanical parameters measured by ORA are corneal hysteresis (CH) and corneal resistance factor (CRF), as well as noncontact intraocular pressures, such as the Goldmann-correlated intraocular pressure (IOPg) and corneal-compensated intraocular pressure (IOPcc). Several studies have tried to set biomechanical parameters to help improve prediction of corneal ectasia, refractive surgery pre- and post-operative evaluation, corneal pathologies, and glaucoma. It has been shown that CH is lower after refractive surgery in corneal ectasia, such as in keratoconus, Fuchs' dystrophy, and glaucoma patients [11–15]. Glaucoma is a chronic and progressive optic neuropathy characterized by loss of the retinal nerve fiber layer, progressive optic disc damage, and the development of characteristically evolving visual field defects. It is associated, although not in all cases, with an increase in IOP. The prevalence of glaucoma is 1.5%–2% in individuals over 40 years of age and even higher in those over 60 years of age. Glaucoma is an especially relevant ocular pathology, since it is the second cause of irreversible blindness after diabetic retinopathy. The most common type, accounting for 60% of glaucoma cases, is primary open-angle glaucoma (POAG). It is usually bilateral, although frequently asymmetric, and the chamber angle is open and is not related to another ocular disorder. The exact etiology of POAG is unknown, but there are some risk factors, including IOP, family history, increasing age, race, myopia, and cardiovascular status [15,16]. It is currently known that, although an increase in IOP is the most important risk factor for suffering from glaucoma and the only one on which we can act at the moment, it is not the only determining factor. Some facts support these claims, suggesting that other risk factors should be considered: There are patients who present an IOP of over 21 mmHg (even 30 mmHg) but do not present alterations in the optic nerve or in the visual field. They are called ocular hypertensive or glaucoma suspects, and although some develop glaucoma (40% in 10 years), others remain unaffected despite elevated intraocular pressure values. Another group of patients present visual field examination and optic nerve head alterations typical of glaucoma, with normal IOP values or even lower than usual, a circumstance that we call low-tension glaucoma or normal-tension glaucoma [17]. It has been reported that 45% of treated glaucoma patients had glaucomatous progression in visual fields despite an average 25% decrease in IOP [18]. Even so, IOP is the only factor on which we can act to stop the progress of the disease and to which all anti-glaucoma treatments have been directed so far.

In the last decade, the biomechanical properties of the cornea have received increasing attention, particularly corneal hysteresis (CH). Corneal biomechanics provides insight into the behavior of the cornea and could reflect the vulnerability of the optic nerve structures to glaucoma. Thus, CH could become a potential glaucoma biomarker, which could serve as a risk indicator of progression. Besides CH, a new compensated IOP (IOPcc) would show a more real IOP value. The analysis, study, and assessment of corneal biomechanical properties, IOPcc, and corneal thickness obtained with the ORA in normal eyes, in eyes with glaucoma, and in eyes with suspected glaucoma, provide new data that can help identify patients with a higher risk of glaucoma progression.

The purpose of this study was to evaluate and compare CH and central corneal thickness (CCT) measurements between a healthy population (controls), patients diagnosed with glaucoma (DG) in treatment for IOP control, and glaucoma suspect patients due to ocular hypertension (OHT) or other risk factors, such as family history of glaucoma (FHG) or glaucoma-like optic discs (GLD) [19]. Additionally, the corneal resistance factor (CRF), Goldmann-correlated intraocular pressure (IOPg), corneal-compensated IOP (IOPcc), and CCT are evaluated and compared between the different groups of patients. Furthermore, the study of a large control group defines the mean values of corneal biomechanical properties and IOP in the healthy Spanish population.

2. Methods

This is a prospective analytical-observational study that was performed at the Anterior Segment section of the Department of Ophthalmology, Hospital Clínico Universitario Lozano Blesa, Saragossa (Spain). The study was approved by the Institutional Review Board of the University of Saragossa Faculty of Medicine and was conducted in accordance with the Declaration of Helsinki for research involving human subjects. The studywas approved by the Ethics Committee for Clinical Research of Aragon (CEICA 18/2017) and the date of approval was 25 October 2017. Written informed consent was signed by all participants.

2.1. Subjects

Subjects included in this study were healthy persons without a diagnosed ocular pathology (controls), patients diagnosed with glaucoma (DG), and glaucoma suspect patients who were undergoing a study for early diagnosis due to ocular hypertension (OHT), family history of glaucoma (FHG), or glaucoma-like optic discs (GLD).

Subjects excluded from this study were patients with serious general diseases, such as recent surgery, malignant neoplastic pathology, collagen diseases, immunological diseases, metabolic stress due to moderate-severe renal failure, decompensated diabetes mellitus, altered nutritional status, or any general situation of the patient that could compromise the results of the evidence. Further exclusion criteria were patients with other ocular pathologies, such as severe dry eye syndrome, corneal chemical burn, infectious and inflammatory diseases of the cornea, conjunctiva, uvea and sclera; corneal ectasia or dystrophies; acute pathologies and postsurgical states, such as retinal detachment, acute glaucoma, proliferative diabetic retinopathy, iris rubeosis, need for valve implants due to glaucoma, patients undergoing any corneal surgery, or patients who presented signs of corneal pathology.

2.2. Examination Techniques

All participants underwent exhaustive ophthalmologic examination, including a review of medical history, slit-lamp biomicroscopy, best-corrected visual acuity, IOP measurement using Goldmann applanation tonometry (GAT), and retinal ophthalmoscopy examination. The clinical examinations necessary for the diagnosis and evolutionary assessment of the patients were carried out following an action protocol specific to the ocular pathology group to which they belonged. The entire battery of diagnostic devices typical of a hospital ophthalmology department were available to us to perform this study. These included a refractometer, indirect ophthalmoscope, optical coherence tomography (OCT), ORBSCAN ocular topography, endothelial analysis with a non-contact specular microscope, and standard automated perimetry (SAP).

In the group of healthy patients, topographic exploration with ORBSCAN was also performed on those patients with refractive defects (to rule out evident keratoconus or subclinical keratoconus), as was specular microscopy on patients with doubtful biomicroscopy or high corneal thickness suspected of edema. If any corneal pathology was evidenced, the patient was excluded from the study.

In the DG group, functional diagnostic tests with standard automated perimetry (SAP), the Swedish Interactive Threshold Algorithm (SITA), 24–2 testing of the HVS Analyzer II, model 750i (Carl Zeiss Meditec, Inc., Dublin, CA, USA), and structural tests (fiber and papilla OCT) were performed to assess glaucomatous damage.

Examination was completed with gonioscopy, stereoscopic optic disc photography, functional tests with SAP, and structural tests (OCT of fibers and papilla) in the glaucoma suspect groups (OHT, FHG, or GLD). If there was evidence of unknown glaucomatous damage, treatment was prescribed, and the patient was excluded from the study. Ocular hypertension was defined as IOP equal to or higher than 21 mmHg with a normal visual field and optic nerve. Family history of glaucoma was determined as at least one of the parents with diagnosed glaucoma. Glaucoma-like optic discs were defined as having a vertical cup-to-disc ratio greater than 0.5 or asymmetry of cupping between the two eyes in patients with normal IOP and visual fields and open angles.

All patients were explored with Reichert's Ocular Response Analyzer (ORA), both to determine their biomechanical properties (CH, CRF) and to determine their Goldman equivalent IOP (IOPg) and compensated IOP (IOPcc). The central corneal thickness (CCT) was determined from the pachymetry performed with the ultrasonic pachymeter incorporated in the ORA. All ocular examinations, including ORA, were performed on the same day. Four consecutive ORA measurements were determined in both eyes. Then the results were averaged. One eye of each patient was chosen at random.

2.3. Statistical Analysis

A total of 1065 patients (one eye of each) were recruited in this prospective analytical-observational study. Normal subjects comprised the control group ($n = 574$), who were studied alongside the DG ($n = 147$), FHG ($n = 78$), GLD ($n = 90$), and OHT ($n = 176$) diagnosis groups. Microsoft Excel was used to collate data including patient age and gender, diagnosis group, CH, CRF, IOPg, IOPcc, and CCT. The IBM SPSS (version 17) statistical package was used for data analysis. An analysis of variance (ANOVA) was carried out for all the dependent variables according to the different diagnostic categories, with multiple comparisons to distinguish between the diagnostic categories in which there were differences, taking $p < 0.05$ as statistically significant.

3. Results

3.1. Subjects

The study included one eye of each of the 1065 patients. Table 1 summarizes the basic demographic information for the patients included in the five different diagnosis groups. A higher percentage of females was present in the FHG (71.8%) and GLD groups (78.9%) compared to the control (50.7%), OHT (54%), and DG (44.2%) groups. The control group patients were younger, on average, than the patients included in the other four groups. After carrying out a comparative study of the control group with the pathological groups, we found the following results for each variable using the ORA (CH, CRF, IOPg, IOPcc, and CCT), which are summarized in Table 2 and Figures 1 and 2.

Table 1. Demographics of the control and the four diagnosis groups included in the study (DG, FHG, GLD, and OHT). Gender is summarized by frequency and percentage; age by mean ± SD.

	Control (*n* = 574)	DG (*n* = 147)	FHG (*n* = 78)	GLD (*n* = 90)	OHT (*n* = 176)	Total (*n* = 1065)
Female	291 (50.7%)	65 (44.2%)	56 (71.8%)	71 (78.9%)	95 (54%)	578 (54.3%)
Male	283 (49.3%)	82 (55.8%)	22 (28.2%)	19 (21.1%)	81 (46%)	487 (45.7%)
Age (years)	39 ± 15	56 ± 16	47 ± 15	48 ± 14	51 ± 13	46 ± 17

DG—diagnosed glaucoma; FHG—family history of glaucoma; GLD—glaucoma-like optic discs; OHT—ocular hypertension; SD—standard deviation.

Table 2. Descriptive statistics of the control and the four diagnosis groups included in the study (DG, FHG, GLD, and OHT). Variables summarized by mean ± SD.

	Control (*n* = 574)	DG (*n* = 147)	FHG (*n* = 78)	GLD (*n* = 90)	OHT (*n* = 176)
IOPg (mmHg)	15.63 ± 3.1	20.07 ± 3.6	21.01 ± 4.0	18.48 ± 3.6	21.76 ± 3.6
IOPcc (mmHg)	15.72 ± 3.0	20.68 ± 3.7	20.41 ± 3.8	18.30 ± 3.9	21.22 ± 3.8
CH (mmHg)	10.75 ± 1.5	9.69 ± 1.9	10.70 ± 1.7	10.63 ± 1.9	10.54 ± 1.8
CRF (mmHg)	10.75 ± 1.6	11.18 ± 2.0	12.32 ± 1.9	11.50 ± 1.9	12.41 ± 1.8
CCT (μ)	556.8 ± 35.3	562.6 ± 39.6	576.3 ± 38.3	569.5 ± 31.5	570.3 ± 34.7

DG—diagnosed glaucoma; FHG—family history of glaucoma; GLD—glaucoma-like optic discs; OHT—ocular hypertension; SD—standard deviation. IOPg: Goldmann-correlated intraocular pressure, IOPcc: corneal-compensated IOP, CH: Corneal Hysteresis, CRF: Corneal Resistance Factor, CCT: Central Corneal Thickness.

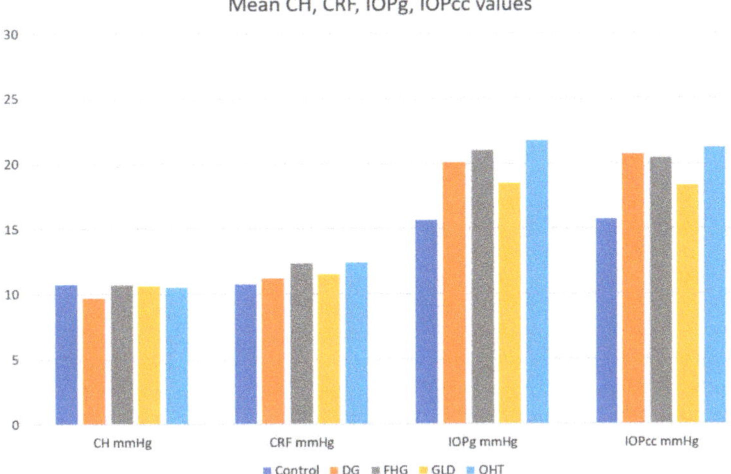

Figure 1. Plot of meanCorneal Hysteresis (CH), Corneal Resistance Factor (CRF), Goldmann-correlated intraocular pressure (IOPg) and corneal-compensated IOP (IOPcc) values in all groups. DG—diagnosed glaucoma; FHG—family history of glaucoma; GLD—glaucoma-like optic discs; OHT—ocular hypertension.

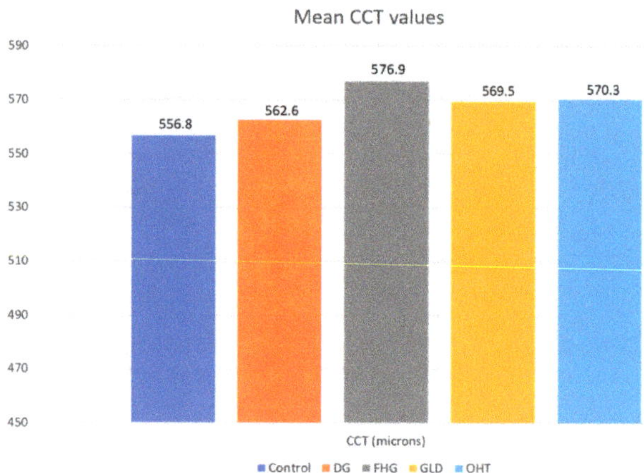

Figure 2. Plot of mean Central Corneal Thickness (CCT) values in all groups. DG—diagnosed glaucoma; FHG—family history of glaucoma; GLD—glaucoma-like optic discs; OHT—ocular hypertension.

3.1.1. CH

The mean CH in DG patients (9.69 ± 1.9 mmHg) was lower than in the control group (10.75 ± 1.5 mmHg). Additionally, the mean CH in DG patients was lower than in all glaucoma suspect groups: FHG, GLD, and OHT (10.70 ± 1.7, 10.63 ± 1.9, and 10.54 ± 1.8 mmHg, respectively). The scatter graphs for the CH variable according to the groups studied show a minimal dispersion in the control group and a greater dispersion in the DG group and in the glaucoma suspect groups (FHG, GLG, and OHT). Figure 3 shows the comparison of the mean values (left) and the scatter graphs (right) of the CH variable in all groups. An inferential statistical study was carried out to verify the significance of these differences, using the ANOVA multiple comparisons test (Table 3), which shows the existence of statistically significant differences ($p < 0.05$) for the CH variable comparing the DG group with the rest of the groups. No significant differences were found between the control group and the glaucoma suspect groups ($p = 1.00$). The FHG, GLD, and OHT groups showed no significant differences between themselves ($p = 1.00$).

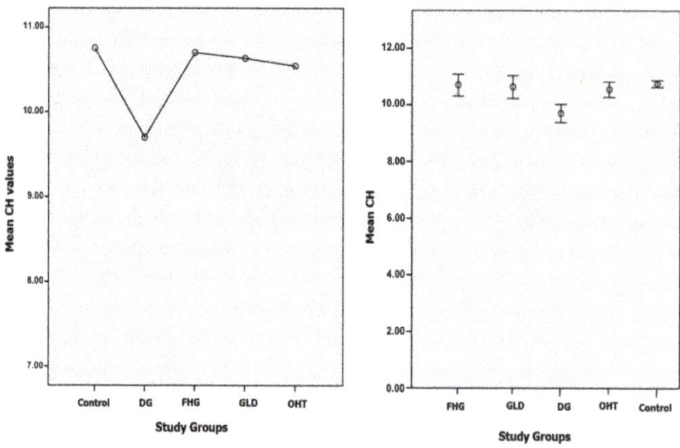

Figure 3. Comparison of mean values (**left**) and the scatter graphs (**right**) of the CH variable in all groups. DG—diagnosed glaucoma; FHG—family history of glaucoma; GLD—glaucoma-like optic discs; OHT—ocular hypertension.

Table 3. Statistical results using ANOVA multiple comparisons test for the CH variable.

Dependent Variable	(I) Pathology	(J) Pathology	Mean Difference (I–J)	SE	*p* Value	95% CI	
						Upper Limit	Lower Limit
CH	Control	DG	1.053 (*)	0.174	0.000 *	0.502	1.604
		FHG	0.052	0.207	1.000	−0.611	0.717
		GLD	0.119	0.216	1.000	−0.572	0.811
		OHT	0.210	0.153	0.995	−0.272	0.693
	DG	Control	−1.053 (*)	0.174	0.000 *	−1.604	−0.502
		FHG	−1.000 (*)	0.254	0.003 *	−1.807	−0.194
		GLD	−0.934 (*)	0.262	0.013 *	−1.763	−0.104
		OHT	−0.842 (*)	0.213	0.003 *	−1.513	−0.172
	FHG	Control	−0.052	0.207	1.000	−0.717	0.611
		DG	1.000 (*)	0.254	0.003 *	0.194	1.807
		GLD	0.066	0.285	1.000	−0.836	0.970
		OHT	0.157	0.240	1.000	−0.605	0.921
	GLD	Control	−0.119	0.216	1.000	−0.811	0.572
		DG	0.934 (*)	0.262	0.013 *	0.104	1.763
		FHG	−0.066	0.285	1.000	−0.970	0.836
		OHT	0.091	0.248	1.000	−0.696	0.879
	OHT	Control	−0.210	0.153	0.995	−0.693	0.272
		DG	0.842 (*)	0.213	0.003 *	0.172	1.513
		FHG	−0.157	0.240	1.000	−0.921	0.605
		GLD	−0.091	0.248	1.000	−0.879	0.696

SE—standard error, * Statistical significance ($p < 0.05$), CI—confidence interval, DG—diagnosed glaucoma; FHG—family history of glaucoma; GLD—glaucoma-like optic discs; OHT—ocular hypertension.

3.1.2. CRF

The glaucoma suspect groups (FHG, GLD, and OHT) showed higher CRF values (12.32 ± 1.9, 11.50 ± 1.9, and 12.41 ± 1.8 mmHg, respectively) than the control group (10.75 ± 1.6 mmHg) with statistically significant differences ($p < 0.001$, $p < 0.05$, and $p < 0.001$, respectively). No statistically significant differences were found between the DG group and the control group. In the comparative study of the DG group versus the glaucoma suspect groups (FHG, GLD, and OHT), the FHG and OHT groups presented higher CRF values and the differences were significant ($p < 0.05$ and $p < 0.001$, respectively) (Table 4).

3.1.3. IOPg

The DG group and the glaucoma suspect groups (FHG, GLD, and OHT) presented higher IOPg values (20.07 ± 3.6, 21.01 ± 4.0, 18.48 ± 3.6, and 21.76 ± 3.6 mmHg, respectively) than the control group (15.63 ± 3.1 mmHg) with statistically significant differences ($p < 0.001$). The DG group had significantly lower IOPg than the OHT group ($p < 0.05$) and significantly higher IOPg than the GLD group ($p < 0.05$). The GLD group presented significantly lower IOPg values than the DG ($p < 0.05$), FHG ($p < 0.001$), and OHT ($p < 0.001$) groups (Table 5).

3.1.4. IOPcc

The DG group and the glaucoma suspect groups (FHG, GLD, and OHT) presented higher IOPcc values (20.68 ± 3.7, 20.41 ± 3.8, 18.30 ± 3.9, and 21.22 ± 3.8 mmHg, respectively) than the control group (15.72 ± 3.0) with statistically significant differences ($p < 0.001$). When comparing the DG group with the glaucoma suspect groups, the IOPcc values were found to be significantly lower in the GLD group ($p < 0.001$). The OHT group presented no differences when compared with the DG group, since the IOPcc values were lower than those of IOPg in this group (Table 6).

Table 4. Statistical results using ANOVA multiple comparisons test for the CRF variable.

Dependent Variable	(I) Pathology	(J) Pathology	Mean Difference (I–J)	SE	*p*-Value	95% CI	
						Upper Limit	Lower Limit
CRF	Control	DG	−0.429	0.180	0.403	−0.998	0.140
		FHG	−1.562 (*)	0.235	0.000 *	−2.317	−0.808
		GLD	−0.745 (*)	0.214	0.020 *	−1.430	−0.060
		OHT	−1.653 (*)	0.155	0.000 *	−2.144	−1.163
	DG	Control	0.429	0.180	0.403	−0.140	0.998
		FHG	−1.133 (*)	0.279	0.002 *	−2.018	−0.249
		GLD	−0.316	0.262	0.999	−1.145	0.511
		OHT	−1.224 (*)	0.216	0.000 *	−1.906	−0.543
	FHG	Control	1.562 (*)	0.235	0.000 *	0.808	2.317
		DG	1.133 (*)	0.279	0.002 *	0.249	2.018
		GLD	0.816	0.302	0.193	−0.141	1.775
		OHT	−0.091	0.263	1.000	−0.929	0.747
	GLD	Control	0.745 (*)	0.214	0.020 *	0.060	1.430
		DG	0.316	0.262	0.999	−0.511	1.145
		FHG	−0.816	0.302	0.193	−1.775	0.141
		OHT	−0.908 (*)	0.245	0.008 *	−1.686	−0.129
	OHT	Control	1.653 (*)	0.155	0.000 *	1.163	2.144
		DG	1.224 (*)	0.216	0.000 *	0.543	1.906
		FHG	0.091	0.263	1.000	−0.747	0.929
		GLD	0.908 (*)	0.245	0.008 *	0.129	1.686

SE—standard error, * Statistical significance ($p < 0.05$), CI—confidence interval, DG—diagnosed glaucoma; FHG—family history of glaucoma; GLD—glaucoma-like optic discs; OHT—ocular hypertension.

Table 5. Statistical results using ANOVA multiple comparisons test for the IOPg variable.

Dependent Variable	(I) Pathology	(J) Pathology	Mean Difference (I–J)	SE	*p*-Value	95% CI	
						Upper Limit	Lower Limit
IOPg	Control	DG	−4.435 (*)	0.328	0.000 *	−5.472	−3.397
		FHG	−5.378 (*)	0.474	0.000 *	−6.902	−3.854
		GLD	−2.844 (*)	0.408	0.000 *	−4.149	−1.539
		OHT	−6.130 (*)	0.302	0.000 *	−7.083	−5.177
	DG	Control	4.435 (*)	0.328	0.000 *	3.397	5.472
		FHG	−0.943	0.546	0.921	−2.680	0.792
		GLD	1.590 (*)	0.490	0.039 *	0.038	3.142
		OHT	−1.695 (*)	0.406	0.001 *	−2.974	−0.415
	FHG	Control	5.378 (*)	0.474	0.000 *	3.854	6.902
		DG	0.943	0.546	0.921	−0.792	2.680
		GLD	2.534 (*)	0.598	0.001 *	0.636	4.432
		OHT	−0.751	0.531	0.992	−2.442	0.939
	GLD	Control	2.844 (*)	0.408	0.000 *	1.539	4.149
		DG	−1.590 (*)	0.490	0.039 *	−3.142	−0.038
		FHG	−2.534 (*)	0.598	0.001 *	−4.432	−0.636
		OHT	−3.285 (*)	0.474	0.000 *	−4.785	−1.785
	OHT	Control	6.130 (*)	0.302	0.000 *	5.177	7.083
		DG	1.695 (*)	0.406	0.001 *	0.415	2.974
		FHG	0.751	0.531	0.992	−0.939	2.442
		GLD	3.285 (*)	0.474	0.000 *	1.785	4.785

SE—standard error. * Statistical significance ($p < 0.05$). CI—confidence interval; DG—diagnosed glaucoma; FHG—family history of glaucoma; GLD—glaucoma-like optic discs; OHT—ocular hypertension.

Table 6. Statistical results using ANOVA multiple comparisons test for the IOPcc variable.

Dependent Variable	(I) Pathology	(J) Pathology	Mean Difference (I–J)	SE	*p*-Value	95% CI Upper Limit	95% CI Lower Limit
IOPcc	Control	DG	−4.954 (*)	0.335	0.000 *	−6.014	−3.895
		FHG	−4.686 (*)	0.450	0.000 *	−6.131	−3.241
		GLD	−2.577 (*)	0.434	0.000 *	−3.966	−1.187
		OHT	−5.503 (*)	0.314	0.000 *	−6.494	−4.513
	DG	Control	4.954 (*)	0.335	0.000 *	3.895	6.014
		FHG	0.268	0.531	1.000	−1.416	1.953
		GLD	2.377 (*)	0.518	0.000 *	0.737	4.017
		OHT	−0.548	0.422	0.998	−1.877	0.779
	FHG	Control	4.686 (*)	0.450	0.000 *	3.241	6.131
		DG	−0.268	0.531	1.000	−1.953	1.416
		GLD	2.109 (*)	0.599	0.015 *	0.211	4.007
		OHT	−0.817	0.518	0.969	−2.462	0.828
	GLD	Control	2.577 (*)	0.434	0.000 *	1.187	3.966
		DG	−2.377 (*)	0.518	0.000 *	−4.017	−0.737
		FHG	−2.109 (*)	0.599	0.015 *	−4.007	−0.211
		OHT	−2.926 (*)	0.505	0.000 *	−4.525	−1.327
	OHT	Control	5.503 (*)	0.314	0.000 *	4.513	6.494
		DG	0.548	0.422	0.998	−0.779	1.877
		FHG	0.817	0.518	0.969	−0.828	2.462
		GLD	2.926 (*)	0.505	0.000 *	1.327	4.525

SE—standard error. * Statistical significance ($p < 0.05$). CI—confidence interval. DG—diagnosed glaucoma; FHG—family history of glaucoma; GLD—glaucoma-like optic discs; OHT—ocular hypertension.

3.1.5. CCT

The DG group and the glaucoma suspect groups (FHG, GLD, and OHT) presented higher CCT values (562.6 ± 39.6 μ, 576.3 ± 38.3 μ, 569.51 ± 31.5 μ, and 570.34 ± 34.7 μ, respectively) than the control group (556.8 ± 35.3 μ), but only the FHG and OHT groups exhibited statistically significant differences ($p < 0.05$). No significant differences were found in the comparative analysis of the DG group with respect to the FHG, GLD, and OHT groups (Table 7).

Table 7. Statistical results using ANOVA multiple comparisons test for the CCT variable.

Dependent Variable	(I) Pathology	(J) Pathology	Mean Difference (I–J)	SE	*p*-Value	95% CI Upper Limit	95% CI Lower Limit
CCT	Control	DG	−5.80	4.36	0.997	−19.71	8.10
		FHG	−19.45 *	5.01	0.006 *	−35.64	−3.27
		GLD	−12.64	4.34	0.122	−26.63	1.35
		OHT	−13.47 *	3.52	0.005 *	−24.62	−2.33
	DG	Control	5.80	4.36	0.997	−8.10	19.71
		FHG	−13.64	6.26	0.585	−33.54	6.24
		GLD	−6.83	5.73	0.999	−25.02	11.35
		OHT	−7.67	5.14	0.984	−23.92	8.58
	FHG	Control	19.45 *	5.01	0.006 *	3.27	35.64
		DG	13.64	6.26	0.585	−6.24	33.54
		GLD	6.81	6.24	1.000	−13.07	26.70
		OHT	5.97	5.70	1.000	−12.21	24.16
	GLD	Control	12.64	4.34	0.122	−1.35	26.63
		DG	6.83	5.73	0.999	−11.35	25.02
		FHG	−6.81	6.24	1.000	−26.70	13.07
		OHT	−0.83	5.11	1.000	−17.12	15.44
	OHT	Control	13.47 *	3.52	0.005 *	2.33	24.62
		DG	7.67	5.14	0.984	−8.58	23.92
		FHG	−5.97	5.70	1.000	−24.16	12.21
		GLD	0.83	5.11	1.000	−15.44	17.12

SE—standard error. * Statistical significance ($p < 0.05$). CI—confidence interval. DG—diagnosed glaucoma; FHG—family history of glaucoma; GLD—glaucoma-like optic discs; OHT—ocular hypertension.

4. Discussion

4.1. Control Group

This work provides reference values for corneal biomechanical parameters (CH and CRF), IOPg, IOPcc, and CCT for the healthy Spanish population because it studied such a large control group (574 eyes). It should be noted that the existence of ocular pathologies (clinical or subclinical keratoconus, glaucoma, corneal dystrophies, and so on) in the control group was ruled out, and the study shows the results of a population with a wide age range. The mean age of the group of healthy control patients was 38.7 years, similar to that of other published studies [11,14,20,21]. The standard deviation of 15.54 in the age range (9–84 years) shows an age range of the control group subjects greater than that of other published works [10,22]. Mean values of CH (10.75 mmHg), CRF (10.75 mmHg), CCT (556.8 µ), IOPg (15.63 mmHg), and IOPcc (15.72 mmHg) hwere obtained. Means of the CH values obtained in other studies have ranged from 9.6 to 11.4 mmHg, but it should be taken into account that disparate population groups were studied regarding race and age, and moreover, some of them were carried out on a population of subjects with high refractive errors [23–26]. The mean CH obtained by Shah et al. [13] in healthy subjects was 10.7 ± 2.0, which is similar to that obtained in our work (10.7 ± 1.5). In another European study carried out on the eyes of healthy subjects [27], mean values of 10.7 ± 1.8 mmHg were obtained for the CRF, of 10.6 ± 1.6 mmHg for CH, of 15.9 ± 3.9 mmHg for IOPg, and of 16.2 ± 3.7 mmHg for IOPcc. It can be seen that they are similar to those obtained in our work, although in their study, they did not rule out the existence of possible subclinical keratoconus.

The ORA can determine IOPg values correlated to GAT, as well as IOPcc values, and it is less influenced by corneal biomechanical properties. In our study, we found that the control group of healthy patients, with normal biomechanical properties, presented similar mean IOPg and IOPcc values (15.6 mmHg and 15.7 mmHg, respectively). These values are similar to the GAT means reported in the literature for the healthy population, which are around 15.5 mmHg. We believe that these results, obtained from a large control group, validate the ORA as a tonometer, since the value means were determined in a large group of a healthy population, in which tests, such as topography and pachymetry, were performed that ruled out corneal subclinical alterations. Ping-Bo et al. [28] conducted a study using the ORA on 296 eyes of 158 healthy patients, classified into three groups according to their CCT (<520 µ, 520–580 µ, >580 µ), and found the following mean IOP values (IOPg: 14.95 ± 2.99 mmHg, IOPcc: 15.21 ± 2.77 mmHg, and GAT: 15.22 ± 2.77 mmHg), which are similar to those obtained in the control group of our work. When analyzing the values according to the CCT, they concluded that IOPcc measurements with ORA were only affected to a small extent by CCT, and they are probably much closer to the true value of the IOP than GAT.

The mean values of the CCT of the healthy population, in most of the published studies, are between 528µ and 562µ [29–32], which is similar to those obtained in this study for the healthy control population (556 µ).

4.2. Glaucoma, FHG, and Glaucoma Suspect Groups

In the last 15 years, a large number of articles about corneal biomechanical characterization have been published [33–38]. In the context of corneal biomechanical parameters of patients with glaucoma, we previously observed a significant decrease in CH when compared to healthy subjects [39,40]. This coincides with the results of other authors [14,41–43] who also found a significant decrease in CH in glaucoma, which was particularly evident in cases of congenital glaucoma [22]. The published results of CRF values are not consistent, as some have obtained low values [37] and others have obtained high values [35]. Our study aims to go into greater depth of cases of suspected glaucoma, which are referred to in this study, either owing to a family history of this pathology or to some doubtful sign, such as a suspicious papillary excavation or borderline or high IOP values, but without evident glaucomatous damage that would confirm the diagnosis.

We carried out a statistical study with multiple comparisons in which we obtained results for each group; we compared them with those of the control group, and we also compared them between each other to verify if there were any statistically significant differences. We found no published study that performs a comparative analysis on these groups of patients, so the results may have a special impact on the assessment of this pathology. This study has several limitations, since we did not analyze the evolutionary data of patients with glaucoma, nor did we differentiate pigmentary from pseudoexfoliative glaucoma; we did not include a group of normal-tension glaucoma, nor did we assess cases of angle-closure glaucoma.

4.2.1. CH

In this study, we verified the existence of decreased CH in the DG group compared to the control group; however, we did not find statistically significant differences in CH values in the three groups studied for suspected glaucoma and FHG when compared to the control group. These groups did not present evident glaucomatous lesions in the visual field or in the OCT fiber study. Consequently, CH could be a promising indicator to predict the progression of glaucoma, since it determines a specific biomechanical condition that is found in the cornea, but that could also affect other ocular structures, conditioning a special susceptibility to suffer glaucomatous damage. Recent studies suggest a possible relationship between lower CH values and structural changes in the optic nerve associated with glaucomatous damage. The relationship of low CH values with mean cup depth, linear cup-to-disc ratio, and greater posterior displacement of the lamina cribrosa has been evidenced [44–46]. Corneal hysteresis may provide insight into the biomechanical properties of the optic nerve and its supporting structures.

Some research indicates that eyes with higher IOP have lower CH values, and that the therapeutic manipulation of IOP can induce an inverse response in CH. It has been suggested that it may be due to the effect of prostaglandin therapy. Nevertheless, Meda et al. [47] do not support this hypothesis and suggest that this increase in CH may be due to IOP control. Furthermore, other medical and surgical treatments have shown to increase CH. Sun et al. [48] found that CH was significantly lower in eyes with chronic angle-closure glaucoma (CACG) compared to the contralateral eye and the control group of normal eyes. On the other hand, in this prospective study, it was found that trabeculectomy decreased the mean IOP from 31.5 to 11.5 mmHg, and that CH increased from 6.8 to 9.2 mmHg in the same period, although CH remained lower than in the contralateral eye without CACG. This study reflects the apparent dependence of CH according to IOP, and the probability that the regression of high IOP increases the mean of CH in this type of patients.

4.2.2. CRF

In this study, the values of CRF in the DG group showed higher values than the control group, but we found no statistically significant differences ($p > 0.05$). FHG, GLD, and OHT groups showed higher CRF values than the control group, with statistically significant differences. The OHT group showed the highest CRF values. Pillunat et al. [37] found that glaucoma patients had the lowest CRF values (9.07 ± 1.93 mmHg) in comparison to controls (10.2 ± 1.9 mmHg) and OHT patients (CRF: 10.6 ± 2.1 mmHg). However, Kaushik et al. found that CRF was significantly higher in POAG and OHT, which matches our results.

4.2.3. CCT

Regarding CCT, in the DG group we found no differences in the CCT of DG patients compared to those of the control group, which coincides with the results of other authors [14,22,38,42]. Although low CCT influences an underestimation of IOP by GAT [16], our glaucoma patients did not present different CCT values from those of the normal population, and the underestimation of IOP by GAT (IOPcc higher than IOPg) in the DG group could be related to other corneal biomechanical conditions, such as CH.

4.2.4. CH and CCT

Several studies have analyzed the association between CH and the visual field and optic nerve deterioration in glaucomatous patients [46,49,50], but the understanding of the direct importance of CH for glaucoma, and especially its relationship with CCT, is still evolving. Although it is true that low CCT has been related to the risk of OHT progression to glaucoma and to the progression of glaucomatous visual field loss, the results of our study agree with those of other authors, such as Congdon et al. [49], who found an association of low CH values with greater progression of the glaucomatous visual field, regardless of the CCT values, in their retrospective observational clinical study. It should be taken into account that CH is a direct estimate of an aspect of ocular biomechanics measured in the cornea, while CCT represents only one parameter that affects biomechanics. Wells et al. [46] found a relationship between low CH and the existence of greater deformation of the optic nerve after hyperpressure caused by suction in patients with glaucoma, but not with CCT.

The importance of measurable biomechanical parameters of the cornea has not yet been fully clarified. We know that CCT influences the estimation of a real IOP. In fact, there are structurally strong, thick corneas (high CCT, CH, and CRF), as in cases of hyperopic patients or OHT with high pachymetry values [51–53], where the IOPcc values are lower than the GAT or IOPg. There are also structurally weak, thick corneas, as in cases of endothelial dystrophy, bullous keratopathy, or rejection in keratoplasties [12,54]. In Fuchs' endothelial dystrophy, it has been shown that, when a high CCT value is due to corneal edema, there is a decrease in the CH and CRF biomechanical parameters. In these cases, there is no overestimation of IOP due to the increase in CCT, quite the opposite. The GAT in these patients underestimates the IOP and the IOPcc values show a higher real IOP [12].

The ORA can provide additional interesting information in the study of glaucoma patients. On the one hand, it provides an IOPcc value that is less influenced by the biomechanical properties of the cornea, which helps assess each case and, furthermore, it indicates CH values that can give guidance in the control of patients. The existence of a low CH value can be considered a risk factor for glaucoma progression. Likewise, in cases of OHT, the presence of high biomechanical values of CH, CRF, and CCT may indicate a low risk of progression to glaucoma; these cases usually present lower IOPcc values (in the normal range) than those of IOPg and GAT.

The present study provides the following conclusions on corneal biomechanics and IOP with the ORA:

1. A mean CH and CRF value of 10.75 mmHg was established in the healthy control population, which can be a reference for the Spanish population. The mean IOPg (15.63 mmHg) and IOPcc (15.72) values estimated by the ORA, in patients without ocular pathology, were similar to the mean GAT values. IOPg and IOPcc values were similar when the biomechanical properties of the cornea were within normal limits.

2. The IOPg and IOPcc means were significantly higher than those of the control group in all glaucoma and glaucoma suspect groups. There was a significant decrease in CH in the DG group compared to the control group, and with respect to the three glaucoma suspect groups. However, the CH values in the three glaucoma suspect groups (FHG, GLD, and OHT) did not show statistically significant differences between them, or with respect to the control group. No statistically significant differences in CRF values between the DG group and the control group were found. However, elevated CRF values in all the glaucoma suspect groups were found, such differences being statistically significant with respect to the control group. There was no CCT alteration in the DG group. POAG showed its own biomechanical profile (normal or high CCT, normal or high CRF, and low CH with IOPcc > IOPg).

3. The OHT and FHG suspect groups presented higher CRF values than the DG group and the differences were statistically significant. The mean CCT values were higher than the control group in all groups, although there were no statistically significant differences. Ocular hypertension suspect cases showed the highest CCT values. OHT

showed its own biomechanical profile (high CCT, high CRF, and normal or high CH with IOPcc < IOPg).

Finally, future studies could be performed to compare the biomechanical characterization of the cornea by two different devices, namely ORA and CORVIS-ST. To date, no study has found a relationship between the parameters they report. The contribution to diagnosis of CORVIS-ST has been studied mainly for corneal ectasia, but there is a lack of data about the differential role of CORVIS parameters in the glaucoma spectrum.

Author Contributions: Conceptualization, Mª.Á.d.B.-S., M.D.P.-D., P.C.-F. and C.P.-M.; methodology, P.C.-F., E.L.-S. and M.D.P.-D.; formal analysis, Mª.Á.d.B.-S., E.L.-S., P.C.-F., M.D.P.-D. and C.P.-M.; writing—original draft preparation, C.P.-M., Mª.Á.d.B.-S. and E.L.-S.; writing—review and editing, C.P.-M., P.C.-F., E.L.-S., M.D.P.-D. and Mª.Á.d.B.-S. supervision, C.P.-M. and Mª.Á.d.B.-S. All authors have read and agreed to the published version of the manuscript.

Funding: This research received no external funding.

Institutional Review Board Statement: The study was conducted according to the guidelines of the Declaration of Helsinki and approved by the local Ethics Committee for Clinical Research of Aragon (CEICA 18/2017) and the date of approval was 25 October 2017.

Informed Consent Statement: Informed consent was obtained from all subjects involved in the study.

Data Availability Statement: Data available on request due to restrictions of privacy.

Conflicts of Interest: The authors declare no conflict of interest.

References

1. Fung, Y.C. The mechanical properties of living tissues. In *Biomechanics*; Springer: New York, NY, USA, 1981; pp. 221–230.
2. Ruiz–De-Gopegui, E.; Ascaso, F.; Del Buey, M.; Cristóbal, J. Effects of encircling scleral buckling on the morphology and biomechanical properties of the cornea. *Arch. Soc. Española Oftalmol. (Engl. Ed.)* **2011**, *86*, 363–367. [CrossRef] [PubMed]
3. Del Buey, M.A.; Casas, P.; Caramello, C.; Lopez, N.; de la Rica, M.; Subiron, A.B.; Lanchares, E.; Huerva, V.; Grzybowski, A.; Ascaso, F.J. An Update on Corneal Biomechanics and Architecture in Diabetes. *J. Ophthalmol.* **2019**, *2019*, 7645352. [CrossRef] [PubMed]
4. Del Buey, M.A.; Lavilla, L.; Ascaso, F.J.; Lanchares, E.; Huerva, V.; Cristóbal, J.A. Assessment of corneal biomechanical properties and intraocular pressure in myopic Spanish healthy population. *J. Ophthalmol.* **2014**, *2014*, 905129. [CrossRef] [PubMed]
5. Ma, J.; Wang, Y.; Wei, P.; Jhanji, V. Biomechanics and structure of the cornea: Implications and association with corneal disor-ders. *Surv. Ophthalmol.* **2018**, *63*, 851–861. [CrossRef] [PubMed]
6. Cristóbal, J.A.; del Buey, M.A.; Ascaso, F.J.; Lanchares, E.; Calvo, B.; Doblaré, M. Effect of Limbal Relaxing Incisions During Phacoemulsification Surgery Based on Nomogram Review and Numerical Simulation. *Cornea* **2009**, *28*, 1042–1049. [CrossRef]
7. Lanchares, E.; Calvo, B.; Del Buey, M.A.; Cristóbal, J.A.; Doblaré, M. The Effect of Intraocular Pressure on the Outcome of Myopic Photorefractive Keratectomy: A Numerical Approach. *J. Heal. Eng.* **2010**, *1*, 461–476. [CrossRef]
8. Lanchares, E.; Del Buey, M.A.; Cristóbal, J.A.; Lavilla, L.; Calvo, B. Biomechanical property analysis after corneal collagen cross-linking in relation to ultraviolet A irradiation time. *Graefe's Arch. Clin. Exp. Ophthalmol.* **2011**, *249*, 1223–1227. [CrossRef]
9. Lanchares, E.; Del Buey, M.A.; Cristóbal, J.A.; Calvo, B.; Ascaso, F.J.; Malvè, M. Computational Simulation of Scleral Buckling Surgery for Rhegmatogenous Retinal Detachment: On the Effect of the Band Size on the Myopization. *J. Ophthalmol.* **2016**, *2016*, 1–10. [CrossRef]
10. Luce, D.A. Determining in vivo biomechanical properties of the cornea with an ocular response analyzer. *J. Cataract. Refract. Surg.* **2005**, *31*, 156–162. [CrossRef]
11. Ortiz, D.; Piñero, D.; Shabayek, M.H.; Arnalich-Montiel, F.; Alió, J.L. Corneal biomechanical properties in normal, post-laser in situ keratomileusis, and keratoconic eyes. *J. Cataract. Refract. Surg.* **2007**, *33*, 1371–1375. [CrossRef]
12. Del Buey, M.A.; Cristóbal, J.A.; Ascaso, F.J.; Lavilla, L.; Lanchares, E. Biomechanical properties of the cornea in Fuchs' corneal dys-trophy. *Investig. Ophthalmol. Vis. Sci.* **2009**, *50*, 3199–3202. [CrossRef]
13. Shah, S.; Laiquzzaman, M.; Bhojwani, R.; Mantry, S.; Cunliffe, I. Assessment of the Biomechanical Properties of the Cornea with the Ocular Response Analyzer in Normal and Keratoconic Eyes. *Investig. Opthalmology Vis. Sci.* **2007**, *48*, 3026–3031. [CrossRef]
14. Touboul, D.; Roberts, C.; Kérautret, J.; Garra, C.; Maurice-Tison, S.; Saubusse, E.; Colin, J. Correlations between corneal hysteresis, intraocular pressure, and corneal central pachymetry. *J. Cataract. Refract. Surg.* **2008**, *34*, 616–622. [CrossRef]
15. Susanna, C.N.; Diniz-Filho, A.; Daga, F.B.; Susanna, B.N.; Zhu, F.; Ogata, N.G.; Medeiros, F.A. A Prospective Longitudinal Study to Investigate Corneal Hysteresis as a Risk Factor for Predicting Development of Glaucoma. *Am. J. Ophthalmol.* **2018**, *187*, 148–152. [CrossRef] [PubMed]

16. Gordon, M.O.; Beiser, J.A.; Brandt, J.D.; Heuer, D.K.; Higginbotham, E.J.; Johnson, C.A.; Keltner, J.L.; Miller, J.P.; Parrish, R.K.; Wilson, M.R. The ocular hypertension treatment study: Baseline factors that predict the onset of primary open-angle glaucoma. *Arch. Ophthalmol.* **2002**, *120*, 714–720. [CrossRef]

17. Murphy, M.L.; Pokrovskaya, O.; Galligan, M.; O'Brien, C. Corneal hysteresis in patients with glaucoma-like optic discs, ocular hypertension and glaucoma. *BMC Ophthalmol.* **2017**, *17*, 1. [CrossRef] [PubMed]

18. Susanna, B.N.; Ogata, N.G.; Jammal, A.A.; Susanna, C.N.; Berchuck, S.I.; Medeiros, F.A. Corneal Biomechanics and Visual Field Progression in Eyes with Seemingly Well-Controlled Intraocular Pressure. *Ophthalmology* **2019**, *126*, 1640–1646. [CrossRef] [PubMed]

19. Stein, J.D.; Khawaja, A.P.; Weizer, J.S. Glaucoma in Adults—Screening, Diagnosis, and Management. *JAMA* **2021**, *325*, 164–174. [CrossRef] [PubMed]

20. Kamiya, K.; Hagishima, M.; Fujimura, F.; Shimizu, K. Factors affecting corneal hysteresis in normal eyes. *Graefe's Arch. Clin. Exp. Ophthalmol.* **2008**, *246*, 1491–1494. [CrossRef]

21. Shen, M.; Fan, F.; Xue, A.; Wang, J.; Zhou, X.; Lu, F. Biomechanical properties of the cornea in high myopia. *Vis. Res.* **2008**, *48*, 2167–2171. [CrossRef]

22. Kirwan, C.; O'Keefe, M.; Lanigan, B. Corneal Hysteresis and Intraocular Pressure Measurement in Children Using the Reichert Ocular Response Analyzer. *Am. J. Ophthalmol.* **2006**, *142*, 990–992. [CrossRef]

23. Haseltine, S.J.; Pae, J.; Ehrlich, J.R.; Shammas, M.; Radcliffe, N.M. Variation in corneal hysteresis and central corneal thickness among black, hispanic and white subjects. *Acta Ophthalmol.* **2012**, *90*, 626–631. [CrossRef]

24. Strobbe, E.; Cellini, M.; Barbaresi, U.; Campos, E.C. Influence of Age and Gender on Corneal Biomechanical Properties in a Healthy Italian Population. *Cornea* **2014**, *33*, 968–972. [CrossRef]

25. Celebi, A.R.C.; Kilavuzoglu, A.E.; Altiparmak, U.E.; Yurteri, C.B.C. Age-related change in corneal biomechanical parameters in a healthy Caucasian population. *Ophthalmic Epidemiol.* **2017**, *25*, 55–62. [CrossRef]

26. Al-Arfaj, K.; Yassin, S.A.; Al-Dairi, W.; Al-Shamlan, F.; Al-Jindan, M. Corneal biomechanics in normal Saudi individuals. *Saudi J. Ophthalmol.* **2016**, *30*, 180–184. [CrossRef]

27. Kopito, R.; Gaujoux, T.; Montard, R.; Touzeau, O.; Allouch, C.; Borderie, V.; Laroche, L. Reproducibility of viscoelastic property and intraocular pressure measurements obtained with the Ocular Response Analyzer. *Acta Ophthalmol.* **2010**, *89*, e225–e230. [CrossRef] [PubMed]

28. Ouyang, P.-B.; Li, C.-Y.; Zhu, X.-H.; Duan, X.-C. Assessment of intraocular pressure measured by Reichert Ocular Response Analyzer, Goldmann Applanation Tonometry, and Dynamic Contour Tonometry in healthy individuals. *Int. J. Ophthalmol.* **2012**, *5*, 102–107. [CrossRef] [PubMed]

29. Pakravan, M.; Javadi, M.A.; Yazdani, S.; Ghahari, E.; Behroozi, Z.; Soleimanizad, R.; Moghimi, S.; Nilforoushan, N.; Zarei, R.; Eslami, Y.; et al. Distribution of intraocular pressure, central corneal thickness and vertical cup-to-disc ratio in a healthy Iranian population: The Yazd Eye Study. *Acta Ophthalmol.* **2016**, *95*. [CrossRef] [PubMed]

30. Peyman, M.; Tai, L.Y.; Khaw, K.W.; Ng, C.M.; Win, M.M.; Subrayan, V. Accutome PachPen handheld ultrasonic pachymeter: Intraobserver repeatability and interobserver reproducibility by personnel of different training grades. *Int. Ophthalmol.* **2015**, *35*, 651–655. [CrossRef] [PubMed]

31. Gros-Otero, J.; Arruabarrena-Sánchez, C.; Teus, M. Espesor corneal central en una población sana española [Central corneal thickness in a healthy Spanish population]. *Arch. Soc. Esp. Oftalmol.* **2011**, *86*, 73–76. [CrossRef]

32. Muir, K.W.; Duncan, L.; Enyedi, L.B.; Freedman, S.F. Central Corneal Thickness in Children: Racial Differences (Black vs. White) and Correlation With Measured Intraocular Pressure. *J. Glaucoma* **2006**, *15*, 520–523. [CrossRef]

33. Mansouri, K.; Leite, M.T.; Weinreb, R.N.; Tafreshi, A.; Zangwill, L.M.; Medeiros, F.A. Association between cor-neal biomechanical properties and glaucoma severity. *Am. J. Ophthalmol.* **2012**, *153*, 419–427. [CrossRef] [PubMed]

34. Ang, G.S.; Bochmann, F.; Townend, J.; Azuara-Blanco, A. Corneal Biomechanical Properties in Primary Open Angle Glaucoma and Normal Tension Glaucoma. *J. Glaucoma* **2008**, *17*, 259–262. [CrossRef]

35. Kaushik, S.; Pandav, S.S.; Banger, A.; Aggarwal, K.; Gupta, A. Relationship Between Corneal Biomechanical Properties, Central Corneal Thickness, and Intraocular Pressure Across the Spectrum of Glaucoma. *Am. J. Ophthalmol.* **2012**, *153*, 840–849.e2. [CrossRef]

36. Park, J.H.; Jun, R.M.; Choi, K.-R. Significance of corneal biomechanical properties in patients with progressive normal-tension glaucoma. *Br. J. Ophthalmol.* **2015**, *99*, 746–751. [CrossRef]

37. Pillunat, K.R.; Hermann, C.; Spoerl, E.; Pillunat, L.E. Analyzing biomechanical parameters of the cornea with glaucoma severity in open-angle glaucoma. *Graefe's Arch. Clin. Exp. Ophthalmol.* **2016**, *254*, 1345–1351. [CrossRef]

38. Detry-Morel, M.; Jamart, J.; Hautenauven, F.; Pourjavan, S. Comparison of the corneal biomechanical properties with the Ocular Response Analyzer® (ORA) in African and Caucasian normal subjects and patients with glaucoma. *Acta Ophthalmol.* **2011**, *90*, e118–e124. [CrossRef] [PubMed]

39. Del Buey, M.A.; Cristóbal, J.; Lavilla, L.; Palomino, C.; Lanchares, E. The use of the Reichert Ocular Response Analyser to establish the relationship between bomechanical properties and ocular pathology. *Investig. Ophthalmol. Vis. Sci.* **2008**, *49*, 653.

40. Del Buey, M.A.; Lavilla, L.; Cristóbal, J.A.; Lanchares, E.; Palomino, C.; Calvo, B. Corneal resistance factor (CRF) and corneal hyste-resis (CH) associated with glaucoma damage. In *Book of Abstract XXVI Congress of the ESCRS*; ESCRS: Berlin, Germany, 2008.

41. Spörl, E.; Terai, N.; Haustein, M.; Böhm, A.; Raiskup-Wolf, F.; Pillunat, L.E. Biomechanical condition of the cornea as a new indica-tor for pathological and structural changes. *Ophthalmologe* **2009**, *106*, 512–520. [CrossRef] [PubMed]
42. Wasielica-Poslednik, J.; Berisha, F.; Aliyeva, S.; Pfeiffer, N.; Hoffmann, E.M. Reproducibility of ocular response analyzer meas-urements and their correlation with central corneal thickness. *Graefes Arch. Clin. Exp. Ophthalmol.* **2010**, *248*, 1617–1622. [CrossRef] [PubMed]
43. Detry-Morel, M.; Jamart, J.; Pourjavan, S. Evaluation of corneal biomechanical properties with the Reichert Ocular Response Analyzer. *Eur. J. Ophthalmol.* **2011**, *21*, 138–148. [CrossRef]
44. Prata, T.S.; Lima, V.C.; De Moraes, C.G.V.; Guedes, L.M.; Magalhães, F.P.; Teixeira, S.H.; Ritch, R.; Paranhos, A. Factors associated with topographic changes of the optic nerve head induced by acute intraocular pressure reduction in glaucoma patients. *Eye* **2010**, *25*, 201–207. [CrossRef]
45. Lee, K.M.; Kim, T.W.; Lee, E.J.; Girard, M.J.A.; Mari, J.M.; Weinreb, R.N. Association of corneal hysteresis with lamina cribrosa curva-ture in primary open angle glaucoma. *Investig. Ophthalmol. Vis. Sci.* **2019**, *60*, 4171–4177. [CrossRef]
46. Wells, A.P.; Garway-Heath, D.F.; Poostchi, A.; Wong, T.; Chan, K.C.; Sachdev, N. Corneal hysteresis but not corneal thickness cor-relates with optic nerve surface compliance in glaucoma patients. *Investig. Ophthalmol. Vis. Sci.* **2008**, *49*, 3262–3268. [CrossRef]
47. Meda, R.; Wang, Q.; Paoloni, D.; Harasymowycz, P.; Brunette, I. The impact of chronic use of prostaglandin analogues on the biomechanical properties of the cornea in patients with primary open-angle glaucoma. *Br. J. Ophthalmol.* **2016**, *101*, 120–125. [CrossRef]
48. Sun, L.; Shen, M.; Wang, J.; Fang, A.; Xu, A.; Fang, H.; Lu, F. Recovery of Corneal Hysteresis After Reduction of Intraocular Pressure in Chronic Primary Angle-Closure Glaucoma. *Am. J. Ophthalmol.* **2009**, *147*, 1061–1066.e2. [CrossRef] [PubMed]
49. Congdon, N.G.; Broman, A.T.; Bandeen-Roche, K.; Grover, D.; Quigley, H.A. Central corneal thickness and corneal hysteresis associated with glau-coma damage. *Am. J. Ophthalmol.* **2006**, *141*, 868–875. [CrossRef] [PubMed]
50. Bochmann, F.; Ang, G.S.; Azuara-Blanco, A. Lower corneal hysteresis in glaucoma patients with acquired pit of the optic nerve (APON). *Graefe's Arch. Clin. Exp. Ophthalmol.* **2008**, *246*, 735–738. [CrossRef]
51. Del Buey, M.A.; Cristobal Bescos, J.A.; Lavilla, L.; Ascaso, F.; Mateo-Orobia, A.; Jimenez, B.; Ruiz de Gopegui, E.; Palominio, C. Bio-mechanical properties in healthy subjects with and without refractive errors. A comparative study. *Acta Ophthalmol.* **2010**, *88*. [CrossRef]
52. Roberts, C.J.; Reinstein, D.Z.; Archer, T.J.; Mahmoud, A.M.; Gobbe, M.; Lee, L. Comparison of ocular biomechanical response pa-rameters in myopic and hyperopic eyes using dynamic bidirectional applanation analysis. *J. Cataract Refract. Surg.* **2014**, *40*, 929–936. [CrossRef] [PubMed]
53. Yagci, R.; Eksioglu, U.; Midillioglu, I.; Yalvac, I.; Altiparmak, E.; Duman, S. Central Corneal Thickness in Primary Open Angle Glaucoma, Pseudoexfoliative Glaucoma, Ocular Hypertension, and Normal Population. *Eur. J. Ophthalmol.* **2005**, *15*, 324–328. [CrossRef] [PubMed]
54. Fabian, I.D.; Barequet, I.S.; Skaat, A.; Rechtman, E.; Goldenfeld, M.; Roberts, C.J.; Melamed, S. Intraocular Pressure Measurements and Biomechanical Properties of the Cornea in Eyes After Penetrating Keratoplasty. *Am. J. Ophthalmol.* **2011**, *151*, 774–781. [CrossRef] [PubMed]

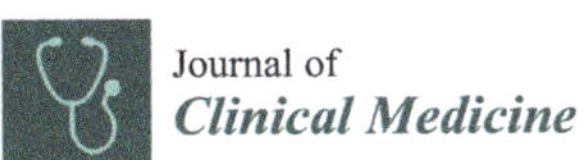

Journal of
Clinical Medicine

Article

Optic Disc Vascular Density in Normal-Tension Glaucoma Eyes with or without Branch Retinal Vessel Occlusion

Jiwon Baek [1], Soo-Ji Jeon [2], Jin-Ho Kim [1], Chan-Kee Park [3] and Hae-Young L. Park [3,*]

1   Department of Ophthalmology, Bucheon St. Mary's Hospital, College of Medicine, The Catholic University of Korea, Bucheon 14647, Korea; md.jiwon@gmail.com (J.B.); dmtko1@naver.com (J.-H.K.)
2   Department of Ophthalmology, Eunpyeong St. Mary's Hospital, College of Medicine, The Catholic University of Korea, Seoul 03312, Korea; sj8801@gmail.com
3   Department of Ophthalmology, Seoul St. Mary's Hospital, College of Medicine, The Catholic University of Korea, Seoul 06591, Korea; ckpark@catholic.ac.kr
*   Correspondence: lopilly@catholic.ac.kr

Abstract: We analyzed the vascular densities (VDs) of the optic disc areas in eyes with normal-tension glaucoma (NTG) according to their branch retinal vessel occlusion (BRVO) status. The VDs of the optic discs and peripapillary areas of 68 NTG patients with BRVO (BRVO group; BRVO eyes and fellow eyes) and 37 patients with NTG alone (control eyes) were measured on angiographic images obtained via swept-source optical coherence tomography angiography. VDs were compared among groups and correlations were assessed. The VD of the optic disc large vessel was the highest in BRVO eyes, followed by the fellow eyes and controls (all $P < 0.05$). Conversely, small and medium vessel VD was in the opposite order (all $P < 0.05$). Large vessel VD was negatively correlated with small and medium vessel VD (r = −0.697, $P < 0.001$). Peripapillary VD was lower in the BRVO eyes than in the control and fellow eyes ($P < 0.001$ and $P = 0.861$, respectively). In conclusion, significant changes in the distribution of VDs for optic disc larger vessel and small and medium vessels were observed in both eyes of NTG patients with BRVO, compared to NTG patients without BRVO.

Keywords: OCTA; vessel density; disc; peripapillary; NTG; BRVO

Citation: Baek, J.; Jeon, S.-J.; Kim, J.-H.; Park, C.-K.; Park, H.-Y.L. Optic Disc Vascular Density in Normal-Tension Glaucoma Eyes with or without Branch Retinal Vessel Occlusion. *J. Clin. Med.* **2021**, *10*, 2574. https://doi.org/10.3390/jcm 10122574

Academic Editor: Emmanuel Andrès

Received: 26 March 2021
Accepted: 2 June 2021
Published: 10 June 2021

Publisher's Note: MDPI stays neutral with regard to jurisdictional claims in published maps and institutional affiliations.

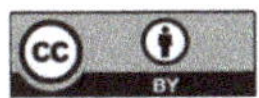

1. Introduction

An association between retinal vein occlusion (RVO) and glaucoma has been documented in many previous studies [1–8]. The prevalence of normal-tension glaucoma (NTG) has been reported to be higher in eyes with RVO than in the general population [1]. This pathogenesis may be explained by abnormal disc anatomy, elevated intraocular pressure (IOP), and the effects of various vascular factors. In the Ocular Hypertension Treatment Study, a greater cup-to-disc ratio was associated with RVO development in patients with elevated IOP [9]. Changes in disc hemodynamics may also link RVO and glaucoma, especially in eyes with NTG; such changes play pathogenic roles in both diseases [10–12].

Recently, optical coherence tomography angiography (OCTA) has been extensively used to analyze the vascular structures of the retina and disc area; OCTA facilitates the detailed, noninvasive evaluation of retinal and choroidal microvascular structures. The results of OCTA studies have supported the notion that hemodynamic changes may trigger glaucoma. Such studies have revealed reduced vascular densities (VDs) in the optic disc and peripapillary area in eyes with glaucoma, including NTG [13–17]. The recent publication of a meta-analysis of OCTA VDs in glaucoma patients confirmed a significant reduction in the mean peripapillary, whole optic disc, and inside-disc VDs [18]. Reduced VD has been associated with disease severity and progression [19–21].

Given that pathogenic hemodynamic parameters are shared by eyes with NTG and eyes with RVO, an analysis of vessel structures around the disc in patients with these diseases might afford useful insights into the roles played by vascular changes. Here, we

135

identified changes in the vascular structures of the optic disc and peripapillary area and we used OCTA to quantitatively analyze the VDs of eyes with NTG, according to their branch retinal vein occlusion (BRVO) status.

2. Materials and Methods

This observational case-control study was performed using medical records. The study was approved by the Institutional Review Board of Seoul St. Mary's Hospital (KC18RESI0852). Patients were informed of the study, but the requirement for written informed consent was waived because of the retrospective nature of the study. The study was conducted in accordance with the tenets of the Declaration of Helsinki.

2.1. Patients

Consecutive patients with NTG (with or without BRVO) in both eyes who visited Seoul St. Mary's Hospital (Seoul, Korea) between March 2018 and March 2020 were enrolled. The number of patients in each group was decided using a two-tailed trial for 80% power and 5% significance. NTG diagnostic criteria were: (1) glaucomatous optic disc change (i.e., rim thinning, disc hemorrhage, rim notch, or vertical cup-to-disc ratio greater than that of the other eye by $\geq$0.2-fold) and glaucomatous visual field (VF) loss (i.e., pattern standard deviation ($P < 0.05$) or glaucoma hemifield test result ($P < 0.01$) outside the normal limits, exhibiting a consistent pattern in the Bjerrum areas of both VFs); (2) maximum IOP < 22 mm Hg (without glaucoma medications) as determined by repeated measurements performed on different days; and (3) an open angle on gonioscopic examination.

BRVO was defined as retinal venous obstruction in a localized area of the retina, characterized by scattered superficial and deep retinal hemorrhages, venous dilation, intraretinal microvascular abnormalities, and occluded and sheathed retinal venules. BRVO was diagnosed at the time of initial NTG diagnosis or during NTG follow-up.

The exclusion criteria were: (1) spherical refraction > $\pm$6.0 diopters; (2) glaucoma with BRVO in both eyes; (3) history of any retinal disease other than BRVO; (4) history of eye trauma or surgery, with the exception of uncomplicated cataract surgery; and (5) any optic nerve disease other than glaucoma.

All patients underwent a complete ophthalmic examination, including assessment of best-corrected visual acuity (BCVA) and refractive error; slit-lamp biomicroscopy; gonioscopy; IOP measurement using Goldmann applanation tonometry; axial length assessment via ocular biometry (IOLMaster; Carl Zeiss Meditec, Dublin, CA, USA); stereoscopic photography and red-free fundus photography (Canon, Tokyo, Japan); Humphrey VF testing using the Swedish Interactive Thresholding Algorithm Standard 24-2 test (Carl Zeiss Meditec, Dublin, CA, USA); optical coherence tomography (Carl Zeiss Meditec, Dublin, CA, USA) of the retinal nerve fiber layer (RNFL); and OCTA of the disc area (DRI OCT Triton, Topcon Corporation, Tokyo, Japan). OCTA data regarding eyes with BRVO were obtained during the inactive phase of BRVO (i.e., in the absence of edema and active hemorrhage). BCVA was converted into the logarithm of the minimal angle of resolution to allow statistical analysis.

2.2. Image Analysis

En face OCTA images (3×3 mm^2 in area, centered at the optic disc) were obtained for each eye. For eyes with macular edema and hemorrhage, OCTAs were taken after subsidence of fluid and hemorrhage. All images were acquired after confirmation of the flow signal shown on the OCT B-scan. For VD analysis, a combined image was automatically generated by ImageNet software (ImageNet 6, ver. 1.19.11030, Topcon Corporation, Tokyo, Japan) and the superficial and choriocapillaris layers were fused (Figure 1A). VD was quantified as follows using FIJI software (an expanded version of ImageJ ver. 1.51a, available at http://fiji.sc/Fiji, accessed on 10 June 2021). First, all vessels were traced using the Frangi vesselness plugin (Figure 1B). Large vessels were defined as retinal arteries and veins coming from and into the optic disc, and vessel areas were traced using the Tubness plugin (Figure 1C). Then, the total, small and medium, and large vessel VDs were measured in regions of interest of the optic disc and peripapillary area; the final figures were calculated by dividing the vessel area by the total region of interest (Figure 1D,E). Peripapillary VDs were subdivided into four quadrants: superotemporal (ST), superonasal (SN), inferonasal (IN), and inferotemporal (IT) (Figure 1E). The means of two measurements of each VD were used. Cases with media opacities were excluded. Only clear images with signal strength index >40 that did not exhibit blurring or artifacts attributable to motion were analyzed.

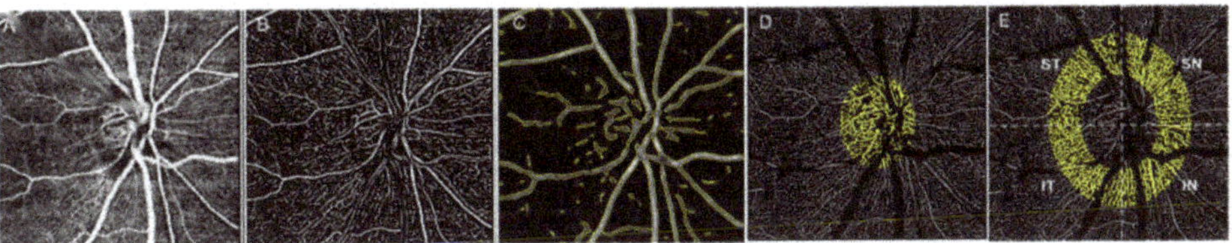

Figure 1. Measurement of vascular density: (**A**) En face, optical coherence tomography angiography image of 3×3-mm^2 disc area showing vessels from two combined layers; (**B**) Vessels were traced using Frangi vesselness plug-in; (**C**) Large vessel areas were selected using Tubness plug-in. Regions of interest were selected in the optic disc (**D**) and peripapillary area (**E**). Vascular density was calculated by dividing vessel area by region of interest.

2.3. Statistical Analysis

Continuous variables were marked as mean $\pm$ standard deviation. Statistical analysis was performed using SPSS Statistics (version 23.0.1; IBM Corp., Armonk, NY, USA). Independent t-test was used for the comparison between unpaired eyes, while paired t-test was used for paired eyes after confirmation of a normal distribution using Kolmogorov–Smirnov test. The Mann–Whitney U test and Wilcoxon signed rank test were employed when a normal distribution could not be confirmed. Categorical variables were compared between groups using the chi-squared test. Standardized adjustment for residuals was used as the post hoc test after the chi-squared test. Effect of treatment modality on VD was assessed using multinomial logistic regression. Correlation analysis was performed with Spearman rank correlation for continuous variables and univariate logistic regression for binary variables. A p-value < 0.05 was considered statistically significant.

3. Results

3.1. Patient Demographics and Clinical Features

In total, 68 NTG patients with BRVO (BRVO group; 68 eyes with BRVO and 68 fellow eyes) and 37 patients with NTG alone (control group; 74 control eyes) were included in this study. Four patients (5.6%) with low image quality were excluded. The mean patient age was 66.97 years. There were no significant differences in age, sex, diabetes mellitus status, cardiovascular disease status, or cerebrovascular disease status between the BRVO group and the control group (all $P > 0.05$). Hypertension was more common in the BRVO group than in the control group ($P < 0.001$). All the NTG patients were on treatment eyedrops: 30 were on prostaglandin analogues, 10 were on beta-blockers, 2 were on alpha-agonist, and 26 were on combination treatment. Patient demographics are summarized in Table 1.

The mean BCVA values were lower in BRVO eyes than in fellow eyes and control eyes (both $P < 0.05$). The mean VF deviation was lower in BRVO eyes compared to control eyes ($P = 0.006$). No other ocular parameters differed significantly between BRVO eyes, fellow eyes, and control eyes (all $P > 0.05$). Ocular parameters are summarized in Table 2.

Table 1. Demographic and clinical parameters of normal-tension glaucoma patients with BRVO and controls.

Variable	Control Group (*n* = 37)	BRVO Group (*n* = 68)	*p*-Value
Age (years), mean ± SD	66.14 ± 10.89	67.81 ± 10.63	0.285 [a]
Sex (male/female), *n*	16/21	22/46	0.118 [b]
Diabetes mellitus, *n* (%)	5 (14)	15 (22)	0.133 [b]
Hypertension, *n* (%)	4 (11)	31 (46)	<0.001 [b] *
CVD (0: no/1: yes)	4 (11)	3 (4)	0.076 [b]

BRVO: branch retinal vein occlusion; SD: standard deviation; CVD: cardio- or cerebrovascular disease. [a] Independent *t*-test between groups. [b] Chi-square test between groups. * *p*-value is significant.

Table 2. Ocular parameters of the groups.

	Control Eyes (*n* = 74)	BRVO Eyes (*n* = 68)	Fellow Eyes (*n* = 68)	*p*-Value [a]	*p*-Value [b]	*p*-Value [c]
BCVA (logMAR), mean ± SD	0.08 ± 0.11	0.21 ± 0.26	0.11 ± 0.18	<0.001 *	0.114	<0.001 *
Refractive error (diopter), mean ± SD	−0.3 ± 2.66	−1.03 ± 2.34	−0.95 ± 2.45	0.071	0.144	0.598
Axial length (mm), mean ± SD	24.3 ± 1.28	24.02 ± 1.43	23.84 ± 1.27	0.0.64	0.052	0.761
IOP (mmHg), mean ± SD	14.34 ± 3.04	14.76 ± 3.4	14.84 ± 3.59	0.448	0.271	0.961
RNFL thickness (μm), mean ± SD	83.01 ± 17.27	80.07 ± 21.51	83.09 ± 20.38	0.863	0.902	0.853
VF mean deviation (dB), mean ± SD	−4.07 ± 5.79	−6.73 ± 7.56	−5.07 ± 6.92	0.006 *	0.075	0.665
Disc hemorrhage, *n* (%)	7 (9)	2 (3)	5 (7)	0.232	0.653	0.564

NTG: normal tension glaucoma; BRVO: branch retinal vein occlusion; BCVA: best-corrected visual acuity; SD: standard deviation; IOP: intraocular pressure; RNFL: retinal nerve fiber layer; VF: visual field. [a] Mann–Whitney U test comparing control eyes and BRVO eyes. [b] Mann–Whitney U test comparing control eyes and fellow eyes. [c] Wilcoxon signed rank test comparing BRVO eyes and fellow eyes. * *p*-value is significant.

3.2. Comparison of VDs Among Groups

Although the total VD of the optic disc area did not differ between the BRVO group and the control group (0.485 ± 0.033 vs. 0.484 ± 0.082; *P* = 0.835), the small and medium vessel and large vessel VDs in the disc area significantly differed between the groups (0.232 ± 0.056 vs. 0.274 ± 0.045 and 0.260 ± 0.068 vs. 0.210 ± 0.053; both *P* < 0.05). Peripapillary VD also significantly differed between the groups (0.282 ± 0.046 vs. 0.296 ± 0.038; *P* = 0.021) (Figure 2). Treatment modality did not affect the VDs of the disc or peripapillary area (both *P* = 0.999).

When eyes were divided into control eyes, BRVO eyes, and fellow eyes, the large vessel VD was highest in BRVO eyes, followed by the fellow eyes and control eyes; the small and medium vessel VD exhibited the opposite order (all *P* < 0.05). The BRVO eyes exhibited lower small and medium vessel and peripapillary VDs, and higher large vessel VDs, compared to both the control eyes and fellow eyes (all *P* < 0.05). The fellow eyes exhibited a higher large vessel VD and a lower small and medium vessel VD than did the control eyes (*P* < 0.001 and = 0.020, respectively) (Table 3).

Table 3. Vessel densities of the groups.

Vascular Density	Control Eyes (*n* = 74)	BRVO Eyes (*n* = 68)	Fellow Eyes (*n* = 68)	*p*-Value [a]	*p*-Value [b]	*p*-Value [c]
Disc total VD	0.485 ± 0.033	0.469 ± 0.101	0.499 ± 0.051	0.835	0.031 *	0.007 *
Disc small and medium vessel VD	0.274 ± 0.045	0.212 ± 0.051	0.252 ± 0.054	<0.001 *	0.020 *	<0.001 *
Disc large vessel VD	0.210 ± 0.053	0.272 ± 0.075	0.248 ± 0.059	<0.001 *	<0.001 *	0.003 *
Peripapillary VD	0.296 ± 0.038	0.269 ± 0.045	0.296 ± 0.042	<0.001 *	0.861	0.017 *
Peripapillary VD ST	0.318 ± 0.057	0.277 ± 0.056	0.308 ± 0.051	<0.001 *	0.297	0.019 *
Peripapillary VD SN	0.273 ± 0.053	0.255 ± 0.055	0.286 ± 0.048	0.032 *	0.396	0.023 *
Peripapillary VD IN	0.288 ± 0.034	0.261 ± 0.053	0.278 ± 0.05	0.001 *	0.285	0.387
Peripapillary VD IT	0.316 ± 0.041	0.282 ± 0.054	0.308 ± 0.058	<0.001 *	0.452	0.017 *

BRVO: branch retinal vessel occlusion; VD: vascular density; ST: superotemporal; SN: superonasal; IN: inferonasal; IT: inferotemporal. [a] Mann–Whitney U test comparing control eyes and BRVO eyes. [b] Mann–Whitney U test comparing control eyes and fellow eyes. [c] Wilcoxon signed rank test comparing BRVO eyes and fellow eyes. * *p*-value is significant.

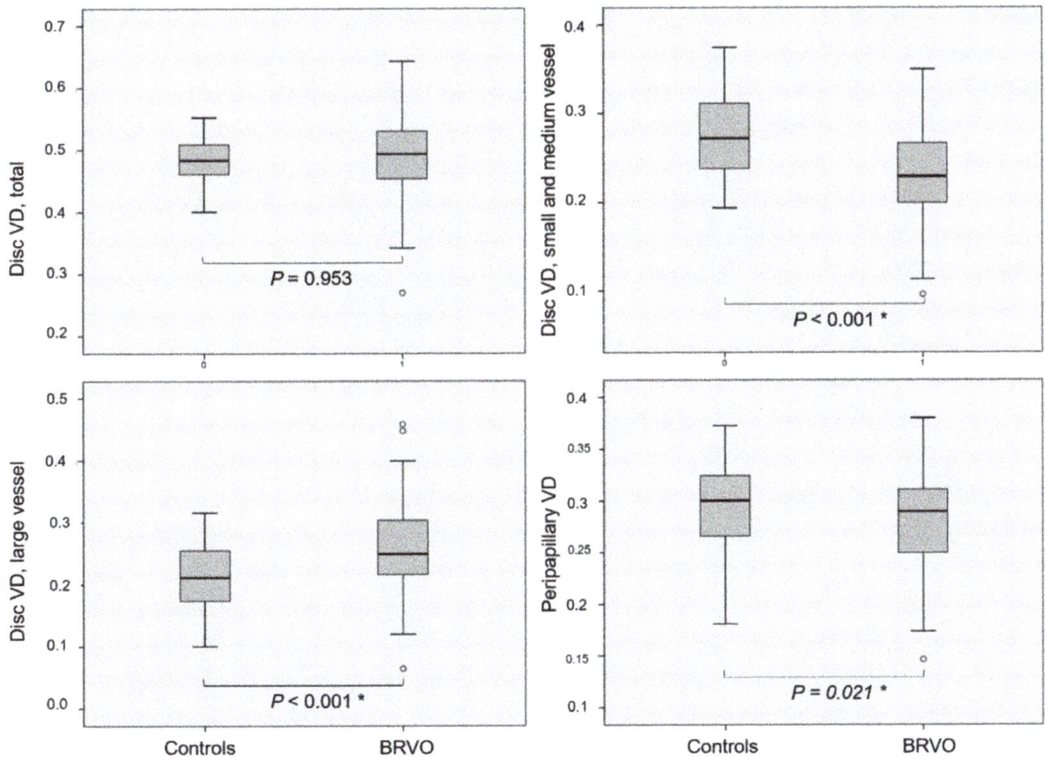

Figure 2. VDs of the disc and peripapillary areas of patients with NTG, according to BRVO status. Small and medium and large vessel VDs in the disc area differed significantly between patients with NTG, according to BRVO status (both $P < 0.001$). Peripapillary VD was lower in BRVO group than in control group ($P = 0.021$).* Statistically significant P-value with Mann–Whitney U test.

3.3. Correlation Analysis of VDs

Total, small and medium vessel, and peripapillary VDs were negatively correlated with BCVA values (r = −0.147, −0.237, and −0.311; P = 0.034, 0.001, and <0.001, respectively). Large vessel VD was positively correlated with BCVA (r = 0.159, P = 0.023). Disc VDs were correlated with refractive error and axial length (all P < 0.05) (Table 4). Large vessel VD was negatively correlated with small and medium vessel VD (r = −0.697, P < 0.001) (Figure 3A). This correlation persisted when eyes were divided into groups (r = −0.775, −0.559, and −0.603; all P < 0.05) (Figure 3B–D). Peripapillary small and medium vessel VDs were positively correlated with the total and small and medium vessel VDs of the optic disc (r = 0.307 and 0.545; both P < 0.05) and negatively correlated with the large vessel VD of the optic disc (r = −0.226; P = 0.001) (Figure 4).

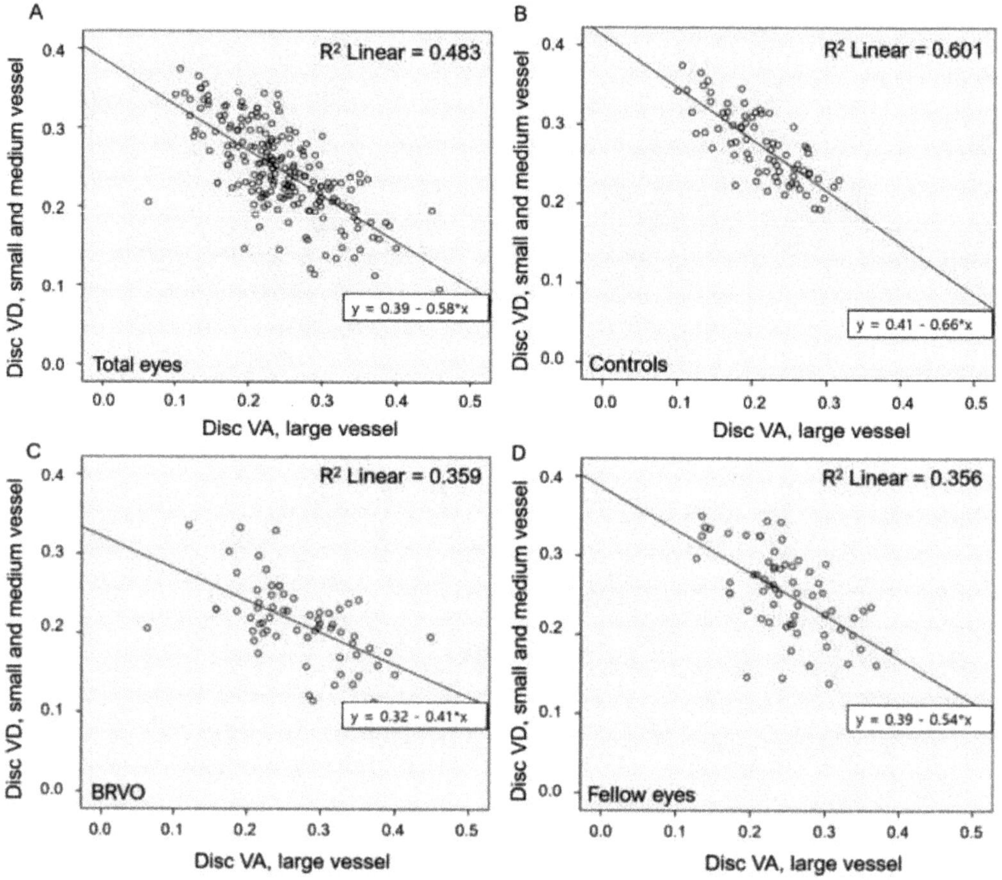

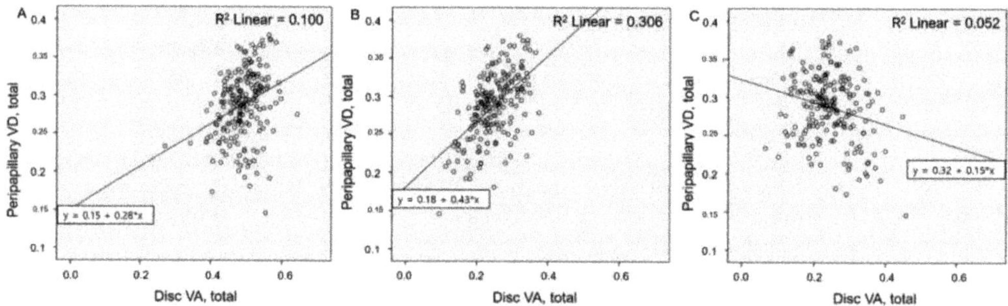

Figure 3. Correlations between large and small and medium vessel VDs in the optic disc area: (**A**) Large vessel VD correlated negatively with small and medium vessel VD; (**B–D**) This correlation remained consistent when patients were divided into groups.

Figure 4. Correlation between disc and peripapillary VDs: (**A,B**) Total and small and medium vessel VDs of the optic disc area were correlated positively with peripapillary VD; (**C**) Larger vessel VD of the optic disc area was correlated negatively with peripapillary VD.

Table 4. Correlation between vascular density and clinical parameters.

Vascular Desity		Age [a]	Sex [b]	DM [b]	HBP [b]	CVD [b]	BCVA [a]
Disc total VD	Coefficient	−0.076	−0.076	−0.038	0.090	0.043	−0.147 *
	p-value	0.274	0.274	0.582	0.196	0.533	0.034
Disc small and medium VD	Coefficient	−0.305 *	−0.058	−0.204 *	−0.111	−0.019	−0.237 *
	p-value	0.000	0.409	0.003	0.111	0.790	0.001
Disc Large VD	Coefficient	0.163 *	0.023	0.096	0.135	0.041	0.159 *
	p-value	0.019	0.738	0.171	0.054	0.558	0.023
Peripapillary VD	Coefficient	−0.206 *	0.125	−0.112	−0.018	0.022	−0.311 *
	p-value	0.003	0.073	0.110	0.799	0.757	0.000
Peripapillary VD ST	Coefficient	−0.198 *	0.102	−0.161 *	−0.070	−0.042	−0.270 *
	p-value	0.004	0.146	0.021	0.320	0.552	0.000
Peripapillary VD SN	Coefficient	−0.166 *	0.038	−0.010	0.134	0.001	−0.319 *
	p-value	0.017	0.585	0.884	0.055	0.989	0.000
Peripapillary VD IN	Coefficient	−0.146 *	0.081	−0.087	−0.053	0.069	−0.244 *
	p-value	0.037	0.247	0.212	0.453	0.326	0.000
Peripapillary VD IT	Coefficient	−0.145 *	0.139 *	−0.128	−0.128	0.043	−0.204 *
	p-value	0.038	0.047	0.066	0.068	0.540	0.003

Vascular Desity		Refractive Error [a]	Axial Length [a]	IOP [a]	RNFL Thickness [a]	VF Mean Deviation [a]	Disc Hemorrhage [b]
Disc total VD	Coefficient	0.176 *	−0.211 *	−0.088	0.105	0.183 *	0.016
	p-value	0.011	0.002	0.207	0.132	0.008	0.821
Disc small and medium VD	Coefficient	−0.218 *	0.169 *	−0.047	−0.005	0.109	0.069
	p-value	0.002	0.015	0.505	0.940	0.118	0.326
Disc Large VD	Coefficient	0.236 *	−0.242 *	0.031	0.025	−0.028	−0.060
	p-value	0.001	0.000	0.654	0.716	0.695	0.393
Peripapillary VD	Coefficient	0.034	−0.065	−0.039	0.247 *	0.277 *	0.027
	p-value	0.630	0.356	0.581	0.000	0.000	0.697
Peripapillary VD ST	Coefficient	−0.015	−0.030	−0.044	0.114	0.234 *	0.116
	p-value	0.832	0.668	0.531	0.104	0.001	0.096
Peripapillary VD SN	Coefficient	0.032	−0.037	−0.007	0.254 *	0.162 *	0.057
	p-value	0.646	0.596	0.922	0.000	0.020	0.414
Peripapillary VD IN	Coefficient	0.054	−0.049	−0.029	0.176 *	0.233 *	−0.016
	p-value	0.437	0.486	0.682	0.011	0.001	0.825
Peripapillary VD IT	Coefficient	0.086	−0.092	−0.047	0.208 *	0.256 *	−0.076
	p-value	0.221	0.189	0.505	0.003	0.000	0.275

DM: diabetes mellitus; HTN: hypertension; CVD: cardio- or cerebrovascular disease; BCVA: best-corrected visual acuity; IOP: intraocular pressure; RNFL: retinal nerve fiber layer; VF: visual field; VD: vascular density; ST: superotemporal; SN: superonasal; IN: inferonasal; IT: inferotemporal. [a] Spearman rank correlation. [b] Logistic regression. * $P < 0.01$ (two-tailed).

4. Discussion

An understanding of hemodynamic changes in the optic disc area may yield valuable insights into the pathogenesis of NTG and BRVO. OCTA enables the noninvasive visualization of vessels in the retina and optic disc as well as the quantification of vessel parameters, thus imparting detailed information regarding hemodynamic changes associated with disease. Here, we quantitatively analyzed the VDs of optic disc vessels evident in OCTA images of eyes with NTG, according to their BRVO status; we compared these findings between and among groups. We found differences in the VDs of the optic disc and peripapillary area between eyes with NTG, according to their BRVO status; we also found correlations between the VDs of the large and small and medium vessels in the disc and peripapillary area. Our principal findings were that BRVO was associated with enhanced large vessel VD and reduced small and medium vessel VD in the optic disc. This was evident in both eyes with BRVO and fellow eyes. Furthermore, the large vessel and small and medium vessel VDs differed significantly between fellow eyes with NTG alone and control eyes, suggesting that such changes may contribute to NTG development in patients with BRVO. Peripapillary VD was significantly reduced only in eyes with NTG + BRVO, suggesting that the change may be attributable to BRVO.

The contributions of large and small and medium vessels to the disc VD differed between eyes with NTG, according to their BRVO status. In NTG patients with BRVO, the mean VD of large vessels was higher, whereas the mean VD of small and medium vessels was lower. As factors that might affect disc vasculature (e.g., age, comorbid diabetes, refractive error, and axial length; Table 4) were comparable among the groups, our interpretation may be valid. Considering the negative correlation between large and small and medium vessel densities observed in the current study, the engorgement of large vessels (especially veins) may be followed by the attenuation of small and medium vessels in eyes with BRVO. The peripapillary VDs were also lower in eyes with BRVO. The optic disc head occupies a limited space; thus, the enhanced large vessel volume caused by congestion may trigger the mechanical compression of small and medium vessels. However, the details of this underlying mechanism requires further investigation.

The fellow eyes in patients with BRVO exhibited a greater large vessel VD and a lower small and medium vessel VD compared to the control eyes, suggesting that underlying systemic factors affect both eyes in patients with BRVO. Hypertension is a possible contributing factor: this demographic differed between patients with BRVO and the control group. In a previous study, we showed that patients with BRVO exhibited more rapid glaucoma progression in their fellow eyes compared to patients with glaucoma who did not develop BRVO [22]. The difference in fellow eye hemodynamics between patients with BRVO and the control group, observed in the present study, might be relevant in this context.

Here, we also found that the fellow eyes of patients with BRVO exhibited a significantly lower small and medium vessel VD in the optic disc, compared with the control eyes. The peripapillary VD parameters did not differ between the fellow eyes in the patients with BRVO and the control eyes, suggesting that a small and medium vessel VD change in the optic disc may accelerate glaucoma progression in the glaucomatous fellow eyes of patients with BRVO [19]. Systemic factors may trigger changes in the disc VDs of both eyes, thereby increasing the proportion of large vessels in patients who develop BRVO, followed by more prominent changes. As this was a cross-sectional study, we could not determine whether the phenomenon was a cause or a result of BRVO.

Blood flows from two principal sources to the optic disc. The superficial layers of the optic nerve head (i.e., the RNFL) are supplied by the central retinal artery; the deeper layers (i.e., the prelaminar, lamina cribrosa, and retrolaminar regions) are supplied by the posterior ciliary artery [23]. Analysis of these respective layers would yield detailed information regarding whether the observed changes reflect alterations in the branches of the central retinal or posterior ciliary arteries. However, the resolution of the current OCTA systems is inadequate for such analysis; it may be achieved in the future by using more powerful angiographic imaging systems.

The peripapillary VDs of the entire region and all four quadrants were lower in eyes with BRVO than in fellow eyes and controls, consistent with the results of a previous study by Shin et al. [24]. Notably, Shin et al. reported that various peripapillary microvascular parameters were lower in the fellow eyes of patients with RVO. Most of the vessels visible on OCTA scans of the peripapillary area are retinal radial peripapillary capillaries [25]. These radial peripapillary capillaries branch from the central retinal artery; thus, a lower peripapillary VD can be largely explained by a reduction of perfusion from the central retinal artery, perhaps attributable to the venous engorgement of eyes with BRVO and the negative correlation between the large vessel VD of the optic disc and the peripapillary VD, despite the weak correlation. However, this may be less important than in the optic disc area, as the peripapillary area is not a limited space. Other possible causes of reduced central retinal artery perfusion include capillary attenuation attributable to vasospasm, atherosclerosis, or shunting.

Our study had the limitations inherent to all cross-sectional retrospective analyses. Systemic factors which are suspected to alter VD, such as blood pressure, were not available due to the retrospective nature of the study. As mentioned above, we could not investigate causal relationships between vessel changes and disease development; we showed only that hemodynamic changes are evident. However, to the best of our knowledge, this study was the first to quantitatively analyze disc vessel density in eyes with NTG, according to their BRVO status. As hemodynamic factors play important pathophysiological roles in both NTG and BRVO, we believe that these results deepen our understanding of the pathogenesis of both diseases. Additionally, although there may be a small chance of inaccurate vessel separation due to the inherent errors of the OCTA system, each step in the VD measurement method used in this study was automatized, therefore yielding high repeatability and reproducibility.

In conclusion, we measured the VDs of the optic disc area of eyes with NTG, according to their BRVO status; in eyes with BRVO, we revealed the enhancement of large vessel VD and reduction of small and medium vessel VD as well as the reduction of peripapillary VD. The large vessel VD was significantly enhanced and the small and medium vessel VD was significantly reduced in fellow eyes (with NTG alone) in patients with BRVO, suggesting that hemodynamic changes may be involved in the progression of NTG or BRVO in these patients. Our results suggest that the hemodynamics around the disc area differ in eyes with NTG, according to their BRVO status, and may be associated with disease development or progression. Prospective follow-up studies with larger samples are required to confirm our findings.

Author Contributions: Contributions were as follows: J.B.: conception and design of the study, writing manuscript text, preparing figures, collection and assembly of data, and data analysis and interpretation; S.-J.J. and J.-H.K.: collection of data; C.-K.P.: conception and design of the study and supervision; H.-Y.L.P.: conception and design of the study, writing manuscript text, preparing figures, collection and assembly of data, data analysis and interpretation, and supervision; All authors reviewed the manuscript. All authors have read and agreed to the published version of the manuscript.

Funding: This research received no external funding.

Institutional Review Board Statement: The study was conducted according to the guidelines of the Declaration of Helsinki, and approved by the Institutional Review Board of Seoul St.Mary's Hospital (KC18RESI0852).

Informed Consent Statement: This study waived the requirement for written informed consent because of the retrospective nature of the study.

Data Availability Statement: The datasets generated and/or analyzed during the current study are available from the corresponding author upon reasonable request.

Conflicts of Interest: The authors declare no competing interests.

Abbreviations

VD	vascular density
NTG	normal-tension glaucoma
RVO	retinal vein occlusion
BRVO	branch retinal vein occlusion
IOP	intraocular pressure
OCTA	optical coherence tomography angiography
VF	visual field
ST	superotemporal
SN	superonasal
IN	inferonasal
IT	inferotemporal

References

1. David, R.; Zangwill, L.; Badarna, M.; Yassur, Y. Epidemiology of retinal vein occlusion and its association with glaucoma and increased intraocular pressure. *Ophthalmologica* **1988**, *197*, 69–74. [CrossRef]

2. Rath, E.Z.; Frank, R.N.; Shin, D.H.; Kim, C. Risk factors for retinal vein occlusions. A case-control study. *Ophthalmology* **1992**, *99*, 509–514. [CrossRef]

3. Klein, R.; Klein, B.E.; Moss, S.E.; Meuer, S.M. The epidemiology of retinal vein occlusion: The Beaver Dam Eye Study. *Trans. Am. Ophthalmol. Soc.* **2000**, *98*, 133–141.

4. Beaumont, P.E.; Kang, H.K. Cup-to-disc ratio, intraocular pressure, and primary open-angle glaucoma in retinal venous occlusion. *Ophthalmology* **2002**, *109*, 282–286. [CrossRef]

5. Hayreh, S.S.; Zimmerman, M.B.; Beri, M.; Podhajsky, P. Intraocular pressure abnormalities associated with central and hemicentral retinal vein occlusion. *Ophthalmology* **2004**, *111*, 133–141. [CrossRef] [PubMed]

6. Klein, B.E.; Meuer, S.M.; Knudtson, M.D.; Klein, R. The relationship of optic disk cupping to retinal vein occlusion: The Beaver Dam Eye Study. *Am. J. Ophthalmol.* **2006**, *141*, 859–862. [CrossRef]

7. Xu, K.; Wu, L.; Ma, Z.; Liu, Y.; Qian, F. Primary angle closure and primary angle closure glaucoma in retinal vein occlusion. *Acta Ophthalmol.* **2019**, *97*, e364–e372. [CrossRef] [PubMed]

8. Kida, T.; Fukumoto, M.; Sato, T.; Oku, H.; Ikeda, T. Clinical Features of Japanese Patients with Central Retinal Vein Occlusion Complicated by Normal-Tension Glaucoma: A Retrospective Study. *Ophthalmologica* **2017**, *237*, 173–179. [CrossRef] [PubMed]

9. Barnett, E.M.; Fantin, A.; Wilson, B.S.; Kass, M.A.; Gordon, M.O. Ocular Hypertension Treatment Study Group. The incidence of retinal vein occlusion in the ocular hypertension treatment study. *Ophthalmology* **2010**, *117*, 484–488. [CrossRef] [PubMed]

10. Flammer, J.; Pache, M.; Resink, T. Vasospasm, its role in the pathogenesis of diseases with particular reference to the eye. *Prog. Retin. Eye Res.* **2001**, *20*, 319–349. [CrossRef]

11. Sin, B.H.; Song, B.J.; Park, S.P. Aqueous vascular endothelial growth factor and endothelin-1 levels in branch retinal vein occlusion associated with normal tension glaucoma. *J. Glaucoma* **2013**, *22*, 104–109. [CrossRef] [PubMed]

12. Yoo, Y.C.; Park, K.H. Disc hemorrhages in patients with both normal tension glaucoma and branch retinal vein occlusion in different eyes. *Korean J. Ophthalmol.* **2007**, *21*, 222–227. [CrossRef] [PubMed]

13. Wang, X.; Jiang, C.; Ko, T.; Kong, X.; Yu, X.; Min, W.; Shi, G.; Sun, X. Correlation between optic disc perfusion and glaucomatous severity in patients with open-angle glaucoma: An optical coherence tomography angiography study. *Graefes Arch. Clin. Exp. Ophthalmol.* **2015**, *253*, 1557–1564. [CrossRef] [PubMed]

14. Akagi, T.; Iida, Y.; Nakanishi, H.; Terada, N.; Morooka, S.; Yamada, H.; Hasegawa, T.; Yokota, S.; Yoshikawa, M.; Yoshimura, N. Microvascular Density in Glaucomatous Eyes with Hemifield Visual Field Defects: An Optical Coherence Tomography Angiography Study. *Am. J. Ophthalmol.* **2016**, *168*, 237–249. [CrossRef] [PubMed]

15. Toshev, A.P.; Schuster, A.K.; Ul Hassan, S.N.; Pfeiffer, N.; Hoffmann, E.M. Optical Coherence Tomography Angiography of Optic Disc in Eyes with Primary Open-angle Glaucoma and Normal-tension Glaucoma. *J. Glaucoma* **2019**, *28*, 243–251. [CrossRef] [PubMed]

16. Yarmohammadi, A.; Zangwill, L.M.; Diniz-Filho, A.; Suh, M.H.; Manalastas, P.I.; Fatehee, N.; Yousefi, S.; Belghith, A.; Saunders, L.J.; Medeiros, F.A.; et al. Optical Coherence Tomography Angiography Vessel Density in Healthy, Glaucoma Suspect, and Glaucoma Eyes. *Investig. Ophthalmol. Vis. Sci.* **2016**, *57*, OCT451–OCT459. [CrossRef]

17. Woo, J.M.; Cha, J.B.; Lee, C.K. Comparison of lamina cribrosa properties and the peripapillary vessel density between branch retinal vein occlusion and normal-tension glaucoma. *PLoS ONE* **2020**, *15*, e0240109. [CrossRef]

18. Miguel, A.I.M.; Silva, A.B.; Azevedo, L.F. Diagnostic performance of optical coherence tomography angiography in glaucoma: A systematic review and meta-analysis. *Br. J. Ophthalmol.* **2019**, *103*, 1677–1684. [CrossRef]

19. Yarmohammadi, A.; Zangwill, L.M.; Diniz-Filho, A.; Suh, M.H.; Yousefi, S.; Saunders, L.J.; Belghith, A.; Manalastas, P.I.; Medeiros, F.A.; Weinreb, R.N. Relationship between Optical Coherence Tomography Angiography Vessel Density and Severity of Visual Field Loss in Glaucoma. *Ophthalmology* **2016**, *123*, 2498–2508. [CrossRef] [PubMed]

20. Moghimi, S.; Zangwill, L.M.; Penteado, R.C.; Hasenstab, K.; Ghahari, E.; Hou, H.; Christopher, M.; Yarmohammadi, A.; Manalastas, P.I.C.; Shoji, T.; et al. Macular and Optic Nerve Head Vessel Density and Progressive Retinal Nerve Fiber Layer Loss in Glaucoma. *Ophthalmology* **2018**, *125*, 1720–1728. [CrossRef]

21. Park, H.Y.; Shin, D.Y.; Jeon, S.J.; Park, C.K. Association Between Parapapillary Choroidal Vessel Density Measured with Optical Coherence Tomography Angiography and Future Visual Field Progression in Patients with Glaucoma. *JAMA Ophthalmol.* **2019**, *137*, 681–688. [CrossRef] [PubMed]

22. Lopilly Park, H.Y.; Jeon, S.; Lee, M.Y.; Park, C.K. Glaucoma Progression in the Unaffected Fellow Eye of Glaucoma Patients Who Developed Unilateral Branch Retinal Vein Occlusion. *Am. J. Ophthalmol.* **2017**, *175*, 194–200. [CrossRef] [PubMed]

23. Hayreh, S.S. Blood supply of the optic nerve head and its role in optic atrophy, glaucoma, and oedema of the optic disc. *Br. J. Ophthalmol.* **1969**, *53*, 721–748. [CrossRef] [PubMed]

24. Shin, Y.I.; Nam, K.Y.; Lee, S.E.; Lim, H.B.; Lee, M.W.; Jo, Y.J.; Kim, J.Y. Changes in Peripapillary Microvasculature and Retinal Thickness in the Fellow Eyes of Patients with Unilateral Retinal Vein Occlusion: An OCTA Study. *Investig. Ophthalmol. Vis. Sci.* **2019**, *60*, 823–829. [CrossRef] [PubMed]

25. Jia, Y.; Wei, E.; Wang, X.; Zhang, X.; Morrison, J.C.; Parikh, M.; Lombardi, L.H.; Gattey, D.M.; Armour, R.L.; Edmunds, B.; et al. Optical coherence tomography angiography of optic disc perfusion in glaucoma. *Ophthalmology* **2014**, *121*, 1322–1332. [CrossRef] [PubMed]

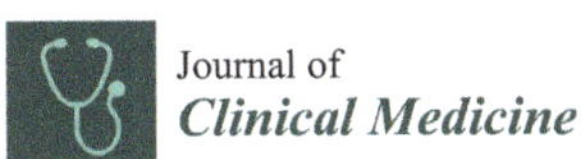

Journal of
Clinical Medicine

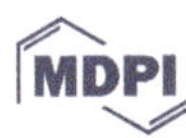

Article

Vessel Density Loss of the Deep Peripapillary Area in Glaucoma Suspects and Its Association with Features of the Lamina Cribrosa

Soo-Ji Jeon [1], Hae-Young Lopilly Park [2] and Chan-Kee Park [2,*]

[1] Apgujeong St. Mary's Eye Center, 859 Eonju-ro, Gangnam-gu, Seoul 06023, Korea; sj8801@gmail.com
[2] Department of Ophthalmology, Seoul St. Mary's Hospital, College of Medicine,
     The Catholic University of Korea, 222 Banpo-daero, Seocho-gu, Seoul 06591, Korea; lopilly@catholic.ac.kr
*   Correspondence: ckpark@catholic.ac.kr; Tel.: +82-2-2258-1188; Fax: +82-2-599-7405

Abstract: Purpose: To investigate the association of decreased vessel density (VD) in the deep peripapillary region and structural features of the lamina cribrosa (LC). Materials and Methods: 70 eyes of glaucoma suspects with enlarged cup-to-disc ratio were scanned and 51 eyes with adequate image quality were included in this study. All subjects had localized VD defects in the deep layer but intact VD in the superficial layer around the peripapillary region using optical coherence tomography angiography (OCTA). Only single-hemizone OCTA results from one eye of each subject had to fulfill the distinctive feature mentioned above to perform inter-eye and inter-hemizone comparisons. The thickness and depth of the LC, and prelaminar thickness were measured using enhanced depth imaging OCT (EDI-OCT). Paired t-tests were performed to evaluate differences in measurements of the LC and prelaminar thickness within each individual. *p*-values lower than 0.05 was considered to be statistically significant. Results: Eyes with deep VD defects in the peripapillary region in OCTA had thinner LC than the fellow eyes. The hemizone with the deep VD defects in the peripapillary region had a thinner LC and a deeper depth of LC than the other hemizone in the same eye. According to logistic regression analysis, a thin LC was a significant factor associated with deep VD defect in the peripapillary region. Conclusions: Glaucoma suspect eyes with deep VD defects in the peripapillary area exhibited structural differences in the LC. The structural changes of the LC was associated with the vessel density in the deep peripapillary layer at the stage of suspected glaucoma.

Keywords: glaucoma suspect; lamina cribrosa; optical coherence tomography angiography; peripapillary vessel density

Citation: Jeon, S.-J.; Park, H.-Y.L.; Park, C.-K. Vessel Density Loss of the Deep Peripapillary Area in Glaucoma Suspects and Its Association with Features of the Lamina Cribrosa. *J. Clin. Med.* **2021**, *10*, 2373. https://doi.org/10.3390/jcm10112373

Academic Editor: Jose Javier Garcia-Medina

Received: 31 March 2021
Accepted: 25 May 2021
Published: 28 May 2021

Publisher's Note: MDPI stays neutral with regard to jurisdictional claims in published maps and institutional affiliations.

1. Introduction

The pathogenesis of glaucoma has been studied continuously, and a number of hypotheses have been proposed to explain glaucomatous damage of retinal ganglion cells (RGCs). The hypotheses have largely been based on two main theories—structural theory and vascular theory [1,2]. According to structural theory, deformation of the lamina cribrosa (LC) is the presumed site of glaucoma-related neural damage. LC compression and the resultative focal LC defects have been reported to be the important structural changes of glaucoma, and associated visual field (VF) and retinal nerve fiber layer (RNFL) loss were noticeable [3,4]. However, the interest of vascular dysregulation has also been investigated consistently as a factor preceding or coinciding with the onset of glaucoma and its progression [5–9].

Owing to recent advances in optical coherence tomography angiography (OCTA), reproducible and non-invasive methods of vascular status measurement are now widely used [10]. The automated layer segmentation allows for en-face imaging of deep vascular details of the macula and peripapillary area, layer by layer, to choroid [11–13].

When analyzing OCTA results by layer, the microvasculature of the superficial retinal layer mainly includes the RNFL, ganglion cell and inner plexiform layer (GCIPL).

145

Glaucomatous damage occurs in the RNFL and ganglion cell layer (GCL); therefore, it is difficult to suggest that decreased vessel density (VD) in the superficial layer could have a causative or resultant relationship with RGC loss. On the other hand, the deep retinal layer including the inner nuclear layer (INL) is relatively less affected by glaucoma, and focusing on changes in vessel density of the deep retinal layer could be useful for monitoring microvasculature changes without the interference of retinal structural thinning in glaucoma patients. The previous studies of our research team have already reported the implications of vessel changes in the deep retinal layer of the macular region [14,15].

In the case of the peripapillary area, we hypothesized that these changes in the deep layer could be meaningful to observe alterations of vessel density without the interference from structural thinning, as occurs in the macula. Sung et al. reported that the peripapillary microvasculature of the deep layer was related to the structural characteristics of optic nerve head (ONH) such as tilt and rotation in myopia [16]. In addition, we detected that there were some patients with localized vessel density defects in the deep layer but intact VD in the superficial layer of peripapillary area among glaucoma suspect subjects in our clinic. These cases raised questions about how deep peripapillary vessel was altered in glaucoma suspect with intact superficial flow.

Therefore, the purpose of this study was to investigate the clinical features to having deep peripapillary VD defects in glaucoma suspect. To minimize the effects of systemic factors on both eyes, we performed inter-eye and intra-eye comparisons.

2. Materials and Methods

2.1. Study Design and Population

This cross-sectional study was performed according to the tenets of the Declaration of Helsinki and was approved by the Institutional Review and Ethics Boards of Seoul St. Mary's Hospital, South Korea. The need for written informed consent was waived by our Review Board. We included 70 subjects with a diagnosis of glaucoma suspect from Seoul St. Mary's Hospital between January 2018 and February 2020.

All subjects underwent comprehensive ophthalmic examinations as in previous OCTA related studies [15]. Examinations included best-corrected visual acuity (BCVA), slit-lamp examination, Goldmann applanation tonometry, gonioscopy, and dilated fundus biomicroscopy. Color fundus and red-free RNFL photographs were obtained with a nonmydriatic retinal camera (Canon, Tokyo, Japan), and standard automated perimetry (SAP) using the Swedish interactive threshold standard algorithm (SITA) 24-2 program (Humphrey Visual Field Analyzer; Carl Zeiss Meditec, Dublin, CA, USA), circumpapillary retinal nerve fiber layer (cpRNFL) and macular GCIPL (mGCIPL) thicknesses were obtained by DRI OCT (Topcon, Tokyo, Japan) for diagnosis of glaucoma suspect. A history of diabetes, hypertension or cerebrovascular disease was documented, and symptoms of hemodynamic instability such as migraine or cold extremities were also recorded. All subjects had open angles on gonioscopy, BCVA of 20/40 or better and intraocular pressure (IOP) of 21 mmHg or lower.

Glaucoma suspect in this study was defined as having normal RNFL thickness in OCT results with only a vertical C/D ratio $\geq$ 0.5 or asymmetric optic discs in both eyes (asymmetry of C/D ratio between two eyes $\geq$ 0.2 that was not caused by the difference in optic disc size or shape). Each photograph was reviewed by two independent glaucoma specialists (SJJ and HYP). In case of disagreement of judgement, a senior reviewer (CKP) adjudicated. RNFL thickness was considered to be normal if it was within 95% of the values within the internally embedded database of healthy, age-matched normal population and it was marked in the green color sector of the temporal-superior-nasal-inferior-temporal (TSNIT) graph. Glaucoma hemifield test results of glaucoma suspect were within normal limits based on a minimum of two reliable visual field measures.

Patients were excluded if they met any of the following criteria: (1) a history of non-glaucomatous optic neuropathy; (2) a history of eye trauma or surgery except for uncomplicated cataract extraction; (3) pathologic myopia (chorioretinal atrophy, intra-choroidal cavitation, choroidal neovascularization, lacquer crack) (4) other retinal diseases including diabetic retinopathy and retinal vascular diseases such as vascular occlusion or uveitis.

2.2. Identification of Study Subjects with VD Defects in the Deep Peripapillary Area Using OCTA

OCTA images were acquired through DRI OCT Triton system (Topcon, Tokyo, Japan) using a swept source laser with a wavelength of 1050 nm and a raster scan protocol. OCTA is based on Topcon OCT angiography ratio analysis (OCTARA) algorithm that could improve the detection of low blood flow by combining ratio analysis from different scanning intervals [17]. An active eye tracker was used to reduce motion artifact during imaging. In the peripapillary region, automated layer segmentation was performed. For the imaging of superficial peripapillary microvasculature, the radial peripapillary capillary segment extending from the internal limiting membrane (ILM) to the RNFL was analyzed. For the imaging of deep peripapillary microvasculature, the embedded segmentation program demarcated the boundary line from 130 μm below the ILM to 390 μm below the basement membrane including the INL, outer plexiform layer (OPL), outer nuclear layer (ONL), and choroid. Highly myopic eyes with a spherical equivalent < −12.0 D or staphyloma were excluded for clear image acquisition around the ONH. The images with image quality scores over 70 were selected.

From OCTA images, we identified the study subjects with VD defects in the deep layer of peripapillary area but with intact superficial VD. Figure 1 represents the subjects meeting these criteria. Systemic vascular factors could function as a confounding factor in assessing the relationship between peripapillary vessel density and the structural change of LC. Therefore, in order to minimize the influence of the systemic factors, we included only subjects with decreased deep peripapillary VD in one eye and normal VD in the opposite eye to perform inter-eye comparison in one subject and inter-hemizone comparison in one eye.

2.3. Lamina Cribrosa Measurements Using Enhanced Depth Imaging OCT

Lamina cribrosa imaging was performed using enhanced depth imaging OCT (EDI-OCT) device (Heidelberg Engineering, Heidelberg, Germany). Radial 2D b-scans centered on the optic disc were obtained with the Heidelberg Spectralis OCT (Spectralis software version 5.1.1.0, Eye Explorer Software 1.6.1.0) using a wavelength of 870 nm providing up to 40,000 A scans/sec, with a depth resolution of 7 μm and a transversal resolution of 14 μm.

The detailed measurement of the lamina cribrosa and prelaminar thickness using EDI-OCT was performed as described previously [18,19]. The thickness and depth of the LC were measured at three different locations; mid-superior, central, and mid-inferior. The LC thickness was defined as the distance between the anterior and posterior borders of the highly reflective region at the vertical center of the ONH in the horizontal cross-sectional B-scans. For LC depth and prelaminar thickness measurements, we drew a reference line connecting both ends of Bruch's membrane opening. A perpendicular line was drawn from the center of the reference line to the anterior border of LC in each B-scan, which we defined as LC depth. Similarly, the prelaminar thickness was measured along the perpendicular line from the anterior border of the reflective region to the anterior border of the highly reflective region, which is the anterior laminar border.

For inter-eye comparisons, the mean of the three measurements (mid-superior, central, and mid-inferior) was defined as the LC thickness, LC depth, and prelaminar thickness. For inter-hemizone comparisons within each eye, three locations of the same interval from each hemizone were measured and the mean of these three measurements was also used as the representative value.

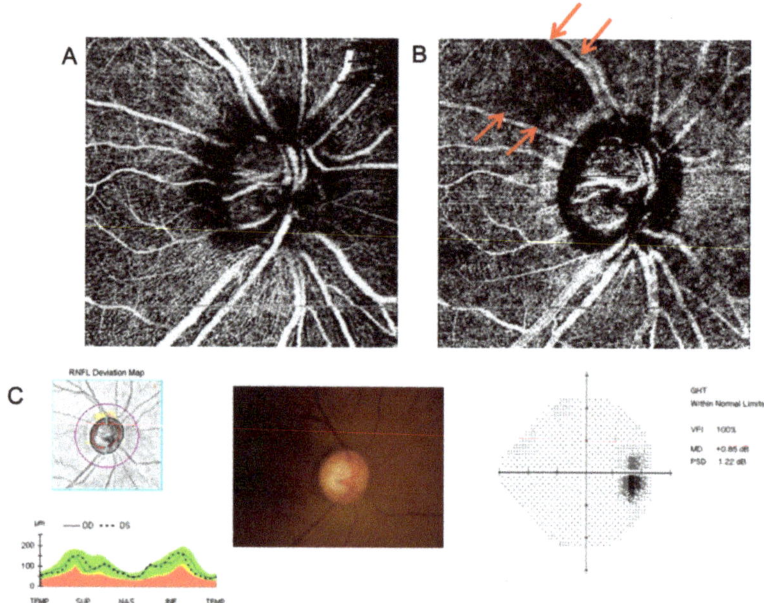

Figure 1. (**A**) Superficial peripapillary OCT angiography in the superficial layer (from the retinal nerve fiber layer (RNFL) to 130 μm below the internal limiting membrane (ILM) including the ganglion cell-inner plexiform (GCIPL) layer). (**B**) Deep peripapillary OCT angiography in the deep layer (from 130 μm below the ILM to the basement membrane including the inner nuclear layer (INL)). (**C**) RNFL OCT and visual field test with increased cup-disc ratio (CDR) which indicate glaucoma suspect. There are subjects among glaucoma suspect patients with wedge-shaped VD defect in the deep layer of peripapillary area (indicated as arrows in **B**), even though the vessel density in the superficial layer is unaffected (intact vascular status in **A**).

Two independent observers (SJJ and HYP) each repeated LC measurements, three times as mentioned above. The values of six results were averaged, and the mean value was used in the analyses. To assess interobserver and intraobserver reproducibility, intraclass correlation coefficient (ICC) was calculated from 15 randomly selected measurements. The interobserver ICC for LC thickness was 0.915, ICC for LC depth was 0.927, and ICC for prelaminar thickness was 0.894. In addition, intraobserver ICC showed excellent agreement of the LC and prelaminar thickness—ICC was 0.975, 0.988 and 0.971 for LC thickness, LC depth and prelaminar thickness, respectively.

Only images with quality scores > 20 were used, and when necessary, the images were re-examined. Each EDI scan included an average of 20 OCT frames; if more than three of the radial scans were unrecognizable, the eye was excluded. We excluded patients with lens opacity that could interfere image quality and localization of lower LC border.

2.4. VF Sensitivity and Macular Vessel Density

VF sensitivity was calculated as the mean value of the threshold in the pattern deviation map of SITA 24-2. Measurement of macular vessel density in OCTA using binary slab images were performed as described in previous studies [14,15,20]. In short, the binarized images created using ImageJ software (National Institutes of Health, Bethesda, MD, USA) were segmented into an area of interest and background after using the "adjust threshold" tool, which automatically sets the lower and upper threshold values. After the white pixels were designated as vessels and the black pixels as background, the vessel density was calculated as a percentage of the total area of the white pixels divided by the total pixel area of the image.

3. Statistical Analysis

All data are presented as means ± standard deviation. The interobserver and intraobserver agreements for LC measurements and prelaminar thickness were assessed by calculation of intraclass correlation coefficients (ICC). Paired t-tests were used for inter-eye and inter-hemizone comparisons of continuous variables. Chi-square tests were used to compare categorical variables between eyes. For logistic regression analyses, variables with p values < 0.3 in univariate analyses were included in the multivariate analysis. p value threshold of 0.1 could include only one variable in the multivariate analysis, we designated p value threshold of 0.3 to include multiple variables. All statistical analyses were performed with SPSS version 24.0 (IBM Corp., Armonk, NY, USA). $p < 0.05$ was considered to be statistically significant.

4. Results

This study initially included 70 subjects with a diagnosis of glaucoma suspect. Among them, there were 19 subjects with poor OCTA or EDI-OCT images that were subsequently excluded from our analyses. Table 1 described the baseline characteristics of study subjects. The number of eyes with a superior location of deep VD defects with our interest in OCTA was greater than those with an inferior location.

Table 1. Comparisons of baseline characteristics of study subjects ($n = 51$).

Age (years)	49.92 (±13.85)
Axial length (mm)	25.13 (±1.60)
Male:Female	21:30
Hypertension (%)	9 (17.64)
Diabetes (%)	4 (7.84)
Systemic vascular dysregulation (%) *	9 (17.64)
Right eye with deep VD defects (%)	14 (27.45)
Superior location of deep VD defects (%)	32 (62.74)

* Systemic vascular dysregulation included history of migraine, cold extremities, cerebrovascular problems, angina or arrhythmia.

Table 2 showed the inter-eye comparisons of study subjects. The eyes with VD defects in the deep peripapillary area had a thinner LC thickness than the fellow eyes with intact VD ($p < 0.001$). However, the cpRNFL thickness, mean deviation (MD) and mean sensitivity of VF were not statistically different.

Table 2. Comparisons between eyes with deep VD defects and fellow eyes without deep VD defects.

	Eyes with Deep VD Defects ($n = 51$)	Fellow Eyes without Deep VD Defects ($n = 51$)	p Value
Disc hemorrhage (%)	3 (5.88)	2 (3.92)	0.647
BCVA (decimal)	0.96 (±0.08)	0.93 (±0.13)	0.245
Intraocular pressure (mmHg)	16.69 (±4.48)	16.43 (±3.89)	0.760
Axial length (mm)	25.10 (±1.55)	25.17 (±1.66)	0.485
RNFL OCT variables			
cpRNFL thickness	89.25 (±8.73)	89.73 (±9.06)	0.790
Rim area	1.12 (±0.27)	1.07 (±0.22)	0.268
Disc area	2.17 (±0.51)	2.07 (±0.45)	0.309
Average C/D ratio	0.66 (±0.12)	0.67 (±0.11)	0.859
Vertical C/D ratio	0.63 (±0.12)	0.63 (±0.11)	0.986
Cup vlume	0.42 (±0.27)	0.41 (±0.25)	0.804

Representative cases are presented in Figures 3 and 4. The eyes of a 60-year-old woman with deep peripapillary VD defect in her left eye showed thinner LC compared with her unaffected right eye (Figure 3). In Figure 4, the left eye of a 47-year-old man showed deep peripapillary VD defect in the superotemporal region. The left EDI-OCT image was from the inferior half with an intact OCTA and the right image was from the superior half with deep VD defect. The LC thickness was thinner and LC depth was deeper in his superior hemizone than the inferior.

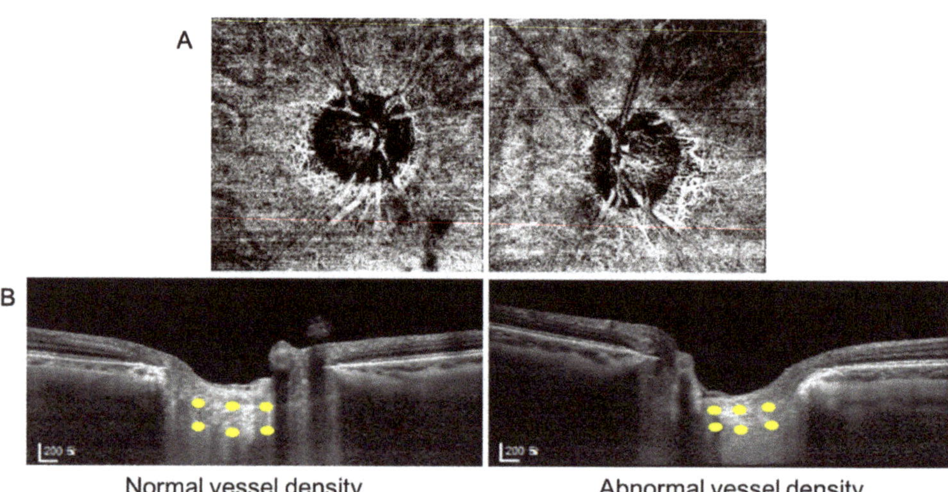

Figure 3. A representative case. (**A**) A 60-year old woman with decreased deep OCTA vessel density of peripapillary area in her left eye. (**B**) The thickness of lamina cribrosa in her left eye with abnormal vessel density was thinner than that in her right eye with normal vessel density.

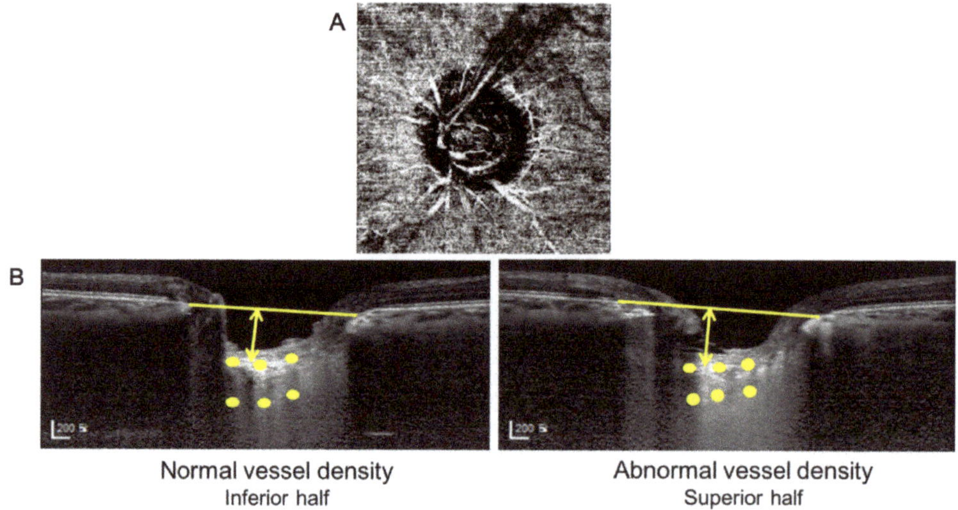

Figure 4. A representative case. (**A**) A 47-year old man with deep VD defect in his superotemporal peripapillary area of left eye. (**B**) The lamina cribrosa of his superior half was thinner and more deeply located than that of his inferior half.

5. Discussion

The present study started with the identification of altered vessel density from the deep peripapillary area including INL, OPL, ONL and choroid among glaucoma suspects. In these cases, the superficial peripapillary vessel density in the RNFL and GCL was intact with normal range of structural thickness of the layer. We tried to search for the distinctive clinical characteristics of those eyes compared to glaucoma suspect eyes without deep peripapillary vessel density alteration. Both structural and functional traits were investigated by comparing bilateral eyes of one subject. The reason we conducted the inter-eye and inter-hemizone comparisons was to minimize the effect of systemic conditions on the vessel density of the ONH.

Tepelus et al. previously suggested the decreased choroidal vascular parameters within the macula and ONH area in glaucoma patients compared with normal controls [21]. The OCTA changes of choriocapillaries located in the deep peripepillary area was called as microvascular dropout and have been focused in glaucoma [22–24]. Likewise, several studies have consistently asserted there should be a focus on the changes occurring in vessels in the deep layer of microvasculature in glaucoma [25–27]. Sung et al. reported that the deep peripapillary microvascular reduction was associated with structural characteristics of the optic disc, such as tilt in myopic eyes [16]. The differential mechanical strain near the ONH could affect the structure of the optic disc and peripapillary microvasculature, and consequently, might affect the eye's susceptibility to glaucoma development.

In the present study, the eyes with deep peripapillary VD defects had thinner LC than the fellow eye. In addition, the hemizone with abnormal deep peripapillary OCTA images showed not only thinner but had a more deeply located LC than the other hemizone. LC thickness was the factor associated with peripapillary VD defects in the deep layer. This finding was consistent with previous reports that structural characteristics of the optic disc were related with microvascular changes in the peripapillary area. To our knowledge, this is the first study investigating microvasculature alterations in glaucoma suspect to consider the changes occurring in the deep peripapillary layer as from the INL to the choroid.

While the mechanism explaining the association between changes in the LC and microvasculature change might not be definite, we have several hypotheses. First, eyes with thin LC may intrinsically have weak structure against mechanical strain on the optic disc. Structural weakness may be consistent in the extracellular matrix (ECM) of microvasculature. The weak ECM would interfere with capillary integrity [28] and, in accordance, could result in increased microvascular vulnerability to vascular dysregulation. Second, it is also possible that the retinal artery within the deep retina (INL, OPL and ONL) could be physically obliterated when the LC itself becomes compressed as a result of increased strain around the ONH. According to Prada et al. [29] the characteristics of the microvasculature around the ONH in the laminar and prelaminar region could affect the blood flow of the deep retina. In other words, strain over the ONH could subsequently effect the small microvasculature of the deep retina piercing the LC and flowing to the deep layer of peripapillary area. Since the vessels of the superficial retina are larger than those of the deep retina [30], it might be possible that only the microvascular change in the deep retina appeared before changes to the superficial retina could occur under the normal range of IOP with gentle strain. From our results, though not statistically significant, the deep macular vessel density of the hemizone with VD defect trended toward decrease compared with the other hemizone (42.71% vs. 45.29%, $p = 0.147$).

Our results also showed that the hemizone with deep VD defect had worse VF mean sensitivity than the unaffected other. Shin et al. previously reported that vessel density was associated with corresponding VF sensitivity [31]. From the study of Arend et al., altitudinal VF asymmetric defects were associated with the different circulation of retina in glaucoma patients [32]. According to Chen et al., reduced microcirculation was found even in the normal hemisphere of glaucoma patients [5]. These studies may partially support our finding of decreased VF sensitivity accompanying microvasculature changes. In the future, after several associated further studies, the deep VD changes could be used as a surrogate implying visual function alterations in glaucoma patients.

This study had several limitations. First, as a cross-sectional study, it was not possible to determine whether a causal relationship existed between structural changes of the LC and alterations in peripapillary vessel density. In the future, a longitudinal study including large populations with various cause and effect possibilities should be performed. Second, since we selected the well performed OCTA images of the deep peripapillary layer, it was mainly the eyes of the subjects who cooperated best with the data acquisition that were included in the analyses; these were mainly young and myopic eyes without lens opacity. It is necessary to study eyes with various age groups and axial lengths to ensure the generalized application of study results. Third, disc tilt could affect the measurements of lamina cribrosa. To minimize the possibility of image distortion, we used b-scan images of 1:1 μm for real measurements. Fourth, subjects with systemic disease such as diabetes or hypertension could have preclinical vascular alteration despite excluding patients with apparent retinopathy to minimize effect of systemic disease. In the future, studies with large populations, and the association between systemic disease and deep peripapillary vascular circulation should be studied. Finally, in this study, we restricted the subjects to those with glaucoma suspect for minimizing the effect of structural thinning of the retina on vascular obliteration. Nevertheless, the VF sensitivity of hemizone showed difference based on the presence of decreased vessel density in the deep peripapillary area. Though the results of this observational study might be a long way from clinical application, if the possibility of glaucoma development from glaucoma suspect is investigated through longitudinal study based on the results of this study, it might be possible to find a novel way of clinical application of OCTA on glaucoma development.

In conclusion, there were eyes with the diagnosis of glaucoma suspect exhibiting VD defect only in the deep layer of peripapillary area and not in the superficial layer. The regions with altered vessel density had different LC structure compared with the other regions. In other words, altered LC structure was associated with decreased vessel density in the deep peripapillary area in glaucoma suspect. Even at the stage of glaucoma suspect with intact RNFL, pre-clinical changes of vessel density accompanied with LC change were detected. Though the causal context between LC structure and vessel density change in the peripapillary area could not be demonstrated in this cross-sectional study, we speculated that the different pattern of lamina structure could affect the vascular status near the optic nerve head. The cause and effect relationship between LC structure and deep vessel density changes around the ONH should be investigated in future study. Further, the progression toward glaucoma from glaucoma suspect with VD defects, or, continuous VD defects change in glaucoma suspect should be studied using longitudinal study to identify the possibility of clinical application of deep VD defects.

Author Contributions: S.-J.J. wrote the main manuscript text. H.-Y.L.P. analyzed the data and prepared tables. C.-K.P. provided the main concept of the study and reviewed all the manuscript. All authors have read and agreed to the published version of the manuscript.

Funding: This research received no external funding.

Institutional Review Board Statement: This cross-sectional study was performed according to the tenets of the Declaration of Helsinki and was approved by the Institutional Review and Ethics Boards of Seoul St. Mary's Hospital, South Korea (protocol code KC21RCSI0368).

Informed Consent Statement: Patient consent was waived by our Review Board because this study was a retrospective chart review that involves no more than minimal risk to the subject and the waiver will not adversely affect the rights and welfare of the subjects.

Conflicts of Interest: The authors report no conflict of interest. The authors alone are responsible for the content and writing of the paper.

References

1. Weinreb, R.N.; Aung, T.; Medeiros, F.A. The pathophysiology and treatment of glaucoma: A review. *JAMA* **2014**, *311*, 1901–1911. [CrossRef]
2. Chan, K.K.W.; Tang, F.; Tham, C.C.Y.; Young, A.L.; Cheung, C.Y. Retinal vasculature in glaucoma: A review. *BMJ Open Ophthalmol.* **2017**, *1*, e000032. [CrossRef]
3. Quigley, H.A.; Addicks, E.M. Regional Differences in the Structure of the Lamina Cribrosa and Their Relation to Glaucomatous Optic Nerve Damage. *Arch. Ophthalmol.* **1981**, *99*, 137–143. [CrossRef]
4. Park, S.C.; Hsu, A.T.; Su, D.; Simonson, J.L.; Al-Jumayli, M.; Liu, Y.; Liebmann, J.M.; Ritch, R. Factors Associated with Focal Lamina Cribrosa Defects in Glaucoma. *Investig. Ophthalmol. Vis. Sci.* **2013**, *54*, 8401–8407. [CrossRef]
5. Chen, C.-L.; Bojikian, K.D.; Wen, J.C.; Zhang, Q.; Xin, C.; Mudumbai, R.C.; Johnstone, M.A.; Chen, P.P.; Wang, R.K. Peripapillary Retinal Nerve Fiber Layer Vascular Microcirculation in Eyes with Glaucoma and Single-Hemifield Visual Field Loss. *JAMA Ophthalmol.* **2017**, *135*, 461–468. [CrossRef]
6. Deokule, S.; Vizzeri, G.; Boehm, A.G.; Bowd, C.; Medeiros, F.A.; Weinreb, R.N. Correlation Among Choroidal, Parapapillary, and Retrobulbar Vascular Parameters in Glaucoma. *Am. J. Ophthalmol.* **2009**, *147*, 736–743. [CrossRef]
7. Moore, N.A.; Harris, A.; Wentz, S.; Vercellin, A.C.V.; Parekh, P.; Gross, J.; Hussain, R.M.; Thieme, C.; Siesky, B. Baseline retrobulbar blood flow is associated with both functional and structural glaucomatous progression after 4 years. *Br. J. Ophthalmol.* **2017**, *101*, 305–308. [CrossRef]
8. Grieshaber, M.C.; Flammer, J. Blood flow in glaucoma. *Curr. Opin. Ophthalmol.* **2005**, *16*, 79–83. [CrossRef] [PubMed]
9. Yanagi, M.; Kawasaki, R.; Wang, J.J.; Wong, T.Y.; Crowston, J.; Kiuchi, Y. Vascular risk factors in glaucoma: A review. *Clin. Exp. Ophthalmol.* **2011**, *39*, 252–258. [CrossRef]
10. Werner, A.C.; Shen, L.Q. A Review of OCT Angiography in Glaucoma. *Semin. Ophthalmol.* **2019**, *34*, 279–286. [CrossRef]
11. Spaide, R.F.; Klancnik, J.M., Jr.; Cooney, M.J. Retinal Vascular Layers Imaged by Fluorescein Angiography and Optical Coherence Tomography Angiography. *JAMA Ophthalmol.* **2015**, *133*, 45–50. [CrossRef]
12. Jia, Y.; Wei, E.; Wang, X.; Zhang, X.; Morrison, J.C.; Parikh, M.; Lombardi, L.H.; Gattey, D.M.; Armour, R.L.; Edmunds, B.; et al. Optical Coherence Tomography Angiography of Optic Disc Perfusion in Glaucoma. *Ophthalmology* **2014**, *121*, 1322–1332. [CrossRef]
13. Lommatzsch, C.; Rothaus, K.; Koch, J.M.; Heinz, C.; Grisanti, S. OCTA vessel density changes in the macular zone in glaucomatous eyes. *Graefe's Arch. Clin. Exp. Ophthalmol.* **2018**, *256*, 1499–1508. [CrossRef]
14. Jeon, S.J.; Park, H.-Y.L.; Park, C.K. Effect of Macular Vascular Density on Central Visual Function and Macular Structure in Glaucoma Patients. *Sci. Rep.* **2018**, *8*, 16009. [CrossRef] [PubMed]
15. Jeon, S.J.; Shin, D.-Y.; Park, H.-Y.L.; Park, C.K. Association of Retinal Blood Flow with Progression of Visual Field in Glaucoma. *Sci. Rep.* **2019**, *9*, 16813. [CrossRef]
16. Sung, M.S.; Lee, T.H.; Heo, H.; Park, S.W. Clinical features of superficial and deep peripapillary microvascular density in healthy myopic eyes. *PLoS ONE* **2017**, *12*, e0187160. [CrossRef]
17. Stanga, P.E.; Tsamis, E.; Papayannis, A.; Stringa, F.; Cole, T.; Jalil, A. Swept-Source Optical Coherence Tomography Angio™ (Topcon Corp, Japan): Technology Review. *Dev. Ophthalmol.* **2016**, *56*, 13–17.
18. Park, H.-Y.L.; Jeon, S.H.; Park, C.K. Enhanced Depth Imaging Detects Lamina Cribrosa Thickness Differences in Normal Tension Glaucoma and Primary Open-Angle Glaucoma. *Ophthalmology* **2012**, *119*, 10–20. [CrossRef]
19. Jung, Y.H.; Park, H.-Y.L.; Jung, K.I.; Park, C.K. Comparison of Prelaminar Thickness between Primary Open Angle Glaucoma and Normal Tension Glaucoma Patients. *PLoS ONE* **2015**, *10*, e0120634. [CrossRef]
20. Parodi, M.B.; Cicinelli, M.V.; Rabiolo, A.; Pierro, L.; Bolognesi, G.; Bandello, F. Vascular abnormalities in patients with Stargardt disease assessed with optical coherence tomography angiography. *Br. J. Ophthalmol.* **2017**, *101*, 780–785. [CrossRef]
21. Tepelus, T.C.; Song, S.; Borrelli, E.; Nittala, M.G.; Baghdasaryan, E.; Sadda, S.R.; Chopra, V. Quantitative Analysis of Retinal and Choroidal Vascular Parameters in Patients with Low Tension Glaucoma. *J. Glaucoma* **2019**, *28*, 557–562. [CrossRef] [PubMed]
22. Akagi, T.; Iida, Y.; Nakanishi, H.; Terada, N.; Morooka, S.; Yamada, H.; Hasegawa, T.; Yokota, S.; Yoshikawa, M.; Yoshimura, N. Microvascular Density in Glaucomatous Eyes with Hemifield Visual Field Defects: An Optical Coherence Tomography Angiography Study. *Am. J. Ophthalmol.* **2016**, *168*, 237–249. [CrossRef]
23. Lee, E.J.; Kim, T.W.; Kim, J.A.; Kim, J.A. Parapapillary Deep-Layer Microvasculature Dropout in Primary Open-Angle Glaucoma Eyes with a Parapapillary gamma-Zone. *Investig. Ophthalmol. Vis. Sci.* **2017**, *58*, 5673–5680. [CrossRef] [PubMed]
24. Park, H.-Y.L.; Jeon, S.J.; Park, C.K. Features of the Choroidal Microvasculature in Peripapillary Atrophy Are Associated with Visual Field Damage in Myopic Patients. *Am. J. Ophthalmol.* **2018**, *192*, 206–216. [CrossRef] [PubMed]
25. Suh, M.H.; Zangwill, L.M.; Manalastas, P.I.C.; Belghith, A.; Yarmohammadi, A.; Medeiros, F.A.; Diniz-Filho, A.; Saunders, L.J.; Weinreb, R.N. Deep Retinal Layer Microvasculature Dropout Detected by the Optical Coherence Tomography Angiography in Glaucoma. *Ophthalmology* **2016**, *123*, 2509–2518. [CrossRef] [PubMed]
26. Rao, H.L.; Pradhan, Z.S.; Suh, M.H.; Moghimi, S.; Mansouri, K.; Weinreb, R.N. Optical Coherence Tomography Angiography in Glaucoma. *J. Glaucoma* **2020**, *29*, 312–321. [CrossRef]
27. Liu, L.; Edmunds, B.; Takusagawa, H.L.; Tehrani, S.; Lombardi, L.H.; Morrison, J.C.; Jia, Y.; Huang, D. Projection-Resolved Optical Coherence Tomography Angiography of the Peripapillary Retina in Glaucoma. *Am. J. Ophthalmol.* **2019**, *207*, 99–109. [CrossRef] [PubMed]

28. Marchand, M.; Monnot, C.; Muller, L.; Germain, S. Extracellular matrix scaffolding in angiogenesis and capillary homeostasis. *Semin. Cell Dev. Biol.* **2019**, *89*, 147–156. [CrossRef]
29. Prada, D.; Harris, A.; Guidoboni, G.; Siesky, B.; Huang, A.M.; Arciero, J. Autoregulation and neurovascular coupling in the optic nerve head. *Surv. Ophthalmol.* **2016**, *61*, 164–186. [CrossRef]
30. Savastano, M.C.; Lumbroso, B.; Rispoli, M. In vivo characterization of retinal vascularization morphology using optical coherence tomography angiography. *Retina* **2015**, *35*, 2196–2203. [CrossRef]
31. Shin, J.W.; Lee, J.; Kwon, J.; Choi, J.; Kook, M.S. Regional vascular density–visual field sensitivity relationship in glaucoma according to disease severity. *Br. J. Ophthalmol.* **2017**, *101*, 1666–1672. [CrossRef] [PubMed]
32. Arend, O.; Remky, A.; Cantor, L.B.; Harris, A. Altitudinal visual field asymmetry is coupled with altered retinal circulation in patients with normal pressure glaucoma. *Br. J. Ophthalmol.* **2000**, *84*, 1008–1012. [CrossRef]

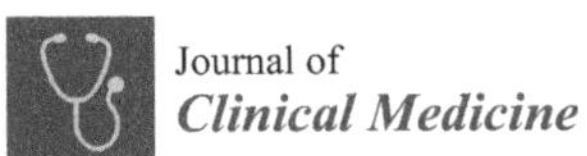

Journal of
Clinical Medicine

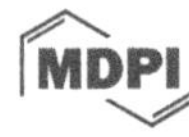

Article

miRNAs and Genes Involved in the Interplay between Ocular Hypertension and Primary Open-Angle Glaucoma. Oxidative Stress, Inflammation, and Apoptosis Networks

Jorge Raga-Cervera [1,†], Jose M. Bolarin [2,†], Jose M. Millan [3,†], Jose J. Garcia-Medina [4,5,6,7], Laia Pedrola [3], Javier Abellán-Abenza [2], Mar Valero-Vello [4], Silvia M. Sanz-González [4,7,8,*], José E. O'Connor [9], David Galarreta-Mira [10], Elena Bendala-Tufanisco [7,11,12], Aloma Mayordomo-Febrer [7,11,13], Maria D. Pinazo-Durán [4,8,‡] and Vicente Zanón-Moreno [4,7,14,‡]

[1] Hospital of Manises, 46940 Valencia, Spain; joracer22@gmail.com
[2] Technological Centre of Information and Communication Technologies (CENTIC), 30100 Murcia, Spain; josemiguel.bolarin@centic.es (J.M.B.); javier.abellan@centic.es (J.A.-A.)
[3] Sequencing Service at the University and Polytechnic Hospital La Fe, 46026 Valencia, Spain; millan_jos@gva.es (J.M.M.); sequencing_service@iislafe.es (L.P.)
[4] Ophthalmic Research Unit "Santiago Grisolía"/FISABIO, 46017 Valencia, Spain; jj.garciamedina@um.es (J.J.G.-M.); vavema@alumni.uv.es (M.V.-V.); dolores.pinazo@uv.es (M.D.P.-D.); vczanon@universidadviu.com (V.Z.-M.)
[5] Department of Ophthalmology, General University Hospital "Morales Meseguer", 30007 Murcia, Spain
[6] Department of Ophthalmology and Optometry, University of Murcia, 30120 Murcia, Spain
[7] Spanish Net of Ophthalmic Research OFTARED RD16/0008/0022, Institute of Health Carlos III, 28029 Madrid, Spain; elena.bendala@uch.ceu.es (E.B.-T.); aloma.mayordomo@uch.ceu.es (A.M.-F.)
[8] Cellular and Molecular Ophthalmobiology Group, Department of Surgery, Faculty of Medicine and Odontology, University of Valencia, 46010 Valencia, Spain
[9] Laboratory of Cytomics, Joint Research Unit Principe Felipe Research Center and University of Valencia, 46010 Valencia, Spain; jose.e.oconnor@uv.es
[10] University Clinic Hospital of Valladolid, 47003 Valladolid, Spain; dgalarreta@saludcastillayleon.es
[11] Mixed Research Unit for Visual Health and Veterinary Ophthalmology CEU/FISABIO, 46020 Valencia, Spain
[12] Physiology Department, Faculty of Health Sciences, CEU University, Alfara del Patriarca, 46115 Valencia, Spain
[13] Animal Medicine and Surgery Department, Veterinary Medicine Faculty, CEU University, Alfara del Patriarca, 46115 Valencia, Spain
[14] Faculty of Health Sciences, Valencian International University, 46002 Valencia, Spain
[*] Correspondence: silsanz5@ext.uv.es
[†] Contributed equally to this work by sharing first place. J.R.-C.; J.M.B.; J.M.M.
[‡] Group Leaders contributing equally to this work by sharing last place. M.D.P.-D., V.Z.-M.

Citation: Raga-Cervera, J.; Bolarin, J.M.; Millan, J.M.; Garcia-Medina, J.J.; Pedrola, L.; Abellán-Abenza, J.; Valero-Vello, M.; Sanz-González, S.M.; O'Connor, J.E.; Galarreta-Mira, D.; et al. miRNAs and Genes Involved in the Interplay between Ocular Hypertension and Primary Open-Angle Glaucoma. Oxidative Stress, Inflammation, and Apoptosis Networks. *J. Clin. Med.* **2021**, *10*, 2227. https://doi.org/10.3390/jcm 10112227

Academic Editor: Kyung Chul Yoon

Received: 21 April 2021
Accepted: 17 May 2021
Published: 21 May 2021

Publisher's Note: MDPI stays neutral with regard to jurisdictional claims in published maps and institutional affiliations.

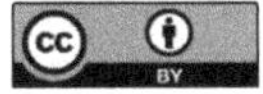

Abstract: Glaucoma has no cure and is a sight-threatening neurodegenerative disease affecting more than 100 million people worldwide, with primary open angle glaucoma (POAG) being the most globally prevalent glaucoma clinical type. Regulation of gene expression and gene networks, and its multifactorial pathways involved in glaucoma disease are landmarks for ophthalmic research. MicroRNAs (miRNAs/miRs) are small endogenous non-coding, single-stranded RNA molecules (18–22 nucleotides) that regulate gene expression. An analytical, observational, case-control study was performed in 42 patients of both sexes, aged 50 to 80 years, which were classified according to: (1) suffering from ocular hypertension (OHT) but no glaucomatous neurodegeneration (ND) such as the OHT group, or (2) have been diagnosed of POAG such as the POAG group. Participants were interviewed for obtaining sociodemographic and personal/familial records, clinically examined, and their tear samples were collected and frozen at 80 °C until processing for molecular-genetic assays. Tear RNA extraction, libraries construction, and next generation sequencing were performed. Here, we demonstrated, for the first time, the differential expression profiling of eight miRNAs when comparing tears from the OHT versus the POAG groups: the miR-26b-5p, miR-152-3p, miR-30e-5p, miR-125b-2-5p, miR-224-5p, miR-151a-3p, miR-1307-3p, and the miR-27a-3p. Gene information was set up from the DIANA-TarBase v7, DIANA-microT-CDS, and TargetScan v7.1 databases. To build a network of metabolic pathways, only genes appearing in at least four of the following databases:

DisGeNet, GeneDistiller, MalaCards, OMIM PCAN, UniProt, and GO were considered. We propose miRNAs and their target genes/signaling pathways as candidates for a better understanding of the molecular-genetic bases of glaucoma and, in this way, to gain knowledge to achieve optimal diagnosis strategies for properly identifying HTO at higher risk of glaucoma ND. Further research is needed to validate these miRNAs to discern the potential role as biomarkers involved in oxidative stress, immune response, and apoptosis for the diagnosis and/or prognosis of OHT and the prevention of glaucoma ND.

Keywords: ocular hypertension; glaucoma; tears; miRNAs; next generation sequencing; biomarkers; genes; signaling pathways; oxidative stress; inflammation; apoptosis; neurodegeneration

1. Introduction

Glaucoma is a neurodegenerative disease and a leading cause of irreversible blindness, affecting over 60 million people worldwide [1]. The number of people with glaucoma will increase to 111.8 million by 2040 [2]. These estimates are important in guiding the designs of glaucoma screening, diagnosis and treatment, research milestones, and related public health strategies.

Primary open-angle glaucoma (POAG) is the most prevalent type of glaucoma, typically characterized by adult onset, chronic intraocular pressure (IOP) elevation, IOP-dependent progressive apoptotic retinal ganglion cell (RGC) death, and visual field loss [1,2]. Main clinical features of glaucomatous optic nerve degeneration include the following: optic disc deepening, papillary hemorrhages, and specific defects of the retinal nerve fiber layer (RNFL) [3].

Diagnosis of POAG underlies a variety of clinical hallmarks such as the IOP elevation (the major risk factor) and the optic nerve head changes, as reflected by the structural/functional imaging techniques to appropriately establish the glaucoma stage [4–6]. Some decades ago, the term ocular hypertension (OHT) arose to catalogue the eyes with elevated IOP but not displaying optic disc damage or altered visual field. In 1977, Shaffer warned professionals about the false sense of security that may involve the managing of these patients that only have OHT, but no signs of neurodegeneration (ND) [7], suggesting that the term glaucoma suspects is preferred to ocular hypertensives. Glaucoma suspects define the group of patients with increased IOP and borderline optic discs (mild-to-moderate alterations), RNFL anomalies and/or visual field changes as well as glaucoma family history and the occurrence of other POAG risk factors. These patients have a higher risk of undergoing optic nerve degeneration (OND) than the normal population [8]. Therefore, classic and emerging technologies are essential for the early detection of POAG damage, but the identification of glaucomatous pre-perimetric changes continues to be a challenging issue for ophthalmologists and researchers. As the elevated IOP is the main risk factor, current knowledge on the etiopathogenic mechanisms for HTO and POAG remains incomplete. Among the cellular and molecular processes underlying these diseases, the following have largely been considered: oxidative/nitrosative stress, mitochondrial failure, inflammation and immune response, autophagy/mitophagy, apoptosis, neurotoxicity, ND, etc. [3–9]. It is imperative that the above processes are individually and integrally addressed.

The regulation of gene expression and gene networks as well as the multifactorial pathways involved in glaucoma disease are high-priority landmarks for ophthalmic research. Recent data have pinpointed potentially interesting routes to mediate glaucomatous RGC dysfunction [9]. Meanwhile, hypotensive therapy (medical, laser, surgical) is the only way to fight against the elevated IOP [10,11]. Despite experimental advances in neuroprotection [12–14], there is no definitive cure for glaucoma ND. Despite great advances in glaucoma, there is still no reliable biomarker that can pre-clinically identify subjects at risk of POAG initiation and progression. Molecular-genetic diagnostic challenges for

POAG are needed to complete the current knowledge in disease pathogenesis as well as to design new diagnostic and therapeutic strategies gathered under the recently proposed term glaucoma theranostics [15] for better eye care.

MicroRNAs (miRNAs) are a family of small endogenous non-coding, single-stranded RNA molecules (18–22 nucleotides) that regulate gene expression by either inhibiting mRNA translation or by degrading mRNA [16,17]. miRNAs are involved in the pathological processes of numerous diseases including eye pathologies [18,19]. Specific miRNAs have also been proposed to regulate IOP [20,21] as well as for use as noninvasive biomarkers for the diagnosis of glaucoma [22–24]. Our group has been widely utilizing tear samples for ophthalmic research with satisfactory results [25,26]. Because of this, we focused on analyzing tear samples that are relatively easy to collect, store, and process, to identify specific miRNAs (and its genetic targets) that differentially express themselves in the clinically silent interface between OHT and glaucoma, and to support their presumable interest as diagnostic biomarkers for individuals at risk of glaucoma ND.

2. Materials and Methods

We performed an analytical, observational, case-control study including 42 patients recruited from the ophthalmological department of the University Hospital Dr. Peset (Valencia, Spain), who agreed to participate in the study and signed the informed consent. Sample size calculation was performed using the ssize.fdr R package (R Core Team, Vienna, Austria) to detect a 1.5-fold change and achieve an 80% statistical power with a false discovery rate of 15% and an estimated proportion of non-differentially expressed miRNAs of 0.85. The study adhered the Declaration of Helsinki (Edinburgh, 2000) and the Ethics Committee standards of the study center (no. 81/16). All requirements for clinical research to maintain the privacy of the data obtained were met. Two ophthalmologists from the glaucoma section performed a systematized examination of the suitable study participants to ensure their appropriated status (Table 1), which were distributed into two groups: (1) patients diagnosed of POAG (n = 20), and (2) patients with OHT (n = 22).

Table 1. Inclusion and exclusion criteria for the study participants.

INCLUSION CRITERIA	
POAG Group	**OHT Group**
Diagnosis of POAG	OHT without signs of neurodegeneration
Ranging 50–80 years	
Both genders	
Capacity to understand and participate in the study	
EXCLUSION CRITERIA	
POAG Group	**OHT Group**
Other GLs different from POAG	With signs of glaucoma neurodegeneration
<40 or >80 years old	
Other ocular diseases or systemic pathologies that may interfere with the study	
Other treatments that may interfere with the study results	
Ocular surgery or laser treatment during the last year	
Contact lenses wearing	
Unable to participate in the study	

POAG: primary open angle glaucoma; OHT: ocular hypertension GL: glaucoma.

Ocular examination included the IOP measurement by Goldman applanation tonometry, morphological [ocular fundus by slit-lamp (IMAGEnet, Topcon Barcelona, Spain), and optical coherence tomography (OCT), and Cirrus Spectral domain OCT (Carl Zeiss Meditec, Inc., Madrid, Spain)], and functional [visual field performance, using the 24-2 Swedish interactive threshold algorithm (Humphrey field analyzer, Carl Zeiss Meditec, Inc., Madrid, Spain)] tests. Classification of the glaucoma staging was done according to the descriptions of Mills et al. [27].

Sampling was done by collecting reflex tears from the inferior meniscus of the eye without instilling anesthetics, as described in our previous work [25,26], using microhematocrite capillary tube, that were appropriately labeled, and immediately transferred into microcentrifuge tubes and stored in an ultra-freezer at −80 °C. On the day of processing, samples were defrosted and prepared for RNA extraction using the miRCURY RNA Isolation Kit-Biofluids (EXIQON Inc., Woburn, MA, USA). This kit is designed to isolate all RNAs sized less than 1000 nucleotides, from mRNA and tRNA to microRNA and small interfering RNA. We carried out the RNA extraction according to the manufacturer's instructions. Briefly, the purification is based on spin column chromatography using a proprietary resin as the separation matrix. Small RNAs are separated from other cellular components such as proteins without the use of phenol or chloroform.

The quality and quantity of total RNA obtained from tears was assessed using a Bioanalyzer 2100 (Agilent® Technologies, Inc., Santa Clara, CA, USA), and the RNA 6000 Nano Kit (Agilent® Technologies, Inc.). RNA libraries were prepared using NEBNext® Multiplex Small RNA Library Prep Set for Illumina® (#E7300 y #7580; New England BioLabs®, Inc., Ipswich, MA, USA), according to the manufacturer's protocol https://international.neb.com/protocols/2018/03/27/protocol-for-use-with-nebnext-small-rna-library-prep-set-for-illumina-e7300-e7580-e7560-e7330 (accessed on 17 May 2021). According to the guidelines for low RNA concentration samples, the adapters and RT primers were diluted 1:2 with nuclease-free water and 15 cycles were used for the amplification by PCR. The indexed libraries were purified using the QIAquick® PCR Purification Kit (#28104, QIAGEN®, Hilden, Germany). Library quality control was assessed using a 4200 TapeStation (Agilent® Technologies, Inc.) and High Sensitivity D1000 Kit (Agilent® Technologies, Inc.). The miRNA fraction of each library (120–200 bp) was collected using the Pippin Prep System (Sage Science, Inc., Beverly, MA, USA) following the manufacturer's guidelines and using 3% agarose dye free gel cassettes with internal standards (Marker P) (Sage Science # CDP3010). miRNAs were quantified using a 4200 TapeStation (Agilent® Technologies, Inc.) and High Sensitivity D1000 Kit (Agilent® Technologies, Inc.) prior to normalization and pooling. Sequencing was performed on a NextSeq 500 System (Illumina, Inc., San Diego, CA, USA) with a Mid-Output flow cell for 150-cycle reads obtaining about 3.5 million reads per sample. FASTQ file quality was assessed using FASTQC tool (https://www.bioinformatics.babraham.ac.uk/projects/fastqc/, accessed on 21 May 2021). Adapters and low liability reads were removed. Non-coding RNAs previously described in the ENSEMBL database were selected and characterized. Statistical analyses (normalization, differential expression, and significance) were performed using Limma and edgeR packages deposited in Bioconductor (www.bioconductor.org). A predictive analysis based on receiver operating characteristic (ROC) curves was performed to select those miRNAs showing an area under the curve (AUC) greater than 0.75. Subsequently, an analysis of the main components (PCA) was performed. Later, the target genes of the selected miRNAs were determined using the R miRFA pipeline [28], which is supported by data from the DIANA-TarBase v7, DIANA-microT-CDS and TargetScan v7.1 databases. Additionally, UniProt and Gene Ontology databases have been used to search for terms associated with the trabecular meshwork functions and the glaucoma pathology [29]. To select all genes needed to build a network of metabolic pathways, we considered only those genes that appeared in at least four of the following databases: DisGeNet, GeneDistiller, MalaCards, OMIM PCAN, UniProt, and GO [30]. These genes also need to have at least seven terms in any of the UniProt categories above-mentioned. Two approaches have been used to build the networks: (1) enrichment of metabolic pathways using the g: Profiler, GSEA, Cytoscape, and EnrichmentMap tools [31], and (2) gene function prediction using the GeneMANIA gene integration tool [32], which can function both as an independent server and as an application in Cytoscape.

For statistical analysis, comparison of two categorical variables was performed using the Pearson Chi square test. We used the Shapiro–Wilk test to check the distribution quantitative variables. The comparison of two means was analyzed by means of the Student t-test for independent samples (normal variables) or the Mann–Whitney U test (non-normal variables). The comparison of more than two means was carried out by the analysis of variance (ANOVA, normal variables) or the Kruskal–Wallis test (non-normal variables). Statistical proceedings were performed using the statistical package ((BM SPSS Statistics for Windows, Version 24.0. Armonk, NY, USA: IBM Corp).

3. Results

3.1. Sociodemographic and Ophthalmologic Data

Mean age of participants was 64.5 ± 1.4 years for the POAG group and 61.1 ± 2.4 years for the OHT group. Comparison between groups did not show statistically significant differences ($p > 0.05$).

Regarding the distribution by gender, both groups showed a greater proportion of women. No statistically significant differences were observed between groups ($p > 0.05$).

Sociodemographic characteristics of the study participants are listed in Table 2. No significant differences were found in any of the study variables.

Table 2. Sociodemographic characteristics of the study participants.

Variables		POAG	OHT	p *
Age (years)		64.5 (1.4)	61.1 (2.4)	0.218
Gender (%, men/women)		47.6/52.4	33.3/66.7	0.366
Height (cm)		165.2 (2.2)	164.0 (2.2)	0.694
Weight (kg)		76.7 (3.7)	70.6 (3.2)	0.217
BMI (kg/m^2)		28.1 (1.2)	26.2 (0.9)	0.238
Smoking (%)		28.6	22.2	0.651
Alcohol consumption (%)		9.5	16.7	0.506
Physical activity (%)	Mild	42.9	61.1	
	Moderate	57.1	33.3	0.225
	High	0.0	5.6	

POAG: primary open-angle glaucoma; OHT: ocular hypertension; BMI: body mass index. Data shows the mean (standard deviation) or percentage. * Significance level was set at 0.05.

The OHT subjects showed elevated IOP but no damage at OCT examination, normal visual fields, and normal ocular fundus. However, POAG patients showed IOP elevation, an increase of optic disc excavation, optic nerve damage, and/or altered visual fields. Ophthalmologic parameters of the study participants are shown in Table 3.

Table 3. Ophthalmological parameters of the study participants.

Variables	POAG	OHT	* p Value
BCVA (decimal)	0.86 ± 0.03	0.90 ± 0.03	0.382
IOP (mmHg)	16.00 ± 0.58	18.17 ± 0.81	0.033
C-D ratio	0.46 ± 0.02	0.046 ± 0.05	0.949
CCT	536.86 ± 6.56	554.42 ± 8.12	0.141
VF-PSD	2.27 ± 0.29	1.33 ± 0.13	0.008
VFI	90.57 ± 2.30	92.22 ± 1.09	0.543
VF-MD	-0.56 ± 0.91	0.98 ± 0.410	0.154
OCT-papillary excavation	0.61 ± 0.04	0.057 ± 0.04	0.439
OCT-fibrillar thickness	84.71 ± 3.13	88.61 ± 2.29	0.334
OCT-rim area	4.58 ± 2.29	1.11 ± 0.05	0.169
RGCs density	68.95 ± 2.23	77.89 ± 2.15	0.008

POAG: primary open-angle glaucoma; OHT: ocular hypertension; BCVA: best corrected visual acuity; IOP: intraocular pressure; C-D: cup-to-disc; CCT: central corneal thickness; VF: visual field; PSD: pattern standard deviation; VFI: visual field index; MD: mean deviation; OCT: optical coherence tomography; RGCs: retinal ganglion cells. * Statistical significance ($p < 0.05$).

3.2. miRNA Identification

After performing all experimental procedures, we were able to identify 95 miRNAs present in tears of OHT and/or POAG patients. Figure 1 shows the PCA plot after the normalization of data. As this figure shows, there was not a good separation between the two groups (POAG in red and OHT in blue) based on the identified miRNAs.

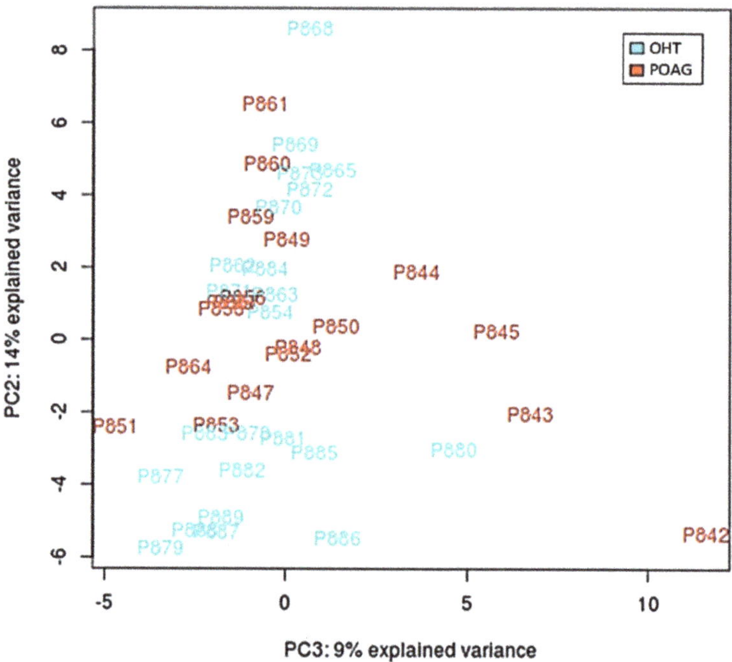

Figure 1. Principal component analysis (PCA) plot after normalization of the data according to the eight differentially expressed miRNAs. Image shows ocular hypertension/ocular hypertension patients (blue marks) and primary open-angle glaucoma (red marks) patients.

The next step was to compare the expression levels of those 95 miRNAs in both study groups (POAG patients vs. OHT subjects). From these 95 miRNAs, 87 showed no significant differences between groups ($p > 0.05$). However, we found six upregulated and two downregulated miRNAs in tears from the POAG patients (Table 4). At this point, we build again the PCA plot, taking into consideration only those eight miRNAs that differentially expressed between groups. The PCA showed a better separation of the miRNAs present in tears from the OHT vs. POAG patients (Figure 2).

Table 4. Differences in miRNA expression between groups.

miRNA ID	Fold Change (POAG vs. OHT) [§]	*p* [*]
hsa-miR-26b-5p	0.855	0.012
hsa-miR-27a-3p	0.774	0.004
hsa-miR-152-3p	0.753	0.004
hsa-miR-30e-5p	0.901	0.005
hsa-miR-125b-2-5p	0.529	0.027
hsa-miR-224-5p	0.745	0.033
hsa-miR-151a-3p	−0.417	0.009
hsa-miR-1307-3p	−1	0.004

POAG: primary open-angle glaucoma; OHT: ocular hypertension. [§] OHT was the reference group. [*] Significance was set at 0.05.

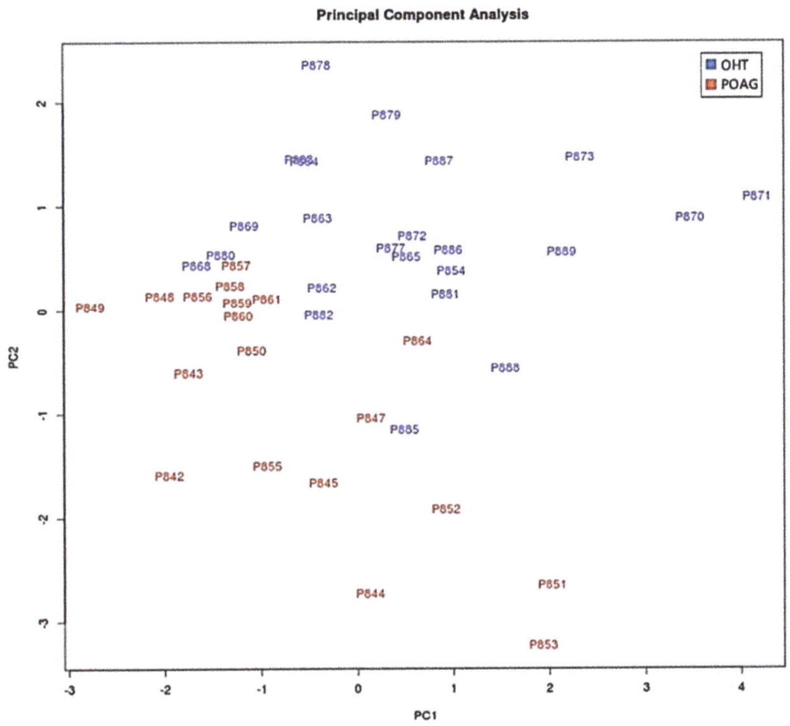

Figure 2. Principal component analysis (PCA) plot comparing the POAG and OHT groups using only miRNAs with statistically significant expression. Red: patients with OHT. Blue: patients with POAG. OHT: ocular hypertension/ocular hypertensives; POAG: primary open angle glaucoma.

In addition, a ROC curve was performed to analyze whether these eight miRNAs could predict POAG in the HTO individuals. Table 5 shows the AUC for each miRNA. The AUC of four of these miRNAs was greater than 0.75, so they could be considered as good predictors of POAG.

Table 5. Area under the curve for the eight miRNAs with significant differential expression between groups.

miRNA	AUC
hsa-miR-26b-5p	0.81693
hsa-miR-152-3p	0.75743
hsa-miR-30e-5p	0.76201
hsa-miR-125b-2-5p	0.67276
hsa-miR-224-5p	0.72082
hsa-miR-151a-3p	0.75972
hsa-miR-1307-3p	0.69565
hsa-miR-27a-3p	0.68192

POAG: primary open-angle glaucoma; OHT: ocular hypertension/hypertensives; AUC: area under the curve.

3.3. Bioinformatic Processing

Using the databases mentioned in the methodology section and combining their predictions, we identified a total of 14,379 potential target genes of the eight miRNAs. Then, these 14,379 genes were searched in four databases (DisGeNet, GeneDistiller, MalaCards, and OMIM PCAN) that collected information on the association between genes and pathologies, finding the presence of 390, 183, 145, and 7 genes in each of them, respectively.

Eleven categories related to trabecular meshwork functions and the glaucoma pathology were selected and the number of genes that had terms in each of them are shown in Table 6. The biological functions marked in bold represent those with the highest number of genes (extracellular matrix and apoptosis processes). In addition, genes related to neurodegeneration, inflammation, and oxidative stress, among others, were also identified.

Table 6. Target genes of the eight miRNAs showing significantly different expression profile between groups.

Biological Function	Number of Genes
IOP, aqueous humor outflow	420
Extracellular matrix	**1143**
Ciliary body functions	593
Focal adhesion	558
Oxidative stress response	272
Apoptosis	**1516**
Neurodegeneration	31
Retinal ganglion cells	27
RHO signaling	213
TGF-β signaling	5
Eye development	420

TM: trabecular meshwork; IOP: intraocular pressure; RHO: Ras homologous protein family; TGFβ: transforming growth factor beta.

We performed the Gene Ontology (GO) Biological Process analysis and found 201 items to which the eight identified miRNAs were significantly associated. Table 7 shows the top 40 biological processes of the above miRNAs. In addition to this GO analysis, we identified 36 reactomes (REACT) significantly associated with the eight miRNAs (Table 8), among them, genes related to apoptosis and extracellular matrix conditions. Additionally, those genes involved in aqueous humor homeostasis, oxidative stress, immune response regulation (TGF-β) and neurodegeneration were identified.

Following the screening criteria detailed in the methodology section, a total of 114 genes were selected to build a network of metabolic pathways (Figure 3). This network shows the clusters involved in apoptosis (blue box), extracellular matrix and collagen concerns (red box), endopeptidase activity (green box) as well as in development pathways (upper left side) among other clusters. Network data are included as Supplementary Materials, as both CYS (Cytoscape session file) and SIF (simple interaction file) formats.

By using the GeneMania program, different maps were created. In these maps, each circle is a node representing a gene. Black nodes belong to the original set of 114 genes studied, while grey circles represent those not present as genes in the original set, but very closely related to them according to the selected network criteria. These diagrams also give information about the number of interactions of each gene (the size of the circle is proportional to this number), and the edges indicate a relationship between genes, meaning that the thicker the line, the more intense the relationship.

With these proceedings, we finally built three maps: the first is a map of genetic interactions between these genes (Figure 4); the second is a map showing the physical interactions (Figure 5); and the third is a map of the metabolic pathways (Figure 6). In these figures, grey circles represent genes not present in the original 114 set, but closely related to them. Circle size is proportional to the number of interactions of each gene. Edges indicate a relationship between genes(a thicker line the more intense relationship). Network data from Figures 4–6 are also included in the Supplementary Materials as both CYS (Cytoscape session file) and SIF (simple interaction file) formats.

Table 7. Top 40 GO Biological Processes associated to POAG and with target miRNAs.

	ID	Name	N	p-Value		ID	Name	N	p-Value
1	GO:0030198	extracellular matrix organization	31	4.63E-25	21	GO:0016043	cellular component organization	75	1.88E-09
2	GO:0043062	extracellular structure organization	31	5.15E-25	22	GO:0008219	cell death	40	1.89E-09
3	GO:0009653	anatomical structure morphogenesis	51	2.36E-15	23	GO:0071840	cellular component organization or biogenesis	76	2.58E-09
4	GO:0150063	visual system development	19	7.78E-15	24	GO:0048592	eye morphogenesis	11	3.22E-09
5	GO:0048880	sensory system development	19	1.36E-14	25	GO:0042981	regulation of apoptosis	33	3.92E-09
6	GO:0001654	eye development	18	1.20E-13	26	GO:0012501	programmed cell death	38	5.16E-09
7	GO:0048513	animal organ development	52	1.29E-13	27	GO:0090596	sensory organ morphogenesis	12	7.97E-09
8	GO:0009887	animal organ morphogenesis	29	2.37E-13	28	GO:0009888	tissue development	35	1.41E-08
9	GO:0007423	sensory organ development	19	1.27E-12	29	GO:0050793	regulation of development	42	2.22E-08
10	GO:0007275	multicellular organism development	65	3.25E-12	30	GO:0072359	circulatory system development	26	4.96E-08
11	GO:0048731	system development	61	3.20E-11	31	GO:0007166	cell surface receptor signaling pathway	48	7.24E-08
12	GO:0030199	collagen fibril organization	10	1.50E-10	32	GO:0042073	intraciliary transport	9	8.63E-08
13	GO:0048646	morphogenesis	29	1.74E-10	33	GO:0097190	apoptotic signaling pathway	20	1.02E-07
14	GO:0032502	development	70	3.01E-10	34	GO:0032501	multicellular organismal process	73	1.22E-07
15	GO:0010941	regulation of cell death	36	4.22E-10	35	GO:0007601	visual perception	12	1.78E-07
16	GO:0043010	anterior chamber eye development	14	4.33E-10	36	GO:0010970	transport along microtubule	12	1.95E-07
17	GO:0048856	anatomical structure development	66	5.22E-10	37	GO:0050953	sensory perception of light stimulus	12	3.29E-07
18	GO:0006915	Apoptosis	37	1.24E-09	38	GO:0032963	collagen metabolic process	10	3.95E-07
19	GO:0043067	Apoptosis regulation	34	1.33E-09	39	GO:0035735	intraciliary transport involved in cilium assembly	8	4.31E-07
20	GO:0006928	movement of cell or subcellular component	42	1.75E-09	40	GO:0098840	protein transport along microtubule	9	4.81E-07

GO: Gene Ontology; POAG: primary open-angle glaucoma; N: number of genes.

Table 8. Reactomes associated with the 8 tear differentially expressed miRNAs.

ID	Name	N	*p*-Value
REAC:R-HSA-1474244	Extracellular matrix organization	29	5.16E-21
REAC:R-HSA-1474228	Extracellular matrix degradation	18	2.59E-14
REAC:R-HSA-1442490	Collagen degradation	13	1.48E-12
REAC:R-HSA-3000178	ECM proteoglycans	13	1.33E-11
REAC:R-HSA-3000171	Non-integrin membrane-ECM interactions	12	1.43E-11
REAC:R-HSA-2022090	Assembly of collagen fibrils (and other multimeric structures)	12	2,21E-11
REAC:R-HSA-8948216	Collagen chain trimerization	10	7.82E-10
REAC:R-HSA-1474290	Collagen formation	12	3.08E-09
REAC:R-HSA-2243919	Crosslinking of collagen fibrils	7	2.62E-08
REAC:R-HSA-216083	Integrin cell surface interactions	11	3.35E-08
REAC:R-HSA-8874081	MET activates PTK2 signaling	8	3.46E-08
REAC:R-HSA-1650814	Collagen biosynthesis and modifying enzymes	10	6.68E-08
REAC:R-HSA-8875878	MET promotes cell motility	8	4.25E-07
REAC:R-HSA-1566948	Elastic fiber formation	8	9.52E-07
REAC:R-HSA-5620924	Intraflagellar transport	8	5.22087E-06
REAC:R-HSA-2129379	Molecules associated with elastic fibers	7	7.44538E-06
REAC:R-HSA-109581	Apoptosis	12	8.49652E-06
REAC:R-HSA-5357801	Apoptosis regulation	12	1.0277E-05
REAC:R-HSA-3000170	Syndecan interactions	6	2.27603E-05
REAC:R-HSA-2214320	Anchoring fibril formation	5	4.00759E-05
REAC:R-HSA-6806834	Signaling by MET	8	8.14274E-05
REAC:R-HSA-109606	Intrinsic Pathway for Apoptosis	7	9.9991E-05
REAC:R-HSA-375165	NCAM signaling for neurite out-growth	7	2.12464E-04
REAC:R-HSA-9006934	Signaling by Receptor Tyrosine Kinases	16	3.8436E-04
REAC:R-HSA-419037	NCAM1 interactions	6	4.6565E-04
REAC:R-HSA-6785807	Interleukin-4 and Interleukin-13 signaling	8	1.40305E-03
REAC:R-HSA-186797	Signaling by PDGF	6	2.114864E-03
REAC:R-HSA-5617833	Cilium Assembly	10	2.548397E-03
REAC:R-HSA-381426	IGF transport & uptake by IGF Binding Proteins (IGFBPs)	8	3.42679E-03
REAC:R-HSA-76009	Platelet Aggregation (Plug Formation)	5	5.752906E-03
REAC:R-HSA-5633008	TP53 Regulates Transcription of Cell Death Genes	5	1.1963399E-02
REAC:R-HSA-76002	Platelet activation, signaling and aggregation	10	2.1334022E-02
REAC:R-HSA-3000157	Laminin interactions	4	4.1196772E-02
REAC:R-HSA-114452	Activation of BH3-only proteins	4	4.1196772E-02
REAC:R-HSA-6803207	TP53 regulation of Caspase activator/Caspases Transcription	3	4.5562937E-02

N: number of genes; REAC: reactome.

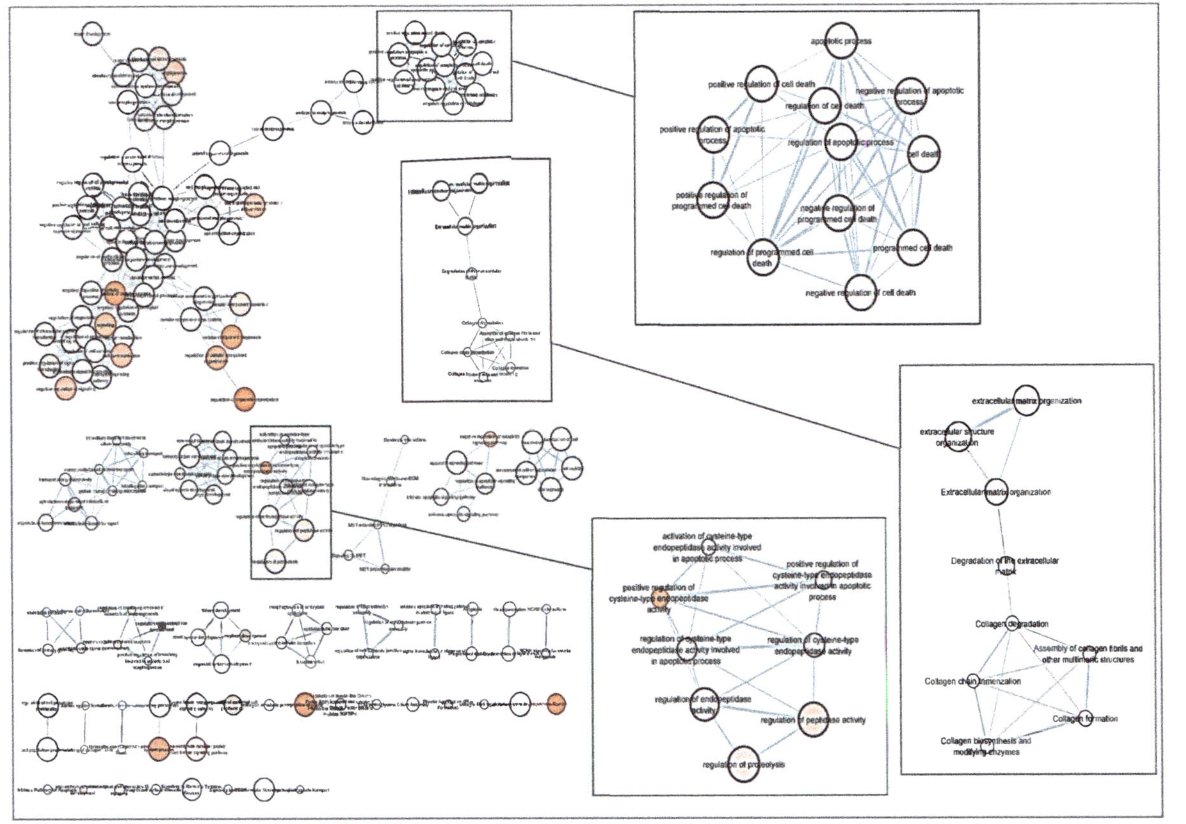

Figure 3. Network of GO terms and Reactome pathways generated with g:Profiler and EnrichmentMap in Cytoscape. Each node (circle) represents a gene set characterized by a particular GO term or reactome pathway. Node fill indicates the enrichment score (FDR q-value). The thickness of blue lines (edges) indicates the number of shared genes (overlap) between two connected nodes. Nodes with high overlap are clustered together, forming groups characterized by similar terms and pathways. Gene clusters involved in apoptosis (blue box), extracellular matrix and collagen concerns (red box), endopeptidase activity (green box) as well as in development pathways (upper left side) have been marked.

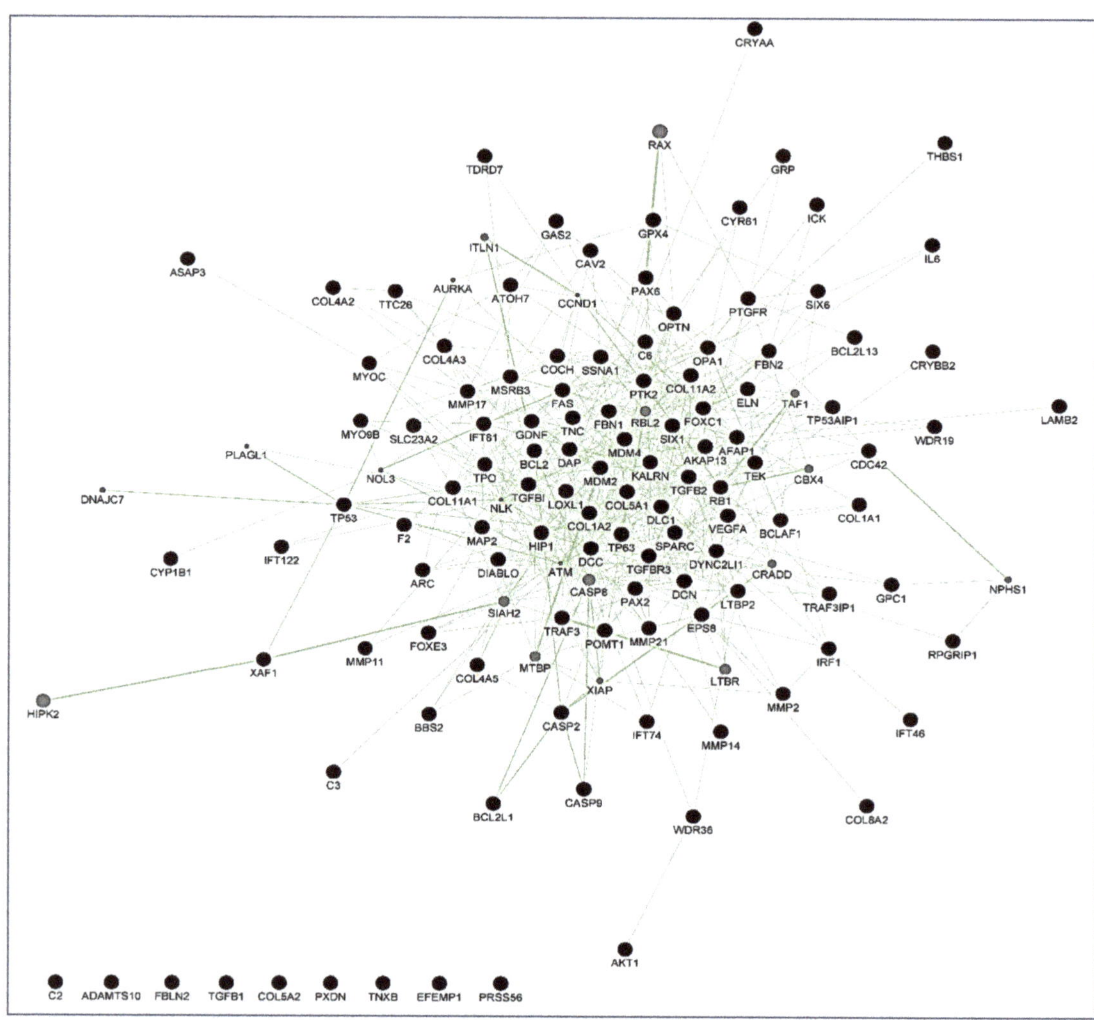

Figure 4. Genetic interaction map created with GeneMania. Black nodes are genes present in the original gene list, grey nodes are genes that are initially not present, but closely related to them. Among the genes, MYOC, OPTN, FOXC1, TGFβ, FAS/TNFR, TP53, CASPs, BCL2, MMPs, and DIABLO were identified. Lines (edges) connecting two genes indicate that they are functionally associated (the effects of perturbing one gene are found to be modified by perturbations to the second gene) using data primary collected from BioGRID. Thicker edges indicate a stronger association.

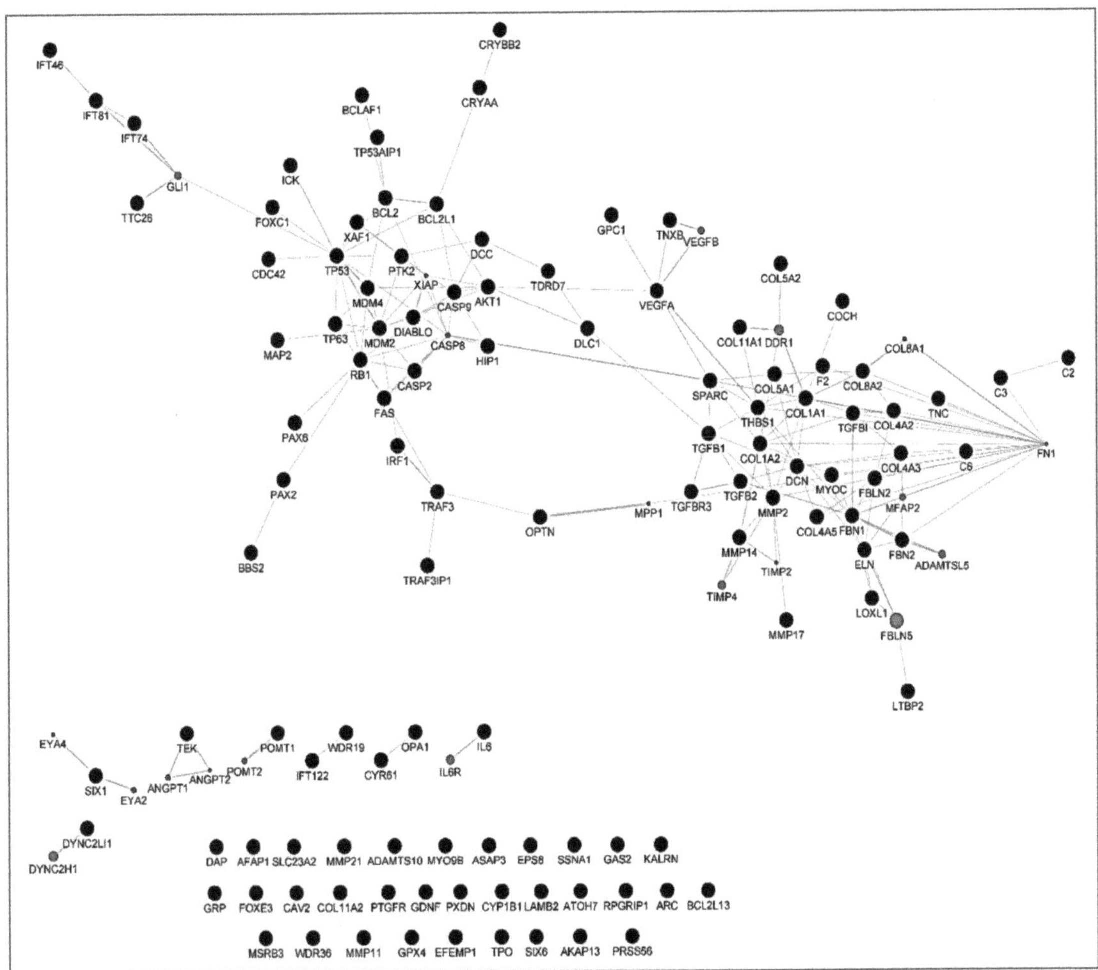

Figure 5. Physical interaction map created with GeneMania. Black nodes are genes present in the original gene list, grey nodes are additional genes that are found interacting with the original ones in a protein–protein interaction study. The genes FOXC1, CASPs, MAP2, TP53, BCL2, DIABLO, IL6, TGFβ, OPTN, MMPs, among others, were identified. Size of grey nodes indicate the likelihood of physical interaction (score), and thicker lines (edges) indicate a stronger interaction. Data are collected from primary studies from protein interaction databases including BioGRID and PathwayCommons.

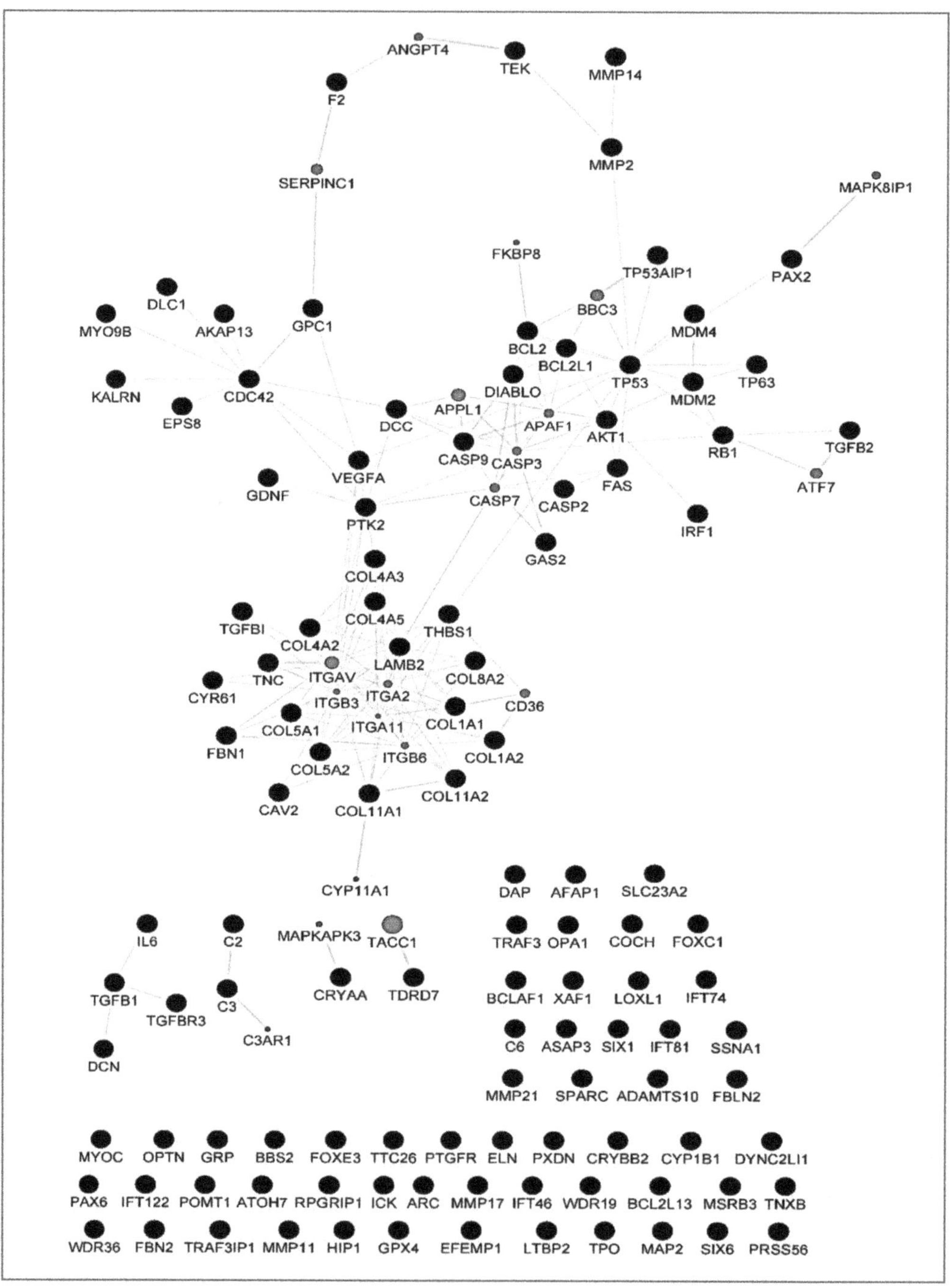

Figure 6. Metabolic pathway map created with GeneMania. Two gene products are linked if they participate in the same reaction within a pathway. Size of gray nodes indicate the likelihood of the gene belonging to the pathway (score), and thicker lines (edges) indicate a stronger relation. Data are collected from various sources such as Reactome and BioCyc, via PathwayCommons.

4. Discussion

In this work, we successfully profiled the tear miRNAs signature from patients with POAG compared to the OHT, as follows: the miR-26b-5p, miR-152-3p, miR-30e-5p, miR-125b-2-5p, miR-224-5p, miR-151a-3p, miR-1307-3p, and the miR-27a-3p. As far as we know, this is the first study in identifying miRNAs in tears from individuals with HTO and glaucoma patients, revealing its potential as molecular-genetic biomarkers of glaucoma suspect.

People more predisposed to glaucoma must be early identified to undertake measures for avoiding optic nerve irreversible damage and vision-threatening consequences [1–6]. Over the years, this concern has continued to shape the thinking of ophthalmologists and researchers worldwide because hypotensive treatment has to be promptly initiated to appropriately control the elevated IOP. In this context, biomarkers might be key diagnostic tools to identify individuals at higher risk for glaucoma such as HTO individuals, just like we did in this report. Our differential expression analysis carried out by NGS led us to identify the tear fingerprint of eight miRNAs that significantly expressed between the POAG patients and HTO individuals. Then, we comprehensively explain the above miRNAs as well as the underlying miRNA-related pathways involved in HTO and POAG, as reflected in Figures 3–6 as well as in the Supplementary Materials.

Specific miRNAs involved in IOP homeostasis and glaucomatous OND were reported by different authors [21–24]. Others have also conducted similar studies to ours in different ophthalmic disorders [33] using different biological samples [34–36]. Liu et al. [37] analyzed the miRNA signature in the aqueous humor of POAG patients and its role in the etiopathogenic mechanisms of glaucomatous OND, reporting 88 miRNAs that differentially expressed between POAG and cataracts. Among them, the miR-151-a-3p was identified in the aqueous humor by these authors, in a similar manner to us in the course of the present work, in which the same miRNA was downregulated in tears of our study participants. Ertekin et al. [38] found miR-26b-5p in plasma from patients with wet macular degeneration. The authors associated this miRNA with oxidative stress occurring in the retinal pigment epithelial cells of the eyes with this disease. We also found the miR-26b-5p in tears of our GPAA patients and OHT individuals. Oxidative/nitrosative stress plays a pivotal role in POAG pathogenesis [12,15,39]; we may hypothesize that in the course of glaucoma, the pro-oxidants may induce the expression of miR-26b-5p, as reflected in this work [39–41]. Interestingly, hsa-miR-26b-5p has recently been involved in pseudoexfoliative glaucoma through interaction with the TGFR1 and TGR2 part of SMAD2 [42].

We also described herein that the miRN-27-a-3p showed a significant differential expression in tears from the POAG patients and the OHT participants. This miRNA has been implicated in cell proliferation and apoptosis in different types of cancer [43,44]. Overexpression of this miRNA promotes proliferation and inhibits apoptosis of cancer cells. Likewise, it has been shown that miR27a-3p induces ischemia-reperfusion injury by triggering oxidative stress [45]. In previous reports, it has been shown that the expression of this miRNA was increased in stretched versus control TM cells [46,47]. Consistent with these findings, we suggest that the miR-27a-3p overexpression in tears from POAG patients may be related to both the apoptotic and oxidative stress processes occurring in the POAG eyes [39–41].

Most target genes corresponding to the eight miRNAs showing significant differential expression profile in tears of the OHT individuals and POAG patients were related to extracellular matrix concerns and apoptosis processes (see the Tables 6–8).

Desjarlais et al. [48] reported the upregulation of miR-152-3p in the choroid during the vasodegenerative phase of an oxygen-induced retinopathy model compared to the control animals. However, these authors did not delve into the role of this miRNA, but just described the differential expression profile between groups. However, Wang et al. [49] pointed out that miR-152-3p may be an interesting molecular target for keloid treatment as a relevant regulator of cell proliferation, invasion, and extracellular matrix expression through targeting FOXF1 in keloid fibroblasts [49]. In this regard, we found the miR-152-3p upregulation in tears from the POAG group, supporting data previously reported by other researchers, emphasizing the importance of this miRNA in the trabecular meshwork changes and elevated IOP occurring in OHT and POAG [47].

The miR-30e-5p was differentially expressed in tears from OHT and POAG participants during the present work. However, only one article dealt with its role at the ocular level, highlighting its possible function as a predictor of the myasthenia gravis through the main ocular manifestation of the disease, the blepharoptosis [50]. No publications on the relationship between miR-30e-50 and glaucoma and/or other degenerative eye diseases have been found. Meng et al. [51] reported significant differential expression of the miR-30e-5p in patients with Alzheimer's disease compared to healthy controls. Additionally, Hardeland et al. [52] reported a negative connection between melatonin availability and neurodegenerative disorders, and in this regard, Scuderi et al. [53] reported that melatonin could protect the eye tissues from free radicals and pro-inflammatory mediators. Taking all these reports into consideration, we may hypothesize that miR-30e-5p may play a role in the ethiopathogenic mechanisms of glaucoma by its negative connection with melatonin.

Toro et al. [54] carried out a recent study in the vitreous humor of patients with different degrees of diabetic proliferative vitreoretinopathy (PVR) in which six miRNAs whose expression significantly increased with disease progression were reported, among them miR-224-5p. Dysregulation of its expression in PVR patients suggests a possible association with certain retinal degenerative processes. In the present study, we also found the upregulation of this miRNA in the POAG patients, pointing to a potential involvement of miR-224-5p in the onset and/or progression of the glaucoma ND.

The miR-151a-3p seems to be associated with a high risk of uveal melanoma [55]. Bianciotto et al. [56] reported that OHT is a risk factor for the development of uveal melanoma. In our OHT participants, a significantly higher expression of this miRNA was seen, suggesting that its downregulation in the POAG patients may be related to the onset of glaucoma ND. Nevertheless, the function of this miRNA in glaucoma needs further investigation.

Oxidative stress, inflammation, and apoptosis are relevant mechanisms involved in POAG [3–8,12,15,39]. In this regard, oxidative stress can trigger a wide spectrum of transcription factors such as p53, Nrf2, NF-κB, AP-1, PPAR-γ, and β-catenin/Wnt, among others [57–60]. When the above molecules undergo activation, they can induce the expression of hundreds of genes such as those related to pro-inflammatory cytokines and chemokines, cell adhesion molecules, metalloproteinases, cell cycle regulators, pro-apoptotic molecules, etc. [60–64]. In the case that the oxidative/inflammatory environment will be prolonged, this can chronically affect the ocular cells and tissues leading to apoptotic cell death and glaucoma ND. Given the target genes of the eight miRNAs with different expression between POAG and OHT, and following the methods explained above, we conducted a bioinformatic work to build several maps that showed the interactions between these genes as well as a connection network between the different metabolic pathways associated with these genes and miRNAs, as reflected in Figures 3–6. Target genes of the eight miRNAs that were identified in tears such as those showing a significant differential expression profile between the OHT and the POAG groups were mainly related to apoptosis and extracellular matrix functions as well as aqueous humor homeostasis, focal adhesion, oxidative stress, inflammation signaling and ND, as reflected in Figures 3–6.

Up to today, genetic testing can help identify people at risk for early-onset glaucoma types in almost 30% of cases [65]. A useful gene-based screening test for adult-onset POAG forms is not yet available [66], but a new test in blood or saliva by multi-trait analyses have found the risk of a person developing glaucoma [67]. Nevertheless, no way exists to predict the risk of a person with OHT to develop glaucoma.

We propose that the miRNAs identified in the present work and their target genes/signaling pathways will allow for a better understanding of the molecular and genetic bases of glaucoma and, in this way, gain knowledge that leads us to develop a better diagnosis strategy for properly identifying HTO at a higher risk of glaucoma ND.

Individuals predisposed to glaucoma such as those suffering OHT should be closely followed to identify early changes to promptly start hypotensive therapy. Top advances in glaucoma genetics have provided an open window for stratifying the risk of glaucoma in HTO cases based on molecular-genetic predictions. Here, we show for the first time a new approach and future avenues dealing with miRNA expression in tears to better diagnose HTO individuals and identify those at highest risk of POAG as well as to better eye/vision care and blindness prevention.

5. Conclusions

In summary, eight miRNAs: **the miR-26b-5p, miR-152-3p, miR-30e-5p, miR-125b-2-5p, miR-224-5p, miR-151a-3p, miR-1307-3p and the miR-27a-3p** were found to be differentially expressed in the tears of patients in the interface between OHT and POAG. We demonstrated that some of these miRNAs, their target genes, and signaling pathways have already been related to **apoptosis, extracellular matrix functions, inflammation, and oxidative stress as well as aqueous humor homeostasis and neurodegeneration.** Further studies are needed to validate our results and deepen the knowledge of these miRNAs to discern its potential as biomarkers for the diagnosis and/or prognosis and future biotherapies for OHT and glaucomatous NDG.

Supplementary Materials: The following are available online at https://www.mdpi.com/article/10.3390/jcm10112227/s1. Supplementary Materials includes network data from Figures 3–6 as both CYS (Cytoscape session file) and SIF (simple interaction file) formats.

Author Contributions: J.R.-C., J.M.B. and J.M.M. share first place authorship because of their equal collaboration in the present study. M.D.P.-D. and V.Z.-M. share the last place as the study coordinators. Conceptualization, S.M.S.-G., J.J.G.-M., V.Z.-M. and M.D.P.-D.; Methodology, M.V.-V., S.M.S.-G., V.Z.-M., J.R.-C., D.G.-M., E.B.-T., A.M.-F., J.M.M., J.E.O., L.P., J.M.B., J.A.-A., J.J.G.-M. and M.D.P.-D.; Software, J.M.B, J.A.-A., D.G.-M., E.B.-T., A.M.-F. and V.Z.-M.; Formal analysis, L.P., J.M.M., J.M.B., J.A.-A., J.E.O., V.Z.-M., S.M.S.-G. and M.D.P.-D.; Writing-Original draft preparation: J.R.-C., S.M.S.-G., J.M.B., V.Z.-M. and M.D.P.-D.; Supervision, V.Z.-M. and M.D.P.-D.; Project administration, M.D.P.-D.; Funding acquisition, J.R.-G., J.M.M. and M.D.P.-D. All authors have read and agreed to the published version of the manuscript.

Funding: This work was done in part with the collaboration of members assigned to the research teams of Valencia (S.M.S.-G., V.Z.-M., J.J.G.-M. and M.D.P.-D.) and Valladolid (D.G.M.) pertaining to the Spanish Network of Ophthalmic Research: OFTARED (RD16-0008) of the Institute of Health Carlos III (ISCIII) of the Spanish Government (Madrid, Spain). This work was funded in part by the VLC-Biomed GLAUMIRNA project (2017-2018) and by the Rare Diseases Networking Biomedical Research Center (CIBERER) of Valencia (J.M.M. and L.P.). Jorge Raga Cervera obtained his PhD in Medicine (University of Valencia, 2018) by this work. S.M.S.-G. received a research fellowship from the Spanish Glaucoma Association for glaucoma patients and families AGAF, Madrid (2020).

Institutional Review Board Statement: The study was conducted according to the guidelines of the Declaration of Helsinki, and approved by the Institutional Review Board (or Ethics Committee) of Dr. Peset Hospital (Valencia, Spain) (protocol code no. 81/16).

Informed Consent Statement: Informed consent was obtained from all subjects involved in the study.

Data Availability Statement: The data is enclosed in the present work. Supplementary Material is also offered through this article. Network data from Figures 4–6 are also included in the Supplementary Materials as both CYS (Cytoscape session file) and SIF (simple interaction file) formats.

Acknowledgments: The authors thank all physicians, ophthalmologists, and researchers who helped us to complete the present study for their work and outstanding interest in glaucoma. We specially wish to thank Julio Escribano (Chairman at the University of Castilla la Mancha, Spain and OFTARED member) for the thoughtful comments and critical reading of the manuscript. We also want to thank Quino Panadero for helping with the bioinformatic analysis during the first part of this work.

Conflicts of Interest: The authors declare no conflict of interest.

References

1. Prum, B.E.; Rosenberg, L.F.; Gedde, S.J.; Mansberger, S.L.; Stein, J.D.; Moroi, S.E.; Herndon, L.W.; Lim, M.C.; Williams, R.D. Primary Open-Angle Glaucoma Preferred Practice Pattern(®) Guidelines. *Ophthalmology* **2016**, *123*, 41–111. [CrossRef]
2. Tham, Y.C.; Li, X.; Wong, T.Y.; Quigley, H.A.; Aung, T.; Cheng, C.Y. Global prevalence of glaucoma and projections of glaucoma burden through 2040: A systematic review and meta-analysis. *Ophthalmology* **2014**, *121*, 2081–2090. [CrossRef] [PubMed]
3. Flammer, J.; Mozaffarieh, M. What is the present pathogenetic concept of glaucomatous optic neuropathy? *Surv. Ophthalmol.* **2007**, *52*, S162–S173. [CrossRef] [PubMed]
4. Kong, Y.X.G.; Coote, A.M.; O'Neill, E.C.; Gurria, L.U.; Xie, J.; Garway-Heath, D.; Medeiros, A.F.; Crowston, J.G. Glaucomatous optic neuropathy evaluation project: A standardized internet system for assessing skills in optic disc examination. *Clin. Exp. Ophthalmol.* **2010**, *39*, 308–317. [CrossRef]
5. Zhang, X.; Dastiridou, A.; Francis, B.A.; Tan, O.; Varma, R.; Greenfield, D.S.; Schuman, J.S.; Huang, D. Comparison of glaucoma progression detection by optical coherence tomography and visual field. *Am. J. Ophthalmol.* **2017**, *184*, 63–74. [CrossRef]
6. Parra-Blesa, A.; Sanchez-Alberca, A.; Garcia-Medina, J.J. Clinical-evolutionary staging system of primary open-angle glaucoma using optical coherence tomography. *J. Clin. Med.* **2020**, *9*, 1530. [CrossRef]
7. Shaffer, R. 'Glaucoma Suspect' or 'Ocular Hypertension'? *Arch. Ophthalmol.* **1977**, *95*, 588. [CrossRef] [PubMed]
8. Adhikari, P.; Zele, A.J.; Thomas, R.; Feigl, B. Quadrant field pupillometry detects melanopsin dysfunction in glaucoma suspects and early glaucoma. *Sci. Rep.* **2016**, *6*, 33373. [CrossRef] [PubMed]
9. Pang, J.-J. Roles of the ocular pressure, pressure-sensitive ion channel, and elasticity in pressure-induced retinal diseases. *Neural Regen. Res.* **2021**, *16*, 68–72. [CrossRef] [PubMed]
10. Heijl, A.; Leske, M.C.; Bengtsson, B.; Hyman, L.; Hussein, M. Reduction of intraocular pressure and glaucoma progression: Results from the Early Manifest Glaucoma Trial. *Arch. Ophthalmol.* **2002**, *120*, 1268–1279. [CrossRef] [PubMed]
11. Lo, K.-J.; Ko, Y.-C.; Hwang, D.-K.; Liu, C.J.-L. The influence of topical non-steroidal anti-inflammatory drugs on the intraocular pressure lowering effect of topical prostaglandin analogues—A systemic review and meta-analysis. *PLoS ONE* **2020**, *15*, e0239233. [CrossRef] [PubMed]
12. Pinazo-Duran, M.D.; Shoaie-Nia, K.; Zanon-Moreno, V.; Sanz-Gonzalez, S.M.; Del Castillo, J.B.; Garcia-Medina, J.J. Strategies to reduce oxidative stress in glaucoma patients. *Curr. Neuropharmacol.* **2018**, *16*, 903–918. [CrossRef] [PubMed]
13. Nucci, C.; Martucci, A. Evidence on neuroprotective properties of coenzyme Q10 in the treatment of glaucoma. *Neural Regen. Res.* **2019**, *14*, 197–200. [CrossRef] [PubMed]
14. Fernández-Albarral, J.A.; De Hoz, R.; Ramírez, A.I.; López-Cuenca, I.; Salobrar-García, E.; Pinazo-Durán, M.D.; Ramírez, J.M.; Salazar, J.J. Beneficial effects of saffron (Crocus sativus L.) in ocular pathologies, particularly neurodegenerative retinal diseases. *Neural Regen. Res.* **2020**, *15*, 1408–1416. [CrossRef]
15. Pinazo-Durán, M.D.; García-Medina, J.J.; Bolarín, J.M.; Sanz-González, S.M.; Valero-Vello, M.; Abellán-Abenza, J.; Zanón-Moreno, V.; Moreno-Montañés, J. Computational analysis of clinical and molecular markers and new theranostic possibilities in primary open-angle glaucoma. *J. Clin. Med.* **2020**, *9*, 3032. [CrossRef] [PubMed]
16. Friedman, R.C.; Farh, K.K.; Burge, C.B.; Bartel, D.P. Most mammalian mRNAs are con-served targets of microRNAs. *Genome. Res.* **2009**, *19*, 92–105. [CrossRef]
17. Shin, S.; Jung, Y.; Uhm, H.; Song, M.; Son, S.; Goo, J.; Jeong, C.; Song, J.J.; Kim, V.N.; Hohng, S. Quantification of purified endogenous miRNAs with high sensitivity and spec-ificity. *Nat. Commun.* **2020**, *11*, 6033. [CrossRef]
18. Zhang, L.-J.; Zhang, Y.; Dong, L.-J.; Li, X.-R. [Expression and function of microRNA in the eye]. *[Zhonghua yan ke za zhi] Chin. J. Ophthalmol.* **2012**, *48*, 1136–1140.
19. Olivares, A.M.; Jelcick, A.S.; Reinecke, J.; Leehy, B.; Haider, A.; Morrison, M.A.; Cheng, L.; Chen, D.F.; DeAngelis, M.M.; Haider, N.B. Multimodal regulation orchestrates normal and complex disease states in the retina. *Sci. Rep.* **2017**, *7*, 690. [CrossRef]
20. Paylakhi, S.H.; Moazzeni, H.; Yazdani, S.; Rassouli, P.; Arefian, E.; Jaberi, E.; Arash, E.H.; Gilani, A.S.; Fan, J.B.; April, C.; et al. FOXC1 in human trabecu-lar meshwork cells is involved in regulatory pathway that includes miR-204, MEIS2, and ITGβ1. *Exp. Eye. Res.* **2013**, *111*, 112–121. [CrossRef]
21. Li, X.; Zhao, F.; Xin, M.; Li, G.; Luna, C.; Li, G.; Zhou, Q.; He, Y.; Yu, B.; Olson, E.; et al. Regulation of intraocular pressure by microRNA cluster miR-143/145. *Sci. Rep.* **2017**, *7*, 915. [CrossRef]
22. Tanaka, Y.; Tsuda, S.; Kunikata, H.; Sato, J.; Kokubun, T.; Yasuda, M.; Nishiguchi, K.M.; Inada, T.; Nakazawa, T. Profiles of extracellular miRNAs in the aqueous humor of glaucoma patients assessed with a microarray system. *Sci. Rep.* **2014**, *4*, 5089. [CrossRef] [PubMed]
23. Hindle, A.G.; Thoonen, R.; Jasien, J.V.; Grange, R.; Amin, K.; Wise, J.; Ozaki, M.; Ritch, R.; Malhotra, R.; Buys, E.S. Identification of candidate miRNA Biomarkers for Glaucoma. *Investig. Ophthalmol. Vis. Sci.* **2019**, *60*, 134–146. [CrossRef]
24. Peng, H.; Sun, Y.B.; Hao, J.L.; Lu, C.W.; Bi, M.C.; Song, E. Neuroprotective effects of overexpressed microRNA-200a on acti-vation of glaucoma-related retinal glial cells and aoptosis of ganglion cells via downregulating FGF7-mediated MAPK signaling pathway. *Cell Signal.* **2019**, *54*, 179–190. [CrossRef]
25. Benitez-Del-Castillo, J.; Cantu-Dibildox, J.; Sanz-González, S.M.; Zanón-Moreno, V.; Pinazo-Duran, M.D. Cytokine expression in tears of patients with glaucoma or dry eye disease: A prospective, observational cohort study. *Eur. J. Ophthalmol.* **2018**, *29*, 437–443. [CrossRef]

26. Benítez Del Castillo, J.M.; Pinazo-Duran, M.D.; Sanz-González, S.; Muñoz-Hernández, A.M.; Garcia-Medina, J.J.; Zanón-Moreno, V. Tear 1H NMR-based metabolomics application to the molecular diagnosis of aqueous tear deficiency and Mei-bomian gland dysfunction. *Ophthalmic Res.* **2020**, *64*, 297–309.

27. Mills, R.P.; Budenz, D.L.; Lee, P.P.; Noecker, R.J.; Walt, J.G.; Siegartel, L.R.; Evans, S.J.; Doyle, J.J. Categorizing the stage of glaucoma from pre-diagnosis to end-stage disease. *Am. J. Ophthalmol.* **2006**, *141*, 24–30. [CrossRef] [PubMed]

28. Borgmästars, E.; De Weerd, H.A.; Lubovac-Pilav, Z.; Sund, M. miRFA: An automated pipeline for microRNA functional analysis with correlation support from TCGA and TCPA expression data in pancreatic cancer. *BMC Bioinform.* **2019**, *20*, 393. [CrossRef]

29. Moazzeni, H.; Mirrahimi, M.; Moghadam, A.; Banaei-Esfahani, A.; Yazdani, S.; Elahi, E. Identification of genes involved in glaucoma pathogenesis using combined network analysis and empirical studies. *Hum. Mol. Genet.* **2019**, *28*, 3637–3663. [CrossRef] [PubMed]

30. Piñero, J.; Bravo, À.; Queralt-Rosinach, N.; Gutiérrez-Sacristán, A.; Deu-Pons, J.; Cen-teno, E.; García-García, J.; Sanz, F.; Furlong, L.I. DisGeNET: A comprehensive platform integrating information on human disease-associated genes and variants. *Nucleic Acids Res.* **2017**, *45*, D833–D839. [CrossRef]

31. Reimand, J.; Isserlin, R.; Voisin, V.; Kucera, M.; Tannus-Lopes, C.; Rostamianfar, A.; Wadi, L.; Meyer, M.; Wong, J.; Xu, C.; et al. Pathway enrichment analysis and visualization of omics data using g:Profiler, GSEA, Cytoscape and EnrichmentMap. *Nat. Protoc.* **2019**, *14*, 482–517. [CrossRef]

32. Franz, M.; Rodriguez, H.; Lopes, C.; Zuberi, K.; Montojo, J.; Bader, G.D.; Morris, Q. GeneMANIA update. *Nucleic Acids Res.* **2018**, *46*, W60–W64. [CrossRef] [PubMed]

33. Su, L.-C.; Xu, W.-D.; Liu, X.-Y.; Fu, L.; Huang, A.-F. Altered expression of circular RNA in primary Sjögren's syndrome. *Clin. Rheumatol.* **2019**, *38*, 3425–3433. [CrossRef] [PubMed]

34. He, M.; Wang, W.; Yu, H.; Wang, D.; Cao, D.; Zeng, Y.; Wu, Q.; Zhong, P.; Cheng, Z.; Hu, Y.; et al. Comparison of expression profiling of circular RNAs in vitreous humour between diabetic retinopathy and non-diabetes mellitus patients. *Acta Diabetol.* **2020**, *57*, 479–489. [CrossRef]

35. Elbay, A.; Ercan, Ç.; Akba, F.; Bulut, H.; Ozdemir, H. Three new circulating microRNAs may be associated with wet age-related macular degeneration. *Scand. J. Clin. Lab. Investig.* **2019**, *79*, 388–394. [CrossRef]

36. Youngblood, H.; Cai, J.; Drewry, M.D.; Helwa, I.; Hu, E.; Liu, S.; Yu, H.; Mu, H.; Hu, Y.; Perkumas, K.; et al. Expression of mRNAs, miRNAs, and lncRNAs in human trabecular meshwork cells upon mechanical stretch. *Investig. Opthalmol. Vis. Sci.* **2020**, *61*, 2. [CrossRef] [PubMed]

37. Liu, Y.; Chen, Y.; Wang, Y.; Zhang, X.; Gao, K.; Chen, S.; Zhang, X. microRNA profiling in glaucoma eyes with varying degrees of optic neuropathy by using next-generation sequencing. *Investig. Opthalmol. Vis. Sci.* **2018**, *59*, 2955–2966. [CrossRef] [PubMed]

38. Ertekin, S.; Yıldırım, O.; Dinç, E.; Ayaz, L.; Fidancı, S.B.; Tamer, L. Evaluation of circulating miRNAs in wet age-related macular degeneration. *Mol. Vis.* **2014**, *20*, 1057–1066.

39. Zanon-Moreno, V.; Marco-Ventura, P.; Lleo-Perez, A.; Pons-Vazquez, S.; Garcia-Medina, J.J.; Vinuesa-Silva, I.; Moreno-Nadal, M.A.; Pinazo-Duran, M.D. Oxidative stress in primary open-angle glaucoma. *J. Glaucoma* **2008**, *17*, 263–268. [CrossRef]

40. Hondur, G.; Göktas, E.; Yang, X.; Al-Aswad, L.; Auran, J.D.; Blumberg, D.M.; Cioffi, G.A.; Liebmann, J.M.; Suh, L.H.; Trief, D.; et al. Oxidative stress-related molecular biomarker candidates for glaucoma. *Investig. Ophthalmol. Vis. Sci.* **2017**, *58*, 4078–4088. [CrossRef]

41. Bagnis, A.; Izzotti, A.; Centofanti, M.; Sacca, S. Aqueous humor oxidative stress proteomic levels in primary open angle glaucoma. *Exp. Eye Res.* **2012**, *103*, 55–62. [CrossRef]

42. Rao, A.; Chakraborty, M.; Roy, A.; Sahay, P.; Pradhan, A.; Raj, N. Differential miRNA Expression: Signature for glaucoma in pseudoexfoliation. *Clin. Ophthalmol.* **2020**, *14*, 3025–3038. [CrossRef] [PubMed]

43. Su, C.; Huang, D.; Liu, J.; Liu, W.; Cao, Y. miR-27a-3p regulates proliferation and apoptosis of colon cancer cells by potentially targeting BTG1. *Oncol. Lett.* **2019**, *18*, 2825–2834. [CrossRef] [PubMed]

44. Ben, W.; Zhang, G.; Huang, Y.; Sun, Y. MiR-27a-3p Regulated the aggressive phenotypes of cervical cancer by targeting FBXW7. *Cancer Manag. Res.* **2020**, *12*, 2925–2935. [CrossRef] [PubMed]

45. Zhao, X.-R.; Zhang, Z.; Gao, M.; Li, L.; Sun, P.-Y.; Xu, L.-N.; Qi, Y.; Yin, L.-H.; Peng, J.-Y. MicroRNA-27a-3p aggravates renal ischemia/reperfusion injury by promoting oxidative stress via targeting growth factor receptor-bound protein 2. *Pharmacol. Res.* **2020**, *155*, 104718. [CrossRef]

46. Gonzalez, P.; Li, G.; Qiu, J.; Wu, J.; Luna, C. Role of MicroRNAs in the Trabecular Meshwork. *J. Ocul. Pharmacol. Ther.* **2014**, *30*, 128–137. [CrossRef]

47. Drewry, M.D.; Cai, J.; Helwa, I.; Hu, E.; Liu, S.; Mu, H.; Hu, Y.; Johnson, W.M.; Gonzalez, P.; Stamer, W.D.; et al. Genome-wide Expression Profiling and Pathway Analysis in Cyclic Stretched Human Trabecular Meshwork. *BioRXiv* **2020**. [CrossRef]

48. DesJarlais, M.; Rivera, J.C.; Lahaie, I.; Cagnone, G.; Wirt, M.; Omri, S.; Chemtob, S. MicroRNA expression profile in retina and choroid in oxygen-induced retinopathy model. *PLoS ONE* **2019**, *14*, e0218282. [CrossRef]

49. Wang, R.; Bai, Z.; Wen, X.; Du, H.; Zhou, L.; Tang, Z.; Yang, Z.; Ma, W. MiR-152-3p regulates cell proliferation, invasion and extracellular matrix expression through by targeting FOXF1 in keloid fibroblasts. *Life Sci.* **2019**, *234*, 116779. [CrossRef]

50. Sabre, L.; Maddison, P.; Wong, S.H.; Sadalage, G.; Ambrose, P.A.; Plant, G.T.; Punga, A.R. miR-30e-5p as predictor of generalization in ocular myasthenia gravis. *Ann. Clin. Transl. Neurol.* **2019**, *6*, 243–251. [CrossRef]

51. Meng, F.; Dai, E.; Yu, X.; Zhang, Y.; Chen, X.; Liu, X.; Wang, S.; Wang, L.; Jiang, W. Constructing and characterizing a bioactive small molecule and microRNA association network for Alzheimer's disease. *J. R. Soc. Interface* **2013**, *18*, 20131057. [CrossRef]
52. Hardeland, R. Neurobiology, Pathophysiology, and treatment of melatonin deficiency and dysfunction. *Sci. World J.* **2012**, *2012*, 640389. [CrossRef]
53. Scuderi, L.; Davinelli, S.; Iodice, C.M.; Bartollino, S.; Scapagnini, G.; Costagliola, C.; Scuderi, G. Melatonin: Implications for ocular disease and therapeutic potential. *Curr. Pharm. Des.* **2019**, *25*, 4185–4191. [CrossRef]
54. Toro, M.D.; Reibaldi, M.; Avitabile, T.; Bucolo, C.; Salomone, S.; Rejdak, R.; Nowomiejska, K.; Tripodi, S.; Posarelli, C.; Ragusa, M.; et al. MicroRNAs in the vitreous humor of patients with retinal detachment and a different grading of proliferative vitreoretinopathy: A pilot study. *Transl. Vis. Sci. Technol.* **2020**, *9*, 23. [CrossRef] [PubMed]
55. Smit, K.N.; Chang, J.; Derks, K.; Vaarwater, J.; Brands, T.; Verdijk, R.M.; Wiemer, E.A.; Mensink, H.W.; Pothof, J.; De Klein, A.; et al. Aberrant MicroRNA expression and its implications for uveal melanoma metastasis. *Cancers* **2019**, *11*, 815. [CrossRef]
56. Bianciotto, C.; Saornil, M.A.; Muiños, Y.; Méndez, Y.; Blanco, G.; Frutos-Baraja, J.M.; López-Lara, F.; Esteban, R. Ocular hypertension as the principal indicator of onset of uveal melanoma. *Arch. Soc. Esp. Oftalmol.* **2005**, *80*, 27–34. [CrossRef] [PubMed]
57. Tezel, G. The immune response in glaucoma: A perspective on the roles of oxidative stress. *Exp. Eye Res.* **2011**, *93*, 178–186. [CrossRef] [PubMed]
58. Yang, X.; Hondur, G.; Li, M.; Cai, J.; Klein, J.B.; Kuehn, M.H.; Tezel, G. Proteomics analysis of molecular risk factors in the ocular hypertensive human retina. *Investig. Opthalmol. Vis. Sci.* **2015**, *56*, 5816–5830. [CrossRef]
59. Batliwala, S.; Xavier, C.; Liu, Y.; Wu, H.; Pang, I.-H. Involvement of Nrf2 in ocular diseases. *Oxidative Med. Cell. Longev.* **2017**, *2017*, 1703810. [CrossRef] [PubMed]
60. Wang, C.; Ren, Y.-L.; Zhai, J.; Zhou, X.-Y.; Wu, J. Down-regulated LAMA4 inhibits oxidative stress-induced apoptosis of retinal ganglion cells through the MAPK signaling pathway in rats with glaucoma. *Cell Cycle* **2019**, *18*, 932–948. [CrossRef]
61. Vernazza, S.; Tirendi, S.; Bassi, A.M.; Traverso, C.E.; Saccà, S.C. Neuroinflammation in primary open-angle glaucoma. *J. Clin. Med.* **2020**, *9*, 3172. [CrossRef]
62. Tabak, S.; Schreiber-Avissar, S.; Beit-Yannai, E. Crosstalk between MicroRNA and oxidative stress in primary open-angle glaucoma. *Int. J. Mol. Sci.* **2021**, *22*, 2421. [CrossRef] [PubMed]
63. Velkovska, M.A.; Goričar, K.; Blagus, T.; Dolžan, V.; Cvenkel, B. Association of genetic polymorphisms in oxidative stress and inflammation pathways with glaucoma risk and phenotype. *J. Clin. Med.* **2021**, *10*, 1148. [CrossRef] [PubMed]
64. Zuo, L.; Prather, E.R.; Stetskiv, M.; Garrison, D.E.; Meade, J.R.; Peace, T.I.; Zhou, T. Inflammaging and oxidative stress in human diseases: From molecular mechanisms to novel treatments. *Int. J. Mol. Sci.* **2019**, *20*, 4472. [CrossRef] [PubMed]
65. Mackey, A.D.; Craig, E.J. Predictive DNA testing for glaucoma: Reality in 2003. *Ophthalmol. Clin. N. Am.* **2003**, *16*, 639–645. [CrossRef]
66. Fan, B.J.; Tam, P.O.S.; Choy, K.W.; Wang, D.Y.; Lam, D.S.C.; Pang, C.P. Molecular diagnostics of genetic eye diseases. *Clin. Biochem.* **2006**, *39*, 231–239. [CrossRef]
67. Craig, J.E.; Han, X.; Qassim, A.; Hassall, M.; Cooke Bailey, J.N.; Kinzy, T.G.; Khawaja, A.P.; An, J.; Marshall, H.; Gharahkhani, P.; et al. Multitrait analysis of glaucoma identifies new risk loci and enables polygenic prediction of disease susceptibility and progression. *Nat. Genet.* **2020**, *52*, 160–166. [CrossRef]

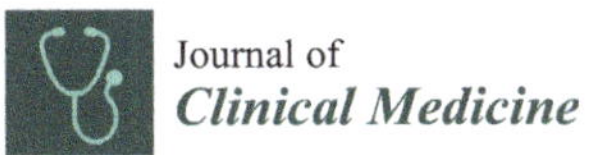

Journal of
Clinical Medicine

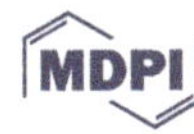

Article

Evaluation of Intraocular Pressure and Other Biomechanical Parameters to Distinguish between Subclinical Keratoconus and Healthy Corneas

Cristina Peris-Martínez [1,2,3,†,‡], María Amparo Díez-Ajenjo [1,4,†], María Carmen García-Domene [1,4], María Dolores Pinazo-Durán [2,‡], María José Luque-Cobija [1,4], María Ángeles del Buey-Sayas [5,‡] and Susana Ortí-Navarro [4,*,‡]

[1] FISABIO Oftalmología Médica (FOM), Anterior Segment and Cornea and External Eye Diseases Unit, Bifurcación Pío Baroja-General Avilés, 12, E-46015 Valencia, Spain; cristinaperismartinez0@gmail.com (C.P.-M.); amparo.diez@uv.es (M.A.D.-A.); m.carmen.garcia-domene@uv.es (M.C.G.-D.); maria.j.luque@uv.es (M.J.L.-C.)

[2] Surgery Department, Ophthalmology, School of Medicine, University of Valencia, Av. Blasco Ibáñez, 15, E-46010 Valencia, Spain; pinazoduran@yahoo.es

[3] Aviño Peris Eye Clinic, Avinguda de l'Oest, 34, E-46001 Valencia, Spain

[4] Optics, Optometry and Vision Sciences Department, School of Physics, University of Valencia, Dr. Moliner, 50, E-46100 Valencia, Spain

[5] Hospital Lozano Blesa, Anterior Segment and Cornea and External Eye Diseases, E-46015 Zaragoza, Spain; madelbuey@gmail.com

* Correspondence: susana.orti@uv.es

† Authors sharing the first place.

‡ Group leaders contributing equally to this work.

Citation: Peris-Martínez, C.; Díez-Ajenjo, M.A.; García-Domene, M.C.; Pinazo-Durán, M.D.; Luque-Cobija, M.J.; del Buey-Sayas, M.Á.; Ortí-Navarro, S. Evaluation of Intraocular Pressure and Other Biomechanical Parameters to Distinguish between Subclinical Keratoconus and Healthy Corneas. *J. Clin. Med.* **2021**, *10*, 1905. https://doi.org/10.3390/jcm10091905

Academic Editors: Vito Romano and Brent Siesky

Received: 21 March 2021
Accepted: 25 April 2021
Published: 28 April 2021

Publisher's Note: MDPI stays neutral with regard to jurisdictional claims in published maps and institutional affiliations.

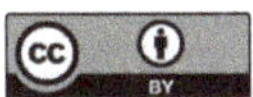

Abstract: (1) Purpose: To assess the main corneal response differences between normal and subclinical keratoconus (SCKC) with a Corvis® ST device. (2) Material and Methods: We selected 183 eyes of normal patients, of a mean age of 33 ± 9 years and 16 eyes of patients with SCKC of a similar mean age. We measured best corrected visual acuity (BCVA) and corneal topography with a Pentacam HD device to select the SCKC group. Biomechanical measurements were performed using the Corvis® ST device. We carried out a non-parametric analysis of the data with SPSS software (Wilcoxon signed rank-test). (3) Results: We found statistically significant differences between the control and SCKC groups in some corneal biomechanical parameters: first and second applanation time ($p = 0.05$ and $p = 0.02$), maximum deformation amplitude ($p = 0.016$), highest concavity radius ($p = 0.007$), and second applanation length and corneal velocity (($p = 0.039$ and $p = 0.016$). (4) Conclusions: Our results show that the use of normalised biomechanical parameters provided by noncontact tonometry, combined with a discriminant function theory, is a useful tool for detecting subclinical keratoconus.

Keywords: intraocular pressure; ocular inflammation; cornea biomechanics; Corvis® ST; subclinical keratoconus

1. Introduction

Knowledge of corneal biomechanics is essential to understand corneal behaviour in certain diseases, surgical procedures, intraocular pressure (IOP) measurements, and in the early detection and treatment of subclinical keratoconus (SCKC).

Keratoconus is a bilateral, inflammatory, asymmetric and progressive corneal ectasia disorder. Bowman's layer in keratoconus patients is impaired, associated changes in the stromal extracellular matrix are brought about [1], and a cycle of thinning and increased strain occurs [2,3]. The collagen network is mostly unorganised, with decreased fibrillar interweaving [3–5]. These changes reduce corneal stiffness [2,5].

The most commonly used device for analysing corneal biomechanical parameters is the Ocular Response Analyzer (ORA®, Reichert Ophthalmic Instruments, Inc., Buffalo, NY,

USA) [4–8]. Some studies found a good correlation between keratoconus and low corneal hysteresis (CH) and corneal resistance factor (CRF) in high grade keratoconus [7–11].

The Corvis® ST device (Oculus Optikgeräte GmbH; Wetzlar, Germany) is a non-contact tonometer system with an ultra-high-speed Scheimpflug camera that provides corneal biomechanical parameters and IOP information [12–26]. It also affords a high degree of repeatability [13,25–27] and gives a correlation between age, corneal thickness, IOP, and some Corvis® ST biomechanical parameters [17,24,28].

Some studies show differences in biomechanical Corvis® ST parameters between keratoconic and healthy corneas [12–23]. More recently, other studies have evaluated SCKC with this device [12,18,19,29,30].

Early SCKC detection is important since treatment with collagen cross-linking can slow the progression of keratoconus effectively. If subtle biomechanical changes in early keratoconus go undetected, advanced keratoconus treatment could be delayed. In addition, proper patient selection (without SCKC) is essential for the success of refractive surgery. Clearly, it is difficult to distinguish between SCKC and eyes with healthy corneas when only using slit-lamp criteria. Topographic values only provide information of static changes and it must be taken into account that air pressure–corneal deformation is affected in keratoconus patients [7,12,15,31].

The main purpose of the present study was to identify the most useful parameters provided by non-contact tonometry for the biomechanical characterization of the cornea and to determine whether it is possible to define an optimized function for SCKC detection.

2. Materials and Methods

This study adheres to the tenets of the Declaration of Helsinki for Research Involving Human Subjects and was approved by our Institutional Review Board. This retrospective, consecutive, non-randomised study analyses 199 eyes of 196 patients using the Corvis® ST tonometer. The eyes were divided into two groups: (a) healthy eyes (183 eyes of 183 patients); and (b) eyes with subclinical keratoconus (16 eyes of 13 patients). The eyes with subclinical keratoconus fulfilled the most widely accepted definition in the literature for this condition [30,32,33]. These eyes had no clinical signs of keratoconus (Vogt's striae, Fleischer rings or corneal scarring), their topography was normal with no asymmetric bowtie, and no focal or inferior steepening pattern. However, they were contralateral eyes of clinically evident keratoconus in the fellow eye [32]. Three of them were considered as bilateral SCKC.

The inclusion criteria for both groups were the non-use of contact lenses during the previous four weeks if such contact lenses were rigid, or two weeks if they were soft, and ages between 18 and 50.

Exclusion criteria were previous ophthalmic surgery, any ocular or systemic disease, corneal scars and/or opacities, chronic use of topical medication, pregnancy or refusal to sign the informed consent form.

We measured the corneal topography of all the patients with a Pentacam HD device (Oculus, Wetzlar, Germany). The corneal status was established by slit-lamp microscopy and analysed and classified by an experienced ophthalmologist. The control patients had no clinical keratoconus symptoms and their corneal topography was within normal limits. Diagnosis of SCKC was made when eyes had no clinical signs of keratoconus (Vogt's striae, Fleischer rings or corneal scarring), their topography was normal with no asymmetric bowtie (with a paracentral inferior–superior dioptric difference less than 1 D), and no focal or inferior steepening pattern. We included patients with the steepest meridian under 47.2 D who did not present clinical signs [30,32,33].

Best corrected visual acuity (BCVA) was measured with an ETDRS chart. The Corvis® ST evaluated corneal biomechanics. This device can identify the applanation time and length and corneal applanation velocity when the air pulse is on (A1time, A1length and A1V, respectively) and off (A2time, A2length and A2V, respectively). It can also identify the highest concavity time (HCtime), the deformation amplitude (DA_{max}), the peak distance (PD) and the curvature radius (R_{HC}) at the highest concavity (HC). All these data are obtained from the dynamic corneal deformation during a defined air pulse. Central corneal thickness (CCT) is also calculated using the horizontal Scheimpflug image at the apex. Intraocular pressure is calculated based on the timing of the first applanation event. The Corvis biomechanical index (CBI) was not evaluated because the updated version was not available on our Corvis® ST device when the measurements were made.

Statistical analysis was performed using the SPSS 26.0 software for Windows (SPSS, Chicago, IL, USA) and principal component analysis (PCA) was carried out with Matlab 2020a (The Mathworks, Inc., Natick, MA, USA). For each variable, values came from the mean of three measurements. The Kolmogorov–Smirnov test was used to check for sample normality. Distributions for the SCKC group failed the normality test, and therefore a non-parametric Wilcoxon signed rank-test was used to compare parameters between the groups. The level of significance used was $p < 0.05$.

3. Results

Table 1 summarizes the demographic data of the patients. There was no significant difference in age between the groups.

Table 1. Demographic data of our sample. Age differences between control and SCKC groups were not significant ($p = 0.55$).

Data	Sex	Control Group	SCKC Group
Age (years)	Men	31 ± 7	26 ± 13
	Women	33 ± 8	31 ± 19
p-value		0.67	0.50
Number of eyes	Men	83	8
	Women	100	5

The control and SCKC group had a BCVA of 0.12 ± 0.20 logMAR and 0.04 ± 0.20 logMAR, respectively ($p = 0.002$). Mean corneal keratometry were 43.0 ± 1.7 D and 44.2 ± 1.9 D for the flattest meridian, in the control and SCKC group, respectively ($p = 0.328$). The steepest meridian was 43.9 ± 1.8 D and 45.0 ± 3.0 D in the control and SCKC group, respectively ($p = 0.006$).

Figures 1a, 2a, 3a and 4a show the values obtained for the first and second applanation, and for the HC. CCT and IOP values were significantly different in the two population samples ($p < 0.05$ for both parameters, with 9.6 ± 2.7 mm Hg and 510 ± 49 μm for the SCKC group and 12.3 ± 2.9 mm Hg and 541 ± 38 μm for the control group). To discount a possible effect of this difference, in Figures 1b, 2b, 3b and 4b, a new control group (n = 53) was defined, matching the CCT and IOP values of the SCKC subjects (517 ± 18 μm and 10.4 ± 1.5 mm Hg). Differences in IOP and CCT between the SCKC and the IOP-CCT matched normals were not significant ($p = 0.57$ and $p = 0.32$ for CCT and IOP, respectively).

The whole control group reached the first applanation significantly later than the SCKC group ($p = 0.001$, see Figure 1a), A1length was greater than the SCKC group ($p = 0.66$, see Figure 2a), and A1V was slower in the control group than in the SCKC group ($p = 0.24$, see Figure 3a), but these changes were not significant.

At HC, DA_{max} (Figure 2a) and the PD (Figure 4a) were smaller in the whole control group than in the SCKC group ($p = 0.0005$ and 0.15, respectively) and R_{HC} (Figure 4) was smaller in the SCKC group than in the whole control group ($p < 0.001$). The HC time was similar in both groups ($p = 0.85$, Figure 1a).

In the second applanation, A2time (Figure 1a) and A2V (Figure 3a) were significantly higher in the SCKC group than in the total control group ($p = 0.02$ and 0.001, respectively), but A2length (Figure 2a) was significantly smaller in the SCKC group than in the control group ($p = 0.01$).

When comparing SCKC with the IOP-CCT matched normals, similar trends are found, but with changes in the significance of the differences. DA_{max} ($p = 0.006$, Figure 2b), A2length ($p = 0.03$, Figure 2b), A2V ($p = 0.006$, Figure 3b), and R_{HC} ($p = 0.05$, Figure 4b) maintained their statistical differences, and differences were also found in A1length ($p = 0.02$, Figure 2b). However, statistical differences were not found in A1time ($p = 0.34$) or A2time ($p = 0.57$) (Figure 1b).

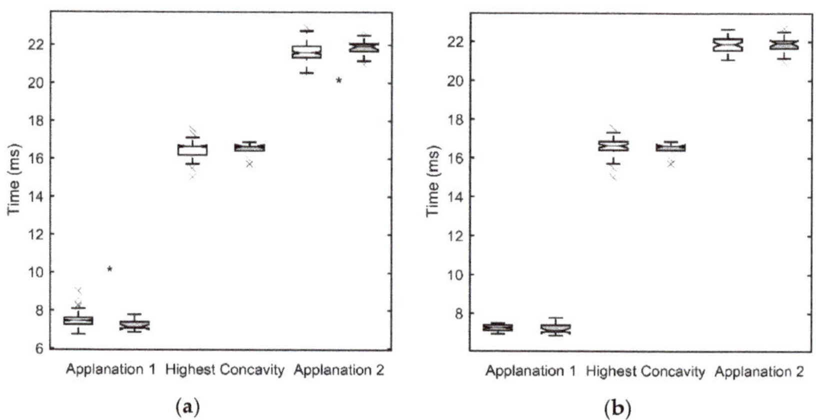

Figure 1. Time to reach first applanation, highest concavity and second applanation for the SCKC (grey) and control groups (white). The middle line of each box is the median of the distribution, the extremes are the first and third quartiles and the whiskers represent 1.5 times the interquartile distance; outliers are plotted with the symbol "x". The notch represents de 95% confidence interval of the mean. "*" indicates statistically significant differences between groups ($p < 0.05$) (**a**) whole control group, (**b**) IOP and CCT matched control group.

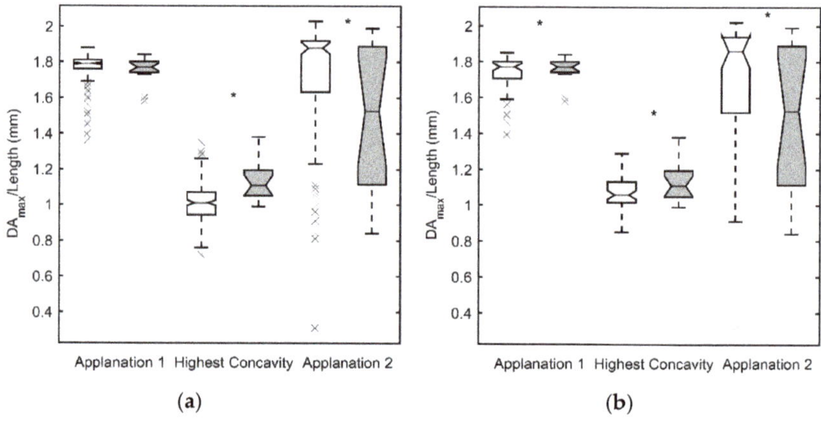

Figure 2. Maximum deformation amplitude (DA_{max}) at highest concavity and length applanation at first and second measurement for the SCKC (grey) and control groups (white). Symbols, as in Figure 1. (**a**) whole control group, (**b**) IOP and CCT matched control group.

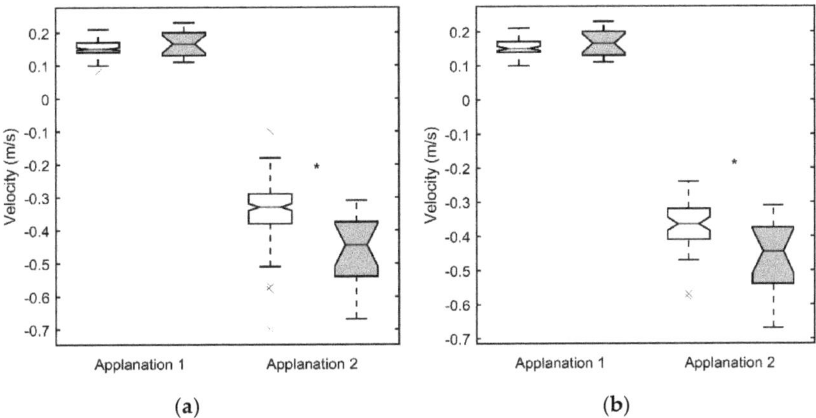

Figure 3. Velocity of deformation at first and second applanation for the SCKC (grey) and control groups (white). Symbols as in Figure 1. (**a**) whole control group, (**b**) IOP and CCT matched control group.

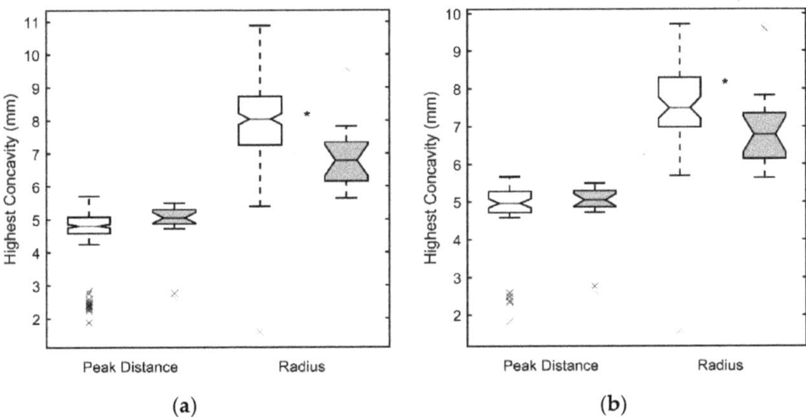

Figure 4. Peak Distance (PD) and radius at highest concavity (R_{HC}) for the SCKC (grey) and control groups (white). Symbols as in Figure 1. (**a**) whole control group, (**b**) IOP and CCT matched control group.

Receiver operating characteristic (ROC) curves were derived, using both the whole normal sample and the IOP and CCT matched normal subjects with the four parameters that yielded significant differences between matched normal and the SCKC group (R_{HC}, A2length, A2V, and DA_{max}). Figure 5 shows the results obtained.

The best result, according to the area under the curve (AUC), is yielded by A2V, but the best sensitivity to specificity ratio is only 25–75%, approximately. To determine whether a combination of these four parameters would improve these results, we performed a principal component analysis (PCA). None of the four principal components achieved a total separation of the normal and SCKC samples, but the first component, explaining 65% of the variance when the total normal sample is used and 59% with the reduced normal sample, yielded a ROC curve that slightly improves the result of the individual variables (see Table 2). The improvement is noticeable only in the specificity at high sensitivity (80% or higher).

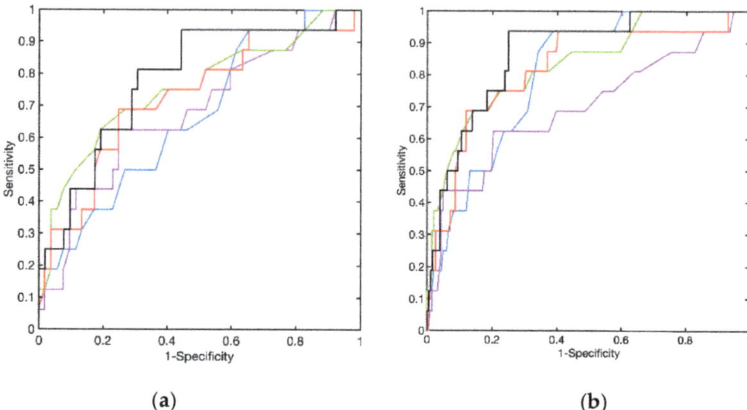

Figure 5. Receiver Operating Characteristic (ROC) curves for High Concavity Radius (red), second applanation length (purple), velocity (green) and maximum amplitude (blue). In black, the curve obtained with the first principal component score of the principal component analysis carried out with these four variables. The dashed line represents the x = y reference line. (**a**) curves obtained with the whole normal sample. (**b**) curves obtained with the IOP and CCP matched normal sample.

Table 2. Area under de ROC curve (AUC) and upper and lower limits of the AUC 95% confidence interval for the different diagnosis parameters computed both with the entire normal sample and the IOP and CCP matched normal sample. DA_{max}, maximum displacement amplitude, second applanation length (A2length) and corneal velocity (A2V), radius at high concavity (Radius) and the first principal component scores of the principal component analysis (1st PCS). '*' marks AUCs significantly different from 0.5 (no discrimination).

	Total Normal Sample			IOP and CCP Matched Normal Sample		
Variable	AUC	Lower ICL	Upper ICL	AUC	Lower ICL	Upper ICL
1st PCS	0.8695 *	0.7452	0.9269	0.7800 *	0.6073	0.8906
A2V	0.8343 *	0.6948	0.9176	0.7524 *	0.5815	0.8814
Radius	0.8203 *	0.6572	0.9142	0.7230 *	0.5662	0.8506
DA_{max}	0.8047 *	0.7052	0.8869	0.6629	0.4710	0.7929
A2length	0.6987 *	0.5244	0.8496	0.6767	0.4970	0.8266

4. Discussion

Detection of corneal ectatic disorders as early on as possible is necessary to prevent, or delay, the progression of keratoconus. Some studies claim to distinguish SCKC from normal eyes using topographic parameters [34–36] and others state that there is an overlap between topographic data obtained from a SCKC group and a normal group [37,38]. As a result, biomechanical data could improve the detection and severity prediction of keratoconus.

There are studies on corneal biomechanics using the ORA device that conclude that the four parameters measured with this device are not enough to detect keratoconus [21,39]. Alternative ORA parameters related to the area under the curve are better for distinguishing SCKC from normal corneas, and when all the parameters are combined, accuracy increases [34,39]. The ORA device has limitations, because it can confuse corneal tissue response with surface response since a specular reflection is required to measure applanation pressure. Central corneal surface irregularities could interfere with the infrared specular reflection beam of the ORA. The Corvis® ST device avoids some of these drawbacks, because a frontal view camera is mounted with a keratometric-type projection system for focusing and aligning the corneal apex to be measured. Moreover, the recording of corneal deformation prevents the specular reflection beam from obtaining reliable corneal response parameters.

If one simply addresses statistical data, our data are consistent with biomechanical corneal properties. The A1time is shorter in the SCKC group than in the control group, and DA_{max} is greater in the SCKC group than in the control group. This agrees with previous studies, in which very similar values of DA_{max} were obtained in the SCKC and control groups [15,16,30,40]. During corneal recovery, A2time and A2V were higher in the SCKC group, and R_{HC} and A2length were higher in controls, in agreement with several studies in the literature [30,40]. Except for A2length, these parameters could be correlated with a decrease in the viscoelastic structure, and abnormal elastic distensibility increased in keratoconic corneas, which is consistent with reduced corneal stiffness [4,41].

Due to the decrease in corneal stiffness, a shorter A1time, a higher DA_{max}, and a lower R_{HC} could be expected in the SCKC group, as well as a longer A2time and A2V, as keratokonic corneas recover more slowly than normal ones, due to higher initial deformation. Although the differences are not significant, the higher PD, A2time, and A1V values in the SCKC group also confirm this hypothesis.

In principle, we could expect greater A2length values in the SCKC group than in the control group as a result of reduced corneal stiffness. It is possible that increased keratoconus cornea distensibility may produce a non-perfect applanation surface, and Corvis® ST only detects a small portion of plane surface. Therefore, it must be taken into account that our study yielded similar results to those obtained in previous studies [16,30,40].

Although we selected patients without clinical signs, BCVA was statistically worse in the SCKC group. This loss of visual acuity may have been due to the wavefront aberrations that can distort visual quality, even at the beginning of the pathology [42].

When the effect of the IOP and CCT parameters are eliminated, Corvis® ST results change. There are parameters that demonstrate their independence of IOP and CCT measurements, such as DA_{max}, A2V, and R_{HC}, so they can be considered as robust parameters. These three parameters can identify SCKC correctly, but parameters determining time to deformation and recovery are greatly dependent on IOP and CCT. This is no surprise, since it is known that higher CCT corneas have more resistance to deformation, and the same result could be expected with higher IOP eyes. In addition, we obtained significant differences in length applanation values by eliminating CCT and IOP effects. This confirms that these parameters also have a great dependence on IOP and CCT values, since higher values in these parameters could lead to smaller applanation length due to the resistance to deformation that the cornea can present.

When we analyse ROC curves with the four parameters that yielded significant differences with the SCKC group, that is, R_{HC}, A2length, A2V and DA_{max}, we can conclude that A2V was the best parameter to diagnose SCKC patients. In this small sample, however, a combination of these four parameters, found by principal component analysis, though improving the AUC under the ROC curve would only improve specificity at high sensitivity.

This study has some limitations. Our SCKC sample was small, and we are aware that a greater number of patients with SCKC would be necessary to obtain more reliable values. To calculate ROC curves with a small SCKC sample could lead to inexact conclusions about the best parameters to detect it. However, a similar number of SCKC eyes (between 12 and 23) were evaluated in previously published studies [12,18,21,22,30], because it is difficult to obtain this sample.

5. Conclusions

We were able to detect biomechanical impairment in SCKC eyes in clinical examinations by using Corvis® ST parameters. Some of them have demonstrated a great dependence on IOP and CCT, so to make a correct diagnosis of these patients, only parameters without IOP and CCT dependence should probably be compared. However, further measurements in SCKC patients are necessary, and the effect of IOP and CCT must be studied in more detail, to confirm the findings of our study and to improve current SCKC screening.

Author Contributions: Conceptualization, M.A.D.-A., M.C.G.-D., M.J.L.-C. and C.P.-M.; methodology, M.C.G.-D., S.O.-N. and M.A.D.-A.; formal analysis, M.C.G.-D., S.O.-N., M.J.L.-C., M.D.P.-D. and M.A.D.-A.; writing—original draft preparation, C.P.-M., S.O.-N. and M.A.D.-A.; writing—review and editing, C.P.-M., M.C.G.-D., S.O.-N. and M.A.D.-A.; supervision, M.J.L.-C., C.P.-M., M.Á.d.B.-S. and M.A.D.-A. All authors have read and agreed to the published version of the manuscript.

Funding: Cátedra FISABIO-Alcon-Universidad de Valencia.

Institutional Review Board Statement: The study was conducted according to the guidelines of the Declaration of Helsinki, and approved by the Institutional Review Board (or Ethics Committee) of FISABIO Oftalmología Médica (Protocol number PI_89, principal investigator Cristina Peris-Martínez, and date of approval: 26 July 2018).

Informed Consent Statement: Informed consent was obtained from all subjects involved in the study.

Data Availability Statement: Data available on request due to restrictions of privacy.

Conflicts of Interest: The authors declare no conflict of interest.

References

1. Brookes, N.; Loh, I.-P.; Clover, G.; Poole, C.; Sherwin, T. Involvement of corneal nerves in the progression of keratoconus. *Exp. Eye Res.* **2003**, *77*, 515–524. [CrossRef]
2. Erie, J.C.; Patel, S.V.; McLaren, J.W.; Nau, C.B.; Hodge, D.O.; Bourne, W.M. Keratocyte density in keratoconus. A confocal microscopy study. *Am. J. Ophthalmol.* **2002**, *134*, 689–695. [CrossRef]
3. Meek, K.M.; Tuft, S.J.; Huang, Y.; Gill, P.S.; Hayes, S.; Newton, R.H.; Bron, A.J. Changes in Collagen Orientation and Distribution in Keratoconus Corneas. *Investig. Opthalmol. Vis. Sci.* **2005**, *46*, 1948–1956. [CrossRef] [PubMed]
4. Esporcatte, L.P.G.; Salomão, M.Q.; Lopes, B.T.; Vinciguerra, P.; Vinciguerra, R.; Roberts, C.; Elsheikh, A.; Dawson, D.G.; Ambrósio, R. Biomechanical Diagnostics of the Cornea. *Int. Ophthalmol. Clin. Summer* **2017**, *57*, 75–86. [CrossRef] [PubMed]
5. Vellara, H.R.; Patel, D.V. Biomechanical properties of the keratoconic cornea: A review. *Clin. Exp. Optom.* **2015**, *98*, 31–38. [CrossRef] [PubMed]
6. Zimmermann, D.R.; Fischer, R.W.; Winterhalter, K.H.; Witmer, R.; Vaughan, L. Comparative studies of collagens in normal and keratoconus corneas. *Exp. Eye Res.* **1988**, *46*, 431–442. [CrossRef]
7. Herber, R.; Ramm, L.; Spoerl, E.; Raiskup, F.; Pillunat, L.E.; Terai, N. Assessment of corneal biomechanical parameters in healthy and keratoconic eyes using dynamic bidirectional applanation device and dynamic Scheimpflug analyzer. *J. Cataract. Refract. Surg.* **2019**, *45*, 778–788. [CrossRef]
8. Luce, D.A. Determining in vivo biomechanical properties of the cornea with an ocular response analyzer. *J. Cataract. Refract. Surg.* **2005**, *31*, 156–162. [CrossRef]
9. Shah, S.; Laiquzzaman, M.; Bhojwani, R.; Mantry, S.; Cunliffe, I. Assessment of the biomechanical properties of the cornea with the ocular re-sponse analyzer in normal and keratoconic eyes. *Investig. Ophthalmol. Vis. Sci.* **2007**, *48*, 3026–3031. [CrossRef]
10. Galletti, J.G.; Pförtner, T.; Bonthoux, F.F. Improved keratoconus detection by ocular response analyzer testing after considera-tion of corneal thickness as a confounding factor. *J. Refract. Surg.* **2012**, *28*, 202–208. [CrossRef]
11. Kara, N.; Altinkaynak, H.; Baz, O.; Goker, Y. Biomechanical Evaluation of Cornea in Topographically Normal Relatives of Patients with Keratoconus. *Cornea* **2013**, *32*, 262–266. [CrossRef]
12. Wu, Y.; Li, X.L.; Yang, S.L.; Yan, X.M.; Li, H.L. Examination and discriminant analysis of corneal biomechanics with Corvis® ST in keratoconus and subclinical keratoconus. *Beijing Da Xue Xue Bao Yi Xue Ban* **2019**, *51*, 881–886.
13. Yang, K.; Xu, L.; Fan, Q.; Zhao, D.; Ren, S. Repeatability and comparison of new Corvis® ST parameters in normal and keratoconus eyes. *Sci. Rep.* **2019**, *9*, 15379. [CrossRef]
14. Yang, K.; Xu, L.; Fan, Q.; Gu, Y.; Song, P.; Zhang, B.; Zhao, D.; Pang, C.; Ren, S. Evaluation of new Corvis® ST parameters in normal, Post-LASIK, Post-LASIK keratectasia and keratoconus eyes. *Sci. Rep.* **2020**, *10*, 5676. [CrossRef]
15. Elham, R.; Jafarzadehpur, E.; Hashemi, H.; Amanzadeh, K.; Shokrollahzadeh, F.; Yekta, A.A.; Khabazkhoob, M. Keratoconus diagnosis using Corvis® ST measured biomechanical parameters. *J. Curr. Ophthalmol.* **2017**, *29*, 175–181. [CrossRef]
16. Zhao, Y.; Shen, Y.; Yan, Z.; Tian, M.; Zhao, J.; Zhou, X. Relationship Among Corneal Stiffness, Thickness, and Biomechanical Parameters Measured by Corvis® ST, Pentacam and ORA in Keratoconus. *Front. Physiol.* **2019**, *10*, 740. [CrossRef]
17. Zhang, M.; Zhang, F.; Li, Y.; Song, Y.; Wang, Z. Early Diagnosis of Keratoconus in Chinese Myopic Eyes by Combining Corvis® ST with Pen-tacam. *Curr. Eye Res.* **2020**, *45*, 118–123. [CrossRef] [PubMed]
18. Koc, M.; Aydemir, E.; Tekin, K.; Inanc, M.; Kosekahya, P.; Kiziltoprak, H. Biomechanical Analysis of Subclinical Keratoconus With Normal Topographic, Topometric, and Tomographic Findings. *J. Refract. Surg.* **2019**, *35*, 247–252. [CrossRef] [PubMed]
19. Chan, T.C.; Wang, Y.M.; Yu, M.; Jhanji, V. Comparison of Corneal Tomography and a New Combined Tomographic Biomechanical Index in Subclinical Keratoconus. *J. Refract. Surg.* **2018**, *34*, 616–621. [CrossRef] [PubMed]

20. Steinberg, J.; Siebert, M.; Katz, T.; Frings, A.; Mehlan, J.; Druchkiv, V.; Bühren, J.; Linke, S.J. Tomographic and Biomechanical Scheimpflug Imaging for Keratoconus Characterization: A Validation of Current Indices. *J. Refract. Surg.* **2018**, *34*, 840–847. [CrossRef]

21. Koh, S.; Ambrósio, R.; Inoue, R.; Maeda, N.; Miki, A.; Nishida, K. Detection of Subclinical Corneal Ectasia Using Corneal Tomographic and Biomechanical Assessments in a Japanese Population. *J. Refract. Surg.* **2019**, *35*, 383–390. [CrossRef]

22. Catalán-López, S.; Cadarso-Suárez, L.; López-Ratón, M.; Cadarso-Suárez, C. Corneal Biomechanics in Unilateral Keratoconus and Fellow Eyes with a Scheimpflug-based Tonometer. *Optom. Vis. Sci.* **2018**, *95*, 608–615. [CrossRef] [PubMed]

23. Song, P.; Yang, K.; Li, P.; Liu, Y.; Liang, D.; Ren, S.; Zeng, Q. Assessment of Corneal Pachymetry Distribution and Morphologic Changes in Subclinical Kerato-conus with Normal Biomechanics. *Biomed. Res. Int.* **2019**, *2019*, 1748579. [CrossRef]

24. Valbon, B.F.; Ambrósio, R., Jr.; Fontes, B.M.; Alves, M.R. Effects of age on corneal deformation by non-contact tonometry integrated with an ultra-high-speed (UHS) Scheimpflug camera. *Arq. Bras. Oftalmol.* **2013**, *76*, 229–232. [CrossRef] [PubMed]

25. Nemeth, G.; Hassan, Z.; Csutak, A.; Szalai, E.; Berta, A.; Modis, J.L. Repeatability of Ocular Biomechanical Data Measurements with a Scheimpflug-Based Noncontact Device on Normal Corneas. *J. Refract. Surg.* **2013**, *29*, 558–563. [CrossRef]

26. Hong, J.; Xu, J.; Wei, A.; Deng, S.X.; Cui, X.; Yu, X.; Sun, X. A New Tonometer—The Corvis® ST Tonometer: Clinical Comparison with Noncontact and Goldmann Applanation Tonometers. *Investig. Opthalmol. Vis. Sci.* **2013**, *54*, 659–665. [CrossRef]

27. Hon, Y.; Lam, A.K. Corneal deformation measurement using Scheimpflug noncontact tonometry. *Optom. Vis. Sci.* **2013**, *90*, e1–e8. [CrossRef]

28. Zhang, Y.; Wang, Y.; Li, L.; Dou, R.; Wu, W.; Wu, D.; Jhanji, V. Corneal Stiffness and Its Relationship with Other Corneal Biomechanical and Nonbiomechan-ical Parameters in Myopic Eyes of Chinese Patients. *Cornea* **2018**, *37*, 881–885. [CrossRef]

29. Vinciguerra, R.; Ambrósio, R., Jr.; Roberts, C.J.; Azzolini, C.; Vinciguerra, P. Biomechanical Characterization of Subclinical Keratoconus Without Topo-graphic or Tomographic Abnormalities. *J. Refract. Surg.* **2017**, *33*, 399–407. [CrossRef]

30. Peña-García, P.; Peris-Martínez, C.; Abbouda, A.; Ruiz-Moreno, J.M. Detection of subclinical keratoconus through non-contacttonometry and the use of discriminant biomechanical functions. *J. Biomech.* **2016**, *49*, 353–363. [CrossRef]

31. Wolffsohn, J.S.; Safeen, S.; Shah, S.; Laiquzzaman, M. Changes of Corneal Biomechanics with Keratoconus. *Cornea* **2012**, *31*, 849–854. [CrossRef]

32. Smadja, D.; Touboul, D.; Cohen, A.; Doveh, E.; Santhiago, M.R.; Mello, G.R.; Krueger, R.R.; Colin, J. Detection of subclinical kerato-conus using an automated decision tree classification. *Am. J. Ophthalmol.* **2013**, *156*, 237–246. [CrossRef]

33. Klyce, S.D. Chasing the suspect: Keratoconus. *Br. J. Ophthalmol.* **2009**, *93*, 845–847. [CrossRef] [PubMed]

34. Ambrósio, R., Jr.; Nogueira, L.P.; Caldas, D.L.; Fontes, B.M.; Luz, A.; Cazal, J.O.; Alves, M.R.; Belin, M.W. Evaluation of corneal shape and biomechanics before LASIK. *Int. Ophthalmol. Clin.* **2011**, *51*, 11–38. [CrossRef] [PubMed]

35. Kamiya, K.; Ishii, R.; Shimizu, K.; Igarashi, A. Evaluation of corneal elevation, pachymetry and keratometry in keratoconic eyes with respect to the stage of Amsler-Krumeich classification. *Br. J. Ophthalmol.* **2014**, *98*, 459–463. [CrossRef] [PubMed]

36. Demir, S.; Ortak, H.; Yeter, V.; Alim, S.; Sayn, O.; Tas, U.; Sönmez, B. Mapping corneal thickness using dual-scheimpflug imaging at different stages of kerato-conus. *Cornea* **2013**, *32*, 1470–1474. [CrossRef] [PubMed]

37. Miháltz, K.; Kovács, I.; Takács, Á.; Nagy, Z.Z. Evaluation of keratometric, pachymetric, and elevation parameters of keratoconus cor-neas with pentacam. *Cornea* **2009**, *28*, 976–980. [CrossRef] [PubMed]

38. De Sanctis, U.; Loiacono, C.; Richiardi, L.; Turco, D.; Mutani, B.; Grignolo, F.M. Sensitivity and specificity of posterior corneal elevation measured by Pentacam in discriminating keratoconus/subclinical keratoconus. *Ophthalmology* **2008**, *115*, 1534–1539. [CrossRef]

39. Ventura, B.V.; Machado, A.P.; Ambrósio, R., Jr.; Ribeiro, G.; Araújo, L.N.; Luz, A.; Lyra, J.M. Analysis of waveform-derived ORA parameters in early forms of kerato-conus and normal corneas. *J. Refract. Surg.* **2013**, *29*, 637–643. [CrossRef]

40. Tian, L.; Huang, Y.-F.; Wang, L.-Q.; Bai, H.; Wang, Q.; Jiang, J.-J.; Wu, Y.; Gao, M. Corneal Biomechanical Assessment Using Corneal Visualization Scheimpflug Technology in Keratoconic and Normal Eyes. *J. Ophthalmol.* **2014**, *2014*, 147516. [CrossRef]

41. Boyce, B.; Jones, R.; Nguyen, T.; Grazier, J. Stress-controlled viscoelastic tensile response of bovine cornea. *J. Biomech.* **2007**, *40*, 2367–2376. [CrossRef] [PubMed]

42. Luz, A.; Fontes, B.M.; Lopes, B.; Ramos, I.; Schor, P.; Ambrósio, R., Jr. ORA waveform-derived biomechanical parameters to distinguish normal from ker-atoconic eyes. *Arq. Bras. Oftalmol.* **2013**, *76*, 111–117. [CrossRef] [PubMed]

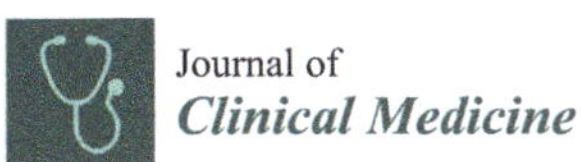

Journal of
Clinical Medicine

Article

Association of Genetic Polymorphisms in Oxidative Stress and Inflammation Pathways with Glaucoma Risk and Phenotype

Makedonka Atanasovska Velkovska [1], Katja Goričar [2], Tanja Blagus [2], Vita Dolžan [2] and Barbara Cvenkel [1,3,*]

[1] Department of Ophthalmology, University Medical Centre Ljubljana, 1000 Ljubljana, Slovenia; atmakedonka@yahoo.com
[2] Pharmacogenetics Laboratory, Institute of Biochemistry and Molecular Genetics, Faculty of Medicine, University of Ljubljana, 1000 Ljubljana, Slovenia; katja.goricar@mf.uni-lj.si (K.G.); tanja.blagus@mf.uni-lj.si (T.B.); vita.dolzan@mf.uni-lj.si (V.D.)
[3] Faculty of Medicine, University of Ljubljana, 1000 Ljubljana, Slovenia
* Correspondence: barbara.cvenkel@gmail.com; Tel.: +386-(40)-233-462

Citation: Atanasovska Velkovska, M.; Goričar, K.; Blagus, T.; Dolžan, V.; Cvenkel, B. Association of Genetic Polymorphisms in Oxidative Stress and Inflammation Pathways with Glaucoma Risk and Phenotype. *J. Clin. Med.* **2021**, *10*, 1148. https://doi.org/10.3390/jcm10051148

Academic Editors: Jose Javier Garcia-Medina and Maria Dolores Pinazo-Duran

Received: 20 January 2021
Accepted: 4 March 2021
Published: 9 March 2021

Publisher's Note: MDPI stays neutral with regard to jurisdictional claims in published maps and institutional affiliations.

Abstract: Oxidative stress and neuroinflammation are involved in the pathogenesis and progression of glaucoma. Our aim was to evaluate the impact of selected single-nucleotide polymorphisms in inflammation and oxidative stress genes on the risk of glaucoma, the patients' clinical characteristics and the glaucoma phenotype. In total, 307 patients with primary open-angle glaucoma or ocular hypertension were enrolled. The control group included 339 healthy Slovenian blood donors. DNA was isolated from peripheral blood. Genotyping was performed for *SOD2* rs4880, *CAT* rs1001179, *GPX1* rs1050450, *GSTP1* rs1695, *GSTM1* gene deletion, *GSTT*1 gene deletion, *IL1B* rs1143623, *IL1B* rs16944, *IL6* rs1800795 and *TNF* rs1800629. We found a nominally significant association of *GSTM1* gene deletion with decreased risk of ocular hypertension and a protective role of *IL1B* rs16944 and *IL6* rs1800629 in the risk of glaucoma. The CT and TT genotypes of *GPX1* rs1050450 were significantly associated with advanced disease, lower intraocular pressure and a larger vertical cup–disc ratio. In conclusion, genetic variability in *IL1B* and *IL6* may be associated with glaucoma risk, while *GPX* and *TNF* may be associated with the glaucoma phenotype. In the future, improved knowledge of these pathways has the potential for new strategies and personalised treatment of glaucoma.

Keywords: glaucoma; inflammation; oxidative stress; phenotype; polymorphism; susceptibility

1. Introduction

There is growing interest in the correlation between oxidative stress, inflammation, apoptosis and primary open-angle glaucoma (POAG) initiation and progression [1–5]. Reactive oxygen species (ROS) are formed in the eyes, following a wide variety of stressors and are largely implicated in glaucoma pathogenesis. Similarly, immune-inflammatory response mediators have recently become a target of interest in glaucoma [6–10].

POAG progression has been linked to an increase in oxidative stress (OS) markers [11,12], and although it has been hypothesised that OS plays an early role in the development of glaucomatous optic neuropathy [13], the link between OS and clinical glaucoma parameters remains to be elucidated [1]. In glaucoma, increased intraocular pressure (IOP), vascular dysregulation and immune system activation can trigger several changes in the retina and optic nerve, including disrupted axonal transport and neurofilament accumulation, microvascular abnormalities, extracellular matrix remodelling and glial cell activation. These alterations can lead to secondary damage such as excitotoxicity, neurotrophin deprivation, oxidative damage, mitochondrial dysfunction and, eventually, retinal ganglion cell death [5,14]. In addition, neurodegeneration extends beyond the retina and optic nerve into the central nervous system [3,15].

Oxidative stress arises due to disturbed equilibrium between the pro-oxidant/antio xidant status that further takes part in the generation of ROS and free radicals, both potentially toxic for neuronal cells. The human body produces oxygen free radicals and other ROS as by-products through numerous physiological and biochemical processes [16]. At the same time, antioxidants, further supported with antioxidant enzymes superoxide dismutase (SOD), catalase (CAT), glutathione reductase and glutathione peroxidase (GPX), help to regulate the level of ROS [17,18]. Decreased antioxidant defence, together with increasing pro-oxidants in the aqueous humour [12,19], ocular tissues [20,21] and blood [22], has been reported in glaucoma. Several antioxidant enzymes such as SOD, CAT and GPX have been found in the aqueous humour [23,24]. The enzyme CAT is the primary scavenger of ROS, and its deficiency and/or genetic variants are associated with a higher risk of diabetes complications and vitiligo [25,26]. GPX has antioxidant effects and catalyses the reduction of hydrogen peroxide by two molecules of glutathione as part of a ROS defence system.

Glaucoma is a neurodegenerative optic neuropathy and, similarly to other neurodegenerative diseases, is also associated with neuroinflammation where astrocytes and microglia play a major role [27]. The presence of reactive astrocytes, microglial activation and the release of inflammatory mediators such as cytokines, ROS, nitric oxide (NO) and tumour necrosis factor-α (TNF-α) cause a state of chronic inflammation that may exert neurotoxic effects [28]. Immune inflammatory response mediators like proteolytic enzymes and pro-inflammatory cytokines (TNF-α, IL-1β, IL-6, IL-12, and NO) have recently become a target of glaucoma research [15,29–40]. TNF-α, a major immunomodulator and inflammatory cytokine, has been suggested to mediate the apoptotic death of retinal ganglion cells in glaucoma patients [34]. Interleukin-1, an inflammatory cytokine, is implicated in ischaemic and excitotoxic damage in the retina [41]. Interleukin-6, a proinflammatory cytokine, modulates neuronal survival and protects retinal ganglion cells from ischaemic and excitotoxic damage [42].

Moreover, further research concerning the functions, effectors and signalling pathways of the above molecules and their interactions may lead to new strategies for the treatment of glaucoma [10,43].

Genetic factors, such as single-nucleotide polymorphisms (SNPs), have been shown to modify these pathways, but their impact on the risk of glaucoma and disease course has not been confirmed yet. Studies evaluating the effect of genetic polymorphisms or alterations in proteins' functions in the oxidative-stress- and inflammation-related genes on the risk of glaucoma have found conflicting results [44,45]. Although the association of genetic variability of inflammation and oxidative stress genes with the risk of glaucoma has already been explored to some extent, the association with patients' clinical characteristics and glaucoma phenotype has not been studied yet.

Therefore, the aim of our study was to investigate the associations of selected SNPs in inflammation and oxidative stress pathways with the risk of glaucoma, as well as the associations between selected SNPs, patients' clinical characteristics and the glaucoma phenotype.

2. Materials and Methods

2.1. Study Participants

The study included patients older than 40 years with POAG or ocular hypertension (OHT) attending the Glaucoma Clinic at the Department of Ophthalmology of the University Medical Centre Ljubljana, Slovenia, from October 2018 until May 2020. The study was approved by the Slovenian Medical Ethics Committee (KME 30/05/11). All subjects signed informed consent in accordance with the Declaration of Helsinki.

Ocular hypertension was defined according to the Guidelines and Terminology of the European Glaucoma Society as IOP higher than 21 mmHg without changes at the optic nerve head and visual field defects [46]. POAG was defined as untreated IOP higher than 21 mmHg, characteristic glaucoma changes at the optic nerve head and/or corresponding visual field defects. Patients with primary juvenile open-angle glaucoma, secondary causes of OHT/glaucoma and non-glaucomatous optic neuropathy and patients after prior intraocular surgery (except non-complicated cataract surgery with more than 6 months after surgery) were excluded. Patients were treated according to the recommendations of the European Glaucoma Society guidelines [47]. Lowering of the IOP was achieved by topical medications, laser trabeculoplasty or surgery, depending on the severity of glaucoma, life expectancy, status of the fellow eye and the rate of progression.

Data on the course of disease and treatment were obtained from medical records. In all patients, the following data were recorded: sex, age, smoking status, a family history of glaucoma, IOP, central corneal thickness (CCT), visual field parameters (with best-corrected visual acuity), vertical cup–disc (C/D) ratio, current ocular diagnosis and systemic diseases. The presence of diabetes, arterial hypertension (AH), hyperlipidaemia and heart disease was also recorded.

The glaucoma phenotype was assessed with the severity of disease, C/D ratio, IOP and CCT. The severity of glaucoma was based on the visual field index mean defect (MD) of the Octopus standard automated perimetry (G program, dynamic strategy) and classified into early (MD < 6 dB), moderate (MD 6–12 dB) and advanced (MD > 12 dB) disease. The IOP was measured by Goldman applanation tonometry. The mean IOP based on all measurements during follow-up was calculated for each eye. CCT values were measured with a manual ultrasound pachymeter (Pachmate-DGH, Tehnology Inc., Exton, PA, USA).

The control group included 339 healthy, unrelated Slovenian blood donors without any systemic disease. For the control group, data about age and sex were available.

2.2. DNA Isolation and Genotyping

Nine candidate genes were selected based on their direct involvement in oxidative stress pathways and signalling cascades of inflammation. Only functional polymorphisms with a minor allele frequency above 5% were included in the study: non-synonymous SNPs in the coding region previously associated with enzyme activity or SNPs in the 5′ untranslated region previously associated with altered gene or protein expression levels were *SOD2* rs4880, *CAT* rs1001179, *GPX1* rs1050450, *GSTP1* rs1695, *IL1B* rs1143623, *IL1B* rs16944, *IL6* rs1800795 and *TNF* rs1800629 (Supplementary Materials Table S1) [48]. We also determined the presence of homozygous *GSTM1* and *GSTT1* gene deletion.

Genomic DNA was isolated from peripheral blood samples using the E.Z.N.A.® SQ II Blood DNA Kit (Omega Bio-tek, Inc., Norcross, GA, USA) following the manufacturer's instructions. *GSTM1* and *GSTT1* were genotyped using multiplex PCR that enabled the detection of homozygous gene deletion. In brief, both genes were simultaneously amplified in a single-step PCR together with the β-globin gene (*HBB*) as the internal positive control, as previously described [49] (Table S2, Figure S1). Genotyping of 8 SNPs was performed with competitive allele-specific PCR (KASP), using the KASP Master mix and custom KASP genotyping assays (all from LGC, Middlesex, UK) according to the manufacturer's instructions (KBiosciences, Herts, UK and LGC Genomics, UK) (Table S2, Figure S2). Ten percent of the samples were genotyped in duplicate as quality control, and all the results were concordant.

2.3. Statistical Analysis

Continuous and categorical variables were described with the median and interquartile range (25–75%) or frequencies, respectively. Fisher's exact test was used to compare the distribution of categorical variables, while nonparametric Mann–Whitney or Kruskal-Wallis tests were used to compare the distribution of continuous variables. Deviation from the Hardy–Weinberg equilibrium (HWE) was evaluated using the standard chi-square test. Both dominant and additive genetic models were used in the analysis. The association of polymorphisms with glaucoma risk was evaluated using logistic regression to calculate non-adjusted and adjusted odds ratios (ORs) and 95% confidence intervals (CIs). For the IOP, CCT and C/D ratio, data from the most affected eye were used in the analysis. If a measurement was available for only one eye, the measurement of that eye was used in the analysis.

All statistical tests were two sided. As 11 SNPs were investigated, the Bonferroni correction was used to account for multiple comparisons: *p*-values below 0.005 were considered statistically significant, while *p*-values between 0.005 and 0.050 were considered nominally significant. All statistical tests were two sided. In risk analysis, for a polymorphism with a minor allele frequency of 0.10, 0.30 and 0.50, this study had 80% power to detect ORs of 1.9, 1.6 and 1.54 or more, respectively. Power calculation was conducted using PS Power and Sample Size Calculation version 3.0 [50]. The statistical analyses were carried out using IBM SPSS Statistics version 21.0 (IBM Corporation, Armonk, NY, USA).

3. Results

A total of 307 patients, 235 with POAG and 72 with OHT, participated in this study. The median age of patients was 70 (interquartile range 64–78) years. Among the patients, 139 (45.3%) were male and 168 (54.7%) were female. The control group consisted of 339 healthy blood donors with the median age of 49 (interquartile range 45–55) years. Among the controls, 251 (74.0%) were male and 88 (26.0%) were female. Patients with POAG or OHT were significantly older than controls (*p* < 0.001). There were more females among patients with POAG or OHT compared to controls (*p* < 0.001). In total, 31.9% of patients reported a family history of glaucoma. Clinical characteristics of all patients, their smoking history and accompanying systemic diseases are presented separately for the OHT and POAG groups in Table 1.

Table 1. Clinical characteristics of patients.

Characteristic		Cases (*n* = 307)	OHT (*n* = 72)	POAG (*n* = 235)	*p*-Value
Sex	Male, *n* (%)	139 (45.3)	34 (47.2)	105 (44.7)	0.787
	Female, *n* (%)	168 (54.7)	38 (52.8)	130 (55.3)	
Age (years)	Median (25–75%)	70 (64–78)	64 (54–69)	72 (66–79)	<0.001
IOP (mmHg)	Right eye, (median (25–75%)	19.71 (16.8–23)	22.6 (20.1–24.2)	18.59 (16.3–22.0)	<0.001
	Left eye, (median (25–75%)	19.78 (16.7–23)	22.5 (19.7–24.2)	18.48 (16.3–22.0)	<0.001
CCT (µm)	Right eye, (median (25–75%)	547 (521–574)	565.5 (533–595)	541 (518–570)	<0.001
	Left eye, (median (25–75%)	548.5 (522.5–577.0) {1}	570.5 (532.3–602.5)	543 (519.5–571.0)	<0.001
C/D ratio	Right eye, (median (25–75%)	0.8 (0.5–0.9)	0.35 (0.3–0.5)	0.9 (0.7–1.0)	<0.001
	Left eye, (median (25–75%)	0.8 (0.5–1)	0.3 (0.3–0.5)	0.9 (0.7–1.0)	<0.001
Family history of glaucoma	No, *n* (%)	209 (68.1)	51 (70.8)	158 (67.2)	0.665
	Yes, *n* (%)	98 (31.9)	21 (29.2)	77 (32.8)	
Arterial hypertension {1}	No, *n* (%)	140 (45.8)	38 (52.8%)	102 (43.6)	0.179
	Yes, *n* (%)	166 (54.2)	34 (47.2%)	132 (56.4)	
Diabetes	No, *n* (%)	280 (91.2)	64 (88.9%)	216 (91.9)	0.476
	Yes, *n* (%)	27 (8.8)	8 (11.1%)	19 (8.1)	
Hyperlipidaemia	No, *n* (%)	209 (68.1)	53 (73.6%)	156 (66.4)	0.312
	Yes, *n* (%)	98 (31.9)	19 (26.4%)	79 (3.6)	
Heart disease {1}	No, *n* (%)	240 (78.4)	63 (87.5%)	177 (75.6)	0.034
	Yes, *n* (%)	66 (21.6)	9 (12.5%)	57 (24.4)	
Smoking	No, *n* (%)	204 (66.4)	40 (55.6%)	164 (69.8)	0.045
	Currently, *n* (%)	26 (8.5)	6 (8.3)	20 (8.5)	
	Former, *n* (%)	77 (25.1)	26 (36.1)	51 (21.7)	

{ }—missing data; OHT—ocular hypertension; POAG—primary open-angle glaucoma; IOP—intraocular pressure; CCT—central corneal thickness; C/D ratio—vertical cup–disc ratio.

Genotypes' distributions for the investigated SNPs in both patient and control groups are presented in Table 2. When susceptibility analysis was performed, *GSTM1* gene deletion was nominally significantly associated with the risk for POAG or OHT. The carriers of *GSTM1* gene deletion had lower odds for developing POAG or OHT (OR = 0.50; 95% CI = 0.30–0.83; *p* = 0.007).

Table 2. Genotype frequencies of the control (*n* = 339) and patient (*n* = 307) groups with the risk of glaucoma or OHT.

SNP	Genotype	Controls *n* (%)	Cases *n* (%)	OR (95% CI) adj.	p_{adj}-Value
SOD2 rs4880	CC	92 (27.1)	78 (25.4)	Reference	
	CT	160 (47.2)	136 (44.3)	1.11 (0.60–2.06)	0.745
	TT	87 (25.7)	93 (30.3)	1.15 (0.58–2.26)	0.690
	CT + TT	247 (72.9)	229 (74.6)	1.12 (0.63–2.00)	0.691
CAT rs1001179	CC	193 (57.1) {1}	184 (59.9)	Reference	
	CT	122 (36.1)	105 (34.2)	0.95 (0.56–1.60)	0.840
	TT	23 (6.8)	18 (5.9)	1.31 (0.42–4.08)	0.642
	CT + TT	145 (42.9)	123 (40.1)	0.99 (0.59–1.63)	0.954
GPX1 rs1050450	CC	170 (50.1)	157 (51.1)	Reference	
	CT	130 (38.3)	125 (40.7)	0.86 (0.51–1.47)	0.592
	TT	39 (11.5)	25 (8.1)	0.49 (0.19–1.28)	0.146
	CT + TT	169 (49.9)	150 (48.9)	0.78 (0.47–1.30)	0.345
GSTP1 rs1695	AA	150 (44.2)	141 (45.9)	Reference	
	AG	152 (44.8)	128 (41.7)	0.98 (0.58–1.67)	0.940
	GG	37 (10.9)	38 (12.4)	1.84 (0.79–4.28)	0.157
	AG + GG	189 (55.8)	166 (54.1)	1.11 (0.67–1.83)	0.686
GSTP1 rs1138272	CC	274 (80.8)	254 (82.7)	Reference	
	CT + TT	65 (19.2)	53 (17.3)	1.25 (0.65–2.41)	0.513
GSTM1 gene deletion	No deletion	136 (40.1)	150 (48.9)	Reference	
	Deletion	203 (59.9)	157 (51.1)	0.50 (0.30–0.83)	**0.007**
GSTT1 gene deletion	No deletion	288 (85)	254 (82.7)	Reference	
	Deletion	51 (15)	53 (17.3)	0.58 (0.30–1.12)	0.103
IL1B rs1143623	GG	174 (51.3)	145 (47.2)	Reference	
	GC	136 (40.1)	135 (44)	1.25 (0.74–2.11)	0.408
	CC	29 (8.6)	27 (8.8)	1.50 (0.61–3.69)	0.378
	GC + CC	165 (48.7)	162 (52.8)	1.29 (0.78–2.12)	0.323
IL1B rs16944	TT	44 (13)	44 (14.3)	Reference	
	TC	145 (42.8)	143 (46.6)	0.69 (0.32–1.47)	0.332
	CC	150 (44.2)	120 (39.1)	0.62 (0.28–1.35)	0.227
	TC + CC	295 (87.0)	263 (85.7)	0.65 (0.32–1.34)	0.248
IL6 rs1800795	GG	120 (35.4)	111 (36.2)	Reference	
	GC	151 (44.5)	154 (50.2)	0.71 (0.41–1.24)	0.226
	CC	68 (20.1)	42 (13.7)	0.67 (0.32–1.39)	0.277
	GC + CC	219 (64.6)	196 (63.8)	0.70 (0.41–1.17)	0.174
TNF rs1800629	GG	228 (67.3)	234 (76.2)	Reference	
	GA + AA	111 (32.7)	73 (23.8)	0.66 (0.38–1.17)	0.156

{ }—missing data; adj–adjusted for age and sex; SNP–single nucleotide polymorphism. Nominally significant values have been marked in bold.

Next, susceptibility analysis was performed separately for patients with POAG (n = 235) and OHT (n = 72), as shown in Table 3. The carriers of *GSTM1* gene deletion had lower odds for developing OHT (OR = 0.43; 95% CI = 0.22–0.81; p = 0.009) but not for developing POAG (OR = 0.61; 95% CI = 0.31–1.18; p = 0.141).

Table 3. Genotype frequencies of selected polymorphisms and their association with the risk of OHT (n = 72) and POAG (n = 235).

SNP	Genotype	OHT			POAG		
		n (%)	OR (95% CI) adj.	p_{adj}-Value	n (%)	OR (95% CI) adj.	p_{adj}-Value
SOD2 rs4880	CC	15 (20.8)	Reference		63 (26.8)	Reference	
	CT	39 (54.2)	1.37 (0.63–3.00)	0.426	97 (41.3)	0.90 (0.41–2.02)	0.806
	TT	18 (25)	1.12 (0.46–2.71)	0.798	75 (31.9)	1.23 (0.51–2.93)	0.643
	CT + TT	57 (79.2)	1.28 (0.61–2.66)	0.515	172 (73.2)	1.02 (0.49–2.14)	0.953
CAT rs1001179	CC	49 (68.1)	Reference		135 (57.4)	Reference	
	CT	20 (27.8)	0.66 (0.33–1.30)	0.230	85 (36.2)	1.36 (0.68–2.69)	0.381
	TT	3 (4.2)	0.40 (0.07–2.19)	0.290	15 (6.4)	3.79 (0.92–15.55)	0.064
	CT + TT	23 (31.9)	0.62 (0.32–1.20)	0.157	100 (42.6)	1.54 (0.80–2.96)	0.201
GPX1 rs1050450	CC	45 (62.5)	Reference		112 (47.7)	Reference	
	CT	22 (30.6)	0.66 (0.33–1.30)	0.228	103 (43.8)	0.93 (0.47–1.85)	0.834
	TT	5 (6.9)	0.36 (0.10–1.26)	0.111	20 (8.5)	0.70 (0.20–2.44)	0.581
	CT + TT	27 (37.5)	0.59 (0.31–1.12)	0.104	123 (52.3)	0.89 (0.46–1.72)	0.725
GSTP1 rs1695	AA	38 (52.8)	Reference		103 (43.8)	Reference	
	AG	26 (36.1)	0.92 (0.47–1.79)	0.800	102 (43.4)	0.92 (0.46–1.84)	0.819
	GG	8 (11.1)	1.37 (0.49–3.83)	0.554	30 (12.8)	2.70 (0.85–8.60)	0.092
	AG + GG	34 (47.2)	0.99 (0.53–1.86)	0.987	132 (56.2)	1.11 (0.58–2.13)	0.747
GSTP1 rs1138272	CC	62 (86.1)	Reference		192 (81.7)	Reference	
	CT + TT	10 (13.9)	1.09 (0.47–2.55)	0.837	43 (18.3)	1.44 (0.60–3.47)	0.410
GSTM1 gene deletion	No deletion	36 (50)	Reference		114 (48.5)	Reference	
	Deletion	36 (50)	0.43 (0.22–0.81)	**0.009**	121 (51.5)	0.61 (0.31–1.18)	0.141
GSTT1 gene deletion	No deletion	60 (83.3)	Reference		194 (82.6)	Reference	
	Deletion	12 (16.7)	0.61 (0.26–1.44)	0.258	41 (17.4)	0.50 (0.22–1.16)	0.107
IL1B rs1143623	GG	38 (52.8)	Reference		107 (45.5)	Reference	
	GC	32 (44.4)	1.16 (0.61–2.19)	0.657	103 (43.8)	1.12 (0.56–2.24)	0.745
	CC	2 (2.8)	0.47 (0.10–2.24)	0.341	25 (10.6)	2.87 (0.95–8.65)	0.061
	GC + CC	34 (47.2)	1.04 (0.56–1.95)	0.893	128 (54.5)	1.34 (0.70–2.57)	0.384
IL1B rs16944	TT	5 (6.9)	Reference		39 (16.6)	Reference	
	TC	34 (47.2)	1.38 (0.45–4.28)	0.574	109 (46.4)	0.34 (0.13–0.90)	**0.030**
	CC	33 (45.8)	1.44 (0.46–4.47)	0.533	87 (37)	0.32 (0.12–0.86)	**0.024**
	TC + CC	67 (93.1)	1.41 (0.48–4.16)	0.536	196 (83.4)	0.33 (0.13–0.82)	**0.017**
IL6 rs1800795	GG	25 (34.7)	Reference		86 (36.6)	Reference	
	GC	36 (50)	0.89 (0.45–1.80)	0.755	118 (50.2)	0.44 (0.21–0.93)	**0.031**
	CC	11 (15.3)	0.77 (0.30–1.96)	0.577	31 (13.2)	0.49 (0.19–1.29)	0.149
	GC + CC	47 (65.3)	0.86 (0.44–1.66)	0.654	149 (63.4)	0.46 (0.23–0.91)	**0.025**
TNF rs1800629	GG	56 (77.8)	Reference		178 (75.7)	Reference	
	GA + AA	16 (22.2)	0.62 (0.30–1.28)	0.196	57 (24.3)	0.67 (0.31–1.41)	0.289

adj—adjusted for age and sex; OHT—ocular hypertension; POAG—primary open-angle glaucoma; SNP—single nucleotide polymorphism. Nominally significant values have been marked in bold.

IL6 and *IL1B* polymorphisms showed nominally significant association with POAG but not with OHT. The carriers of the *IL1B* rs16944 polymorphism had lower odds for developing POAG in the dominant and additive genetic model (OR = 0.33; 95% CI = 0.13–0.82; p = 0.017). *IL6* rs1800795 was associated with lower odds for developing POAG in the dominant genetic model (OR = 0.46; 95% CI = 0.23–0.91; p = 0.025) (Table 3).

The distribution of genotype frequencies for the investigated polymorphisms was compared between groups of patients with OHT without visual field defects and patients with glaucoma of different severity (Table 4). The results showed statistically significant differences among groups only for the distribution of *GPX1* rs1050450 genotypes in the dominant model. The carriers of at least one polymorphic *GPX1* allele had less OHT and more POAG (p = 0.025; Table 4).

Table 4. Association of selected polymorphisms with OHT and POAG severity.

SNP	Genotype	OHT (n = 72)	Early POAG (n = 62)	Moderate POAG (n = 54)	Severe POAG (n = 119)	p-Value *
		n (%)	n (%)	n (%)	n (%)	
SOD2 rs4880	CC	15 (19.2)	15 (19.2)	15 (19.2)	33 (42.3)	Padd = 0.681
	CT	39 (28.7)	27 (19.9)	22 (16.2)	48 (35.3)	
	TT	18 (19.4)	20 (21.5)	17 (18.3)	38 (40.9)	
	CT + TT	57 (24.9)	47 (20.5)	39 (17)	86 (37.6)	Pdom = 0.722
CAT rs1001179	CC	49 (26.6)	31 (16.8)	35 (19)	69 (37.5)	Padd = 0.149
	CT	20 (19)	23 (21.9)	18 (17.1)	44 (41.9)	
	TT	3 (16.7)	8 (44.4)	1 (5.6)	6 (33.3)	
	CT + TT	23 (18.7)	31 (25.2)	19 (15.4)	50 (40.7)	Pdom = 0.158
GPX1 rs1050450	CC	45 (28.7)	33 (21)	19 (12.1)	60 (38.2)	Padd = 0.134
	CT	22 (17.6)	24 (19.2)	29 (23.2)	50 (40)	
	TT	5 (20)	5 (20)	6 (24)	9 (36)	
	CT + TT	27 (18)	29 (19.3)	35 (23.3)	59 (39.3)	**Pdom = 0.025**
GSTP1 rs1695	AA	38 (27)	26 (18.4)	23 (16.3)	54 (38.3)	Padd = 0.628
	AG	26 (20.3)	30 (23.4)	21 (16.4)	51 (39.8)	
	GG	8 (21.1)	6 (15.8)	10 (26.3)	14 (36.8)	
	AG + GG	34 (20.5)	36 (21.7)	31 (18.7)	65 (39.2)	Pdom = 0.570
GSTP1 rs1138272	CC	62 (24.4)	49 (19.3)	41 (16.1)	102 (40.2)	0.299
	CT + TT	10 (18.9)	13 (24.5)	13 (24.5)	17 (32.1)	
GSTM1 gene deletion	No deletion	36 (24)	23 (15.3)	30 (20)	61 (40.7)	0.195
	Deletion	36 (22.9)	39 (24.8)	24 (15.3)	58 (36.9)	
GSTT1 gene deletion	No deletion	60 (23.6)	50 (19.7)	46 (18.1)	98 (38.6)	0.940
	Deletion	12 (22.6)	12 (22.6)	8 (15.1)	21 (39.6)	
IL1B rs1143623	GG	38 (26.2)	27 (18.6)	22 (15.2)	58 (40)	Padd = 0.358
	GC	32 (23.7)	27 (20)	26 (19.3)	50 (37)	
	CC	2 (7.4)	8 (29.6)	6 (22.2)	11 (40.7)	
	GC + CC	34 (21)	35 (21.6)	32 (19.8)	61 (37.7)	Pdom = 0.526
IL1B rs16944	TT	5 (11.4)	14 (31.8)	7 (15.9)	18 (40.9)	Padd = 0.074
	TC	34 (23.8)	30 (21)	30 (21)	49 (34.3)	
	CC	33 (27.5)	18 (15)	17 (14.2)	52 (43.3)	
	TC + CC	67 (25.5)	48 (18.3)	47 (17.9)	101 (38.4)	Pdom = 0.079

Table 4. *Cont.*

SNP	Genotype	OHT (*n* = 72)	Early POAG (*n* = 62)	Moderate POAG (*n* = 54)	Severe POAG (*n* = 119)	*p*-Value *
IL6 rs1800795	GG	25 (22.5)	24 (21.6)	23 (20.7)	39 (35.1)	Padd = 0.862
	GC	36 (23.4)	31 (20.1)	23 (14.9)	64 (41.6)	
	CC	11 (26.2)	7 (16.7)	8 (19)	16 (38.1)	
	GC + CC	47 (24)	38 (19.4)	31 (15.8)	80 (40.8)	Pdom = 0.617
TNF rs1800629	GG	56 (23.9)	46 (19.7)	43 (18.4)	89 (38)	0.873
	GA + AA	16 (21.9)	16 (21.9)	11 (15.1)	30 (41.1)	

* Comparison of all 4 groups using Fisher's exact test; add—additive model; dom—dominant model; OHT—ocular hypertension; POAG—primary open-angle glaucoma; SNP—single nucleotide polymorphism. Statistically significant values have been marked in bold.

We also analysed the association of the investigated polymorphisms with the glaucoma phenotype, such as the IOP, CCT and C/D ratio (Table 5). The results showed a statistically significant association of *GPX1* rs1050450 with the IOP and C/D ratio in the dominant model. The carriers of at least one polymorphic *GPX1* allele had a lower IOP (p = 0.019) and a slightly increased C/D ratio (p = 0.035). In addition, a statistically significant association of *TNF* rs*1800629* with the CCT was found in the dominant model. The carriers of at least one polymorphic *TNF* rs*1800629* allele had a larger CCT (p = 0.001).

Table 5. Association of investigated polymorphisms with the IOP, CCT and C/D ratio.

SNP	Genotype	IOP Max Median (25–75%)	*p*-Value	CCT Min. Median (25–75%)	*p*-Value	C/D Max. Median (25–75%)	*p*-Value
SOD2 rs4880	CC	21 (17.5–26)	Padd = 0.301	539 (520.75–571)	Padd = 0.422	0.85 (0.6–1)	Padd = 0.246
	CT	20.8 (17.5–23.3)		548 (520–577)		0.8 (0.5–1)	
	TT	20.2 (17.3–23)		541 (514.5–573)		0.9 (0.7–1)	
	CT + TT	20.6 (17.5–23)	Pdom = 0.139	544 (518.5–573)	Pdom = 0.590	0.9 (0.6–1)	Pdom = 0.985
CAT rs1001179	CC	20.8 (17.5–23.7)	Padd = 0.574	543 (518.25–573.75)	Padd = 0.331	0.85 (0.6–1)	Padd = 0.517
	CT	20.6 (17.4–23.7)		541 (519.5–571.5)		0.9 (0.6–1)	
	TT	22.5 (17.5–26)		557 (532.5–584.5)		0.8 (0.6–0.9)	
	CT + TT	20.8 (17.5–24)	Pdom = 0.759	544 (520–573)	Pdom = 0.994	0.9 (0.6–1)	Pdom = 0.690
GPX1 rs1050450	CC	21.2 (17.9–24)	Padd = 0.061	551 (520.5–575)	Padd = 0.245	0.8 (0.5–1)	Padd = 0.105
	CT	19.4 (17.2–23)		538 (519–571)		0.9 (0.7–1)	
	TT	19 (17.2–24)		540 (501.5–572)		0.9 (0.6–1)	
	CT + TT	19.3 (17.2–23.2)	**Pdom = 0.019**	538.5 (518–571)	Pdom = 0.094	0.9 (0.675–1)	**Pdom = 0.035**
GSTP1 rs1695	AA	20.5 (17.6–23.5)	Padd = 0.991	546 (519.5–575)	Padd = 0.154	0.8 (0.55–1)	Padd = 0.572
	AG	21 (17.2–24)		537.5 (515.5–570)		0.9 (0.6–1)	
	GG	20.1 (17.7–24.1)		547.5 (531–574.75)		0.9 (0.7–1)	
	AG + GG	20.9 (17.4–24)	Pdom = 0.899	540.5 (520–572.25)	Pdom = 0.598	0.9 (0.6–1)	Pdom = 0.357
GSTP1 rs1138272	CC	20.6 (17.5–24)	0.924	544 (520–573)	0.965	0.9 (0.6–1)	0.846
	CT + TT	21 (17.4–23.7)		540 (519.5–575.5)		0.9 (0.6–1)	
GSTM1 gene deletion	No deletion	21 (17.2–24)	0.967	544 (515–576)	0.894	0.9 (0.6–1)	0.823
	Deletion	20.6 (17.6–23.5)		541 (520–572.5)		0.8 (0.6–1)	

Table 5. *Cont.*

SNP	Genotype	IOP Max Median (25–75%)	*p*-Value	CCT Min. Median (25–75%)	*p*-Value	C/D Max. Median (25–75%)	*p*-Value
GSTT1 gene deletion	No deletion	20.7 (17.4–23.9)	0.354	541.5 (518–573)	0.199	0.9 (0.6–1)	0.994
	Deletion	21 (18–24)		544 (529.5–577)		0.9 (0.6–1)	
IL1B rs1143623	GG	21 (17.6–24)	Padd = 0.268	539 (518–575)	Padd = 0.382	0.9 (0.6–1)	Padd = 0.843
	GC	20.2 (17.2–23)		544 (520–571)		0.8 (0.6–1)	
	CC	21 (17.6–24)		557 (530–573)		0.9 (0.6–1)	
	GC + CC	20.3 (17.3–23)	Pdom = 0.128	547 (521–571.5)	Pdom = 0.383	0.85 (0.6–1)	Pdom = 0.970
IL1B rs16944	TT	20.4 (17.7–23.1)	Padd = 0.411	551 (529.25–570)	Padd = 0.617	0.9 (0.7–1)	Padd = 0.541
	TC	20.4 (17.5–23)		544 (520–574)		0.8 (0.6–1)	
	CC	21 (17.2–25)		538.5 (518–573.75)		0.9 (0.5–1)	
	TC + CC	20.8 (17.4–24)	Pdom = 0.989	541 (519–574)	Pdom = 0.508	0.9 (0.6–1)	Pdom = 0.319
IL6 rs1800795	GG	20 (17.6–23.3)	Padd = 0.184	546 (520–578)	Padd = 0.354	0.8 (0.5–1)	Padd = 0.342
	GC	20.6 (17.2–23.4)		541.5 (520.75–573)		0.9 (0.6–1)	
	CC	21.8 (18.4–26)		534 (502.75–569.25)		0.8 (0.4–1)	
	GC + CC	21 (17.3–24)	Pdom = 0.491	540.5 (518–571)	Pdom = 0.390	0.9 (0.6–1)	Pdom = 0.451
TNF rs1800629	GG	20.5 (17.2–23.2)	0.166	540 (517.75–570)	**0.001**	0.9 (0.6–1)	0.539
	GA + AA	21.7 (17.7–24.1)		564 (529.5–589.5)		0.9 (0.6–1)	

add—additive model; dom—dominant model; IOP—intraocular pressure; CCT—central corneal thickness; C/D ratio—vertical cup–disc ratio; SNP—single nucleotide polymorphism. Statistically significant values have been marked in bold.

We also analysed the association between patients' clinical characteristics and the glaucoma phenotype. Cases with AH had a significantly lower maximal median IOP compared to those without AH ($p < 0.001$) and a greater C/D ratio ($p = 0.008$) (Table 6). Similarly, ischaemic heart disease was significantly associated with lower IOP ($p = 0.002$). However, patients with glaucoma were older compared to OHT subjects ($p < 0.001$) with a higher prevalence of heart disease ($p = 0.034$). Diabetes was significantly associated with a larger CCT ($p = 0.030$).

Table 6. Association of patients' clinical characteristics with the glaucoma phenotype.

Characteristic		IOP Max. Median (25–75%)	*p*-Value	CCT Min. Median (25–75%)	*p*-Value	C/D Ratio Max. Median (25–75%)	*p*-Value
Smoking	No, *n* (%)	20.1 (17.5–23.7)	0.356	541 (520–573)	0.589	0.9 (0.6–1)	**0.019**
	Yes, *n* (%)	21 (17.4–24)		544 (520–573)		0.8 (0.5–1)	
Family history	No, *n* (%)	21 (17.7–24)	0.073	544 (520–574)	0.632	0.9 (0.6–1)	0.695
	Yes, *n* (%)	20 (17.1–23.2)		540.5 (518.8–570.5)		0.9 (0.6–1)	
AH	No, *n* (%)	22 (18.6–24.2)	**<0.001**	548.5 (526.8–575.5)	0.050	0.8 (0.5–1)	**0.008**
	Yes, *n* (%)	19.4 (16.9–22.8)		538 (512–570.3)		0.9 (0.6–1)	
Diabetes	No, *n* (%)	20.6 (17.2–23.7)	0.071	541 (518.3–573)	**0.030**	0.9 (0.6–1)	0.543
	Yes, *n* (%)	22 (19.3–24)		558 (540–580)		0.9 (0.4–1)	
Hyperlipidaemia	No, *n* (%)	21 (17.6–24)	0.078	543 (518.5–574)	0.959	0.8 (0.6–1)	0.541
	Yes, *n* (%)	19.7 (17.2–23.1)		543.5 (520–570)		0.9 (0.6–1)	

Table 6. *Cont.*

Characteristic		IOP Max. Median (25–75%)	*p*-Value	CCT Min. Median (25–75%)	*p*-Value	C/D Ratio Max. Median (25–75%)	*p*-Value
Heart disease	No, *n* (%)	21 (17.7–24)	**0.002**	544.5 (520–575.5)	0.173	0.8 (0.6–1)	0.485
	Yes, *n* (%)	19 (16.7–21.5)		536.5 (515.8–562.3)		0.9 (0.6–1)	

AH—arterial hypertension; IOP—intraocular pressure; CCT—central corneal thickness; C/D ratio—vertical cup–disc ratio. Statistically significant values have been marked in bold.

In the multivariable analysis including *GPX1* rs1050450, AH and diabetes, both *GPX1* rs1050450 ($p = 0.014$) and patients' clinical characteristics remained significantly associated with the IOP ($p < 0.001$ and $p = 0.019$, respectively). In the multivariable analysis including *GPX1* rs1050450, AH and smoking, only *GPX1* rs1050450 remained significantly associated with the C/D ratio ($p = 0.027$). In the multivariable model including *TNF* rs1800629 and diabetes, both variables were significantly associated with the CCT ($p < 0.001$ and $p = 0.015$).

4. Discussion

In this study, we evaluated the associations of selected SNPs in antioxidative and inflammation pathways with the risk of glaucoma and the glaucoma phenotype. Our main finding was that in the antioxidative pathways, *GSTM1* gene deletion may play a protective role in the development of OHT, while inflammatory pathway polymorphisms such as *IL1B* rs16944 and *IL6* rs1800795 may play a protective role in the development of POAG. Interestingly, *GPX1* rs1050450 polymorphism was mainly associated with the severity of POAG and with the phenotype such as the IOP and C/D ratio.

In our study, we observed that the carriers of *GSTM1* gene deletion had lower odds for developing OHT, but we found no association between *GSTT1* gene deletion and the risk of OHT or POAG. GSTs play an important role in cellular protection against oxidative stress. Homozygous *GSTM1* and *GSTT1* deletion results in the absence of the encoded enzymes and may thus impair detoxification and inactivation of reactive metabolites generated during oxidative stress. *GSTM1* and *GSTT1* gene deletion was extensively investigated with regard to glaucoma risk. Whereas some studies have found a significantly higher frequency of the *GSTM1* null genotype in patients with POAG, especially in smokers compared to controls [51–53], others have reported increased risk with a *GSTM1* positive phenotype, or in combination with a *GSTT1* null genotype, [54,55] or did not find any association with the risk of glaucoma [56–58]. Many factors might account for the differences in results between similar studies, such as differences in sample size, types of glaucoma and ethnic and geographical *GSTM1* null and *GSTT1* null distribution in populations. A recent meta-analysis suggested that there might be a significant association between *GSTM1* polymorphisms and increased susceptibility to glaucoma [57].

In our study, *GPX1* rs1050450 was not associated with the risk of glaucoma. We also found no association between the *CAT* rs1001179 promoter variant and the risk of glaucoma. CAT and GPX1 directly participate in the inactivation of hydrogen peroxide, while GPX1 also participates in the detoxification of reactive secondary metabolites of oxidative stress, such as various lipid hydroperoxides. The most common *GPX1* rs1050450 polymorphism codes for Pro198Leu substitution and leads to decreased enzyme activity; therefore, the capacity for antioxidant defence may also be decreased [59]. Defence capacity against ROS may also be decreased in carriers of a common functional *CAT* rs1001179 polymorphism that influences transcription factor binding in the promoter region and is associated with decreased catalase levels [60]. Associations of *GPX1* polymorphisms have only been studied in other neurodegenerative diseases such as Alzheimer's disease [61] and Parkinson's disease [48] but not in glaucoma. Likewise, *CAT* rs1001179 genotype frequencies did not differ significantly between cases and controls in previous studies [24,62]. Only the synonymous SNP *CAT* rs769217 was significantly associated with POAG in the Chinese population [62]. We also found no association between *SOD* rs4880 and glaucoma. Similarly, no difference in the allele and genotype frequency in SNPs rs4880 between POAG cases and controls was reported by Zhou et al. [63].

With regard to inflammatory pathway polymorphisms, we found a protective effect of *IL1B* rs16944 and *IL6* rs1800795 on the development of POAG. Both polymorphisms are located in the promoter region and may lead to altered gene expression. In patients with POAG, significantly increased mRNA expression of the *IL1B* gene has been found in blood and significantly increased IL-1B protein expression in the aqueous humour compared to controls [64]. In an animal model of acute glaucoma, upregulation of IL-1B caused an increase in retinal ganglion cell death [65]. Polymorphisms in the *IL1B* promoter region (rs16944 and rs1143634—not analysed in our study) have already been investigated for an association with POAG. Whereas positive associations were reported in Caucasian populations [66,67], associations with POAG were not observed in Asian populations [68–71]. Meta-analysis evaluating the role of these two SNPs of *IL1B* in the susceptibility to glaucoma did not find any association, but the conclusions should be interpreted with caution as only a small number of studies was included [72].

With regard to *IL6*, Zimmermann et al. suggested that the promoter *IL6 rs1800795* polymorphism is unlikely to be a major risk factor for POAG [73]. In addition, a recent systematic review and meta-analysis found a statistically significant glaucoma risk associated only with rs1524107, but not with rs1800795, which was investigated in our study [42]. However, when patients with early to moderate glaucoma were compared to patients with advanced glaucoma, the *IL6* rs1800795 C allele as well as the GC genotype were protective against less severe forms of normal-tension glaucoma [69].

We are not aware of any studies investigating the association of SNPs involved in the inflammatory and oxidative stress pathways with the glaucoma phenotype, including the severity of glaucoma, IOP, C/D ratio and CCT. We found a statistically significant association of *GPX1* rs1050450 with the severity of glaucoma. In the dominant model, the frequency of at least one polymorphic *GPX* allele increased with the severity of glaucoma (19.3% in early, 23.3% in moderate and 39.3% in advanced glaucoma). The *GPX1* rs1050450 CT and TT genotypes were reported to be associated with increased risk of damage caused by oxidative stress, such as in coronary heart disease and cancer [74,75]. The *GPX1* rs1050450 CT and TT genotypes were associated with increased risk of POAG in the Polish population, but the link with glaucoma phenotypes has not been investigated [76]. Antioxidant enzymes, such as GPX, are an important defence system against oxidative stress, which may play a major pathophysiological role in glaucoma. An increase in oxidative stress markers in serum and aqueous humour with a decrease in serum antioxidant stress markers was present in glaucoma patients compared to controls. However, despite a decrease in serum GPX, there was an important increase in GPX in the aqueous humour [11]. This may indicate a protective response of the eye against oxidative stress and may wear off in the long term [19].

Glaucoma is a heritable disease, and siblings of POAG cases have a tenfold-increased risk of developing the disease [77]. The C/D ratio, IOP and CCT used clinically to predict POAG risk are heritable traits related to the disease and may be associated with genetic variability in inflammation and oxidative stress pathways. In our study, carriers of at least one polymorphic *GPX1* rs1050450 allele had statistically lower IOP and a lower C/D ratio. Patients with advanced glaucoma require lower target IOP to prevent progression of disease than those with early glaucoma or ocular hypertension [78]. In our study, approximately 30% of all cases had advanced disease. Therefore, those with lower IOP had presumably advanced glaucoma, which might partly explain the link between *GPX1* polymorphisms and lower IOP and severity of glaucoma. However, the association between this SNP and the C/D ratio is not clear. We found no previous studies analysing the association of the *GPX1* SNP with the glaucoma phenotype.

In the last decade, genome-wide association studies (GWAS) have identified over 50 C/D-ratio-associated loci, but only 9 of these have been associated with POAG [79,80]. Up till now, multiple IOP-associated loci were identified using large and multi-ethnic biobank-based cohorts. Among the significant results were also loci at genes previously associated with POAG but not previously known to influence IOP. This indicates that genetic variation at these genes mediates the increased POAG risk via raised IOP rather than via direct effect on retinal ganglion cells [79,80]. The identified loci explained 17% of the variance of IOP in the EPIC–Norfolk Eye Study [81].

The central corneal thickness has been associated with increased POAG development and progression [82,83], but it is uncertain whether this relationship is caused by IOP measurement artefacts or whether the relationship is biologically causal [84]. In our study, the GG genotype of *TNF* rs1800629 was associated with a low CCT. The link between *TNF* polymorphisms and the CCT has not been investigated. However, recently, the results of GWAS for the CCT have suggested that the CCT may not be a heritable trait for POAG and that the CCT–glaucoma association observed in studies is due to IOP measurement artefacts rather than biological causality [80].

Multiple epidemiological studies have reported the role of hypertension as a risk factor for POAG [85,86]. Treatment of hypertensive patients with beta-blockers results in nocturnal hypotension, which is a potential risk factor for glaucomatous optic neuropathy [87,88]. The mechanisms by which hypertension induces optic nerve damage are still unclear. Whether or not an association exists between diabetes mellitus and glaucoma has been an issue of debate, but findings from several studies in recent years suggest that the risk of glaucoma among diabetic patients may be greater than once believed [89–93]. Patients with POAG may suffer from ischaemic heart disease more often than those without glaucoma [93]. We also analysed the association between clinical characteristics (AH, diabetes, ischaemic heart disease, family history of glaucoma) with the glaucoma phenotype (IOP, C/D ratio, CCT). In our study, patients with AH had significantly lower maximal median IOP and a greater C/D ratio compared to those without AH. A possible explanation is that among cases with AH, there were older patients with advanced glaucoma, requiring lower target IOP compared to cases with OHT. Similarly, in our study, patients with ischaemic heart disease had significantly lower IOP. As patients with glaucoma were older compared to OHT subjects and with a higher prevalence of heart disease, they required lower target IOP to prevent progression, which could explain our results. Diabetes was significantly associated with a larger CCT in our study. Our observation is in line with the findings of a meta-analysis that suggested that diabetes and hyperglycaemia are associated with a thicker cornea [94]. We found no other associations between the glaucoma phenotype or clinical characteristics with the investigated SNPs.

One of the limitations of our study was that the number of control subjects and cases was small compared to larger studies investigating genetic factors. Furthermore, we investigated only a limited number of polymorphisms in the oxidative stress and inflammation pathways. The strength of our study was that we used a pathway-based approach and selected SNPs with a known functional effect that are common in the Caucasian population. Perhaps other polymorphisms of the genes involved in these pathways, not investigated in our study, may have had a potential impact. Another limitation was that only data on age and sex were available for the control group. However, all controls were healthy blood donors without any self-reported systemic disease. Furthermore, the chance of controls having undiagnosed glaucoma was small due to the low prevalence of the disease in this age group, estimated to be between 0.2% and 1.1% in a Caucasian population of the same age [95–97]. Another strength of our study was that all patients attended the same glaucoma unit with the same treatment approach and follow-up, unambiguous diagnostic criteria and classification of phenotype. Furthermore, all patients and controls originated from a genetically homogenous population, thus limiting possible bias due to the population structure [98,99].

Although our findings should be interpreted with caution, there is further perspective to this research. Ganglion cell death in glaucoma is a complex process triggered by different molecular mechanisms, among which oxidative stress and activation of inflammation by retinal glial cells play an important role. Improving antioxidant defence and addressing inflammation pathways might stimulate cell survival and boost the cells' ability to withstand pathological insult. Several studies have shown the potential protective effect of antioxidants on retinal ganglion cells [100–103], while there is experimental evidence that modulation of inflammation reduces retinal ganglion cell death [102]. Therefore, improved knowledge of these pathways might help to establish predictive biomarkers to improve treatment strategies for glaucoma. Patients could be stratified into groups with detectable deficits in oxidative stress and/or inflammation pathways, so supplementary therapy could be more specific and treatment personalised. Our study investigated genes and SNPs with broad implications in glaucoma and other neurodegenerative diseases that share similar biomarkers [104,105]. This type of study on glaucoma and similar diseases may help to design inflammation and oxidative stress pathway gene panels that could be used in testing patients with different but related diseases in order to personalise treatment and potentially improve treatment outcomes.

In conclusion, we used a pathway-based approach to address the relationship between oxidative stress and inflammation polymorphisms, and POAG risk. We found some indications for a possible association of genetic variability in *GSTM1* with OHT. While *IL1B* and *IL6* may be associated with the risk of glaucoma, *GPX* and *TNF* may affect the glaucoma phenotype. However, the evidence presented here is limited and further association and functional studies are required.

Supplementary Materials: The following are available online at https://www.mdpi.com/2077-038 3/10/5/1148/s1, Table S1: Characteristics of investigated polymorphisms, variant allele frequency and agreement with Hardy-Weinberg equilibrium in controls, Table S2: Primers used for multiplex PCR (a) and thermal cycling conditions used for genotyping for multiplex PCR (b) and KASP chemistry (c), Figure S1: Representative gel image of *GSTT1* and *GSTM1* genotyping analysis, Figure S2: Representative cluster image for *IL6* rs1800795 analysis obtained after KASP competitive allele specific PCR. References [106–111] are cited in the supplementary materials.

Author Contributions: Conceptualisation, V.D. and B.C.; methodology, V.D. and B.C.; software, K.G.; validation, M.A.V., V.D., K.G., T.B. and B.C.; formal analysis, M.A.V., K.G. and T.B.; investigation, M.A.V., K.G., V.D. and B.C.; resources, V.D. and B.C.; data curation, M.A.V., K.G. and T.B.; writing—original draft preparation, M.A.V. and B.C.; writing—M.A.V., K.G., V.D. and B.C.; review and editing, V.D. and B.C.; visualisation, M.A.V. and K.G.; supervision, V.D. and B.C.; project administration, M.A.V., K.G., V.D. and T.B.; funding acquisition, none. All authors have read and agreed to the published version of the manuscript.

Funding: This research was funded by the Slovenian Research Agency (ARRS) (grant nos. P1-0170 and P3-0333).

Institutional Review Board Statement: The study was conducted according to the guidelines of the Declaration of Helsinki and approved by the Slovenian Medical Ethics Committee (KME 30/05/11).

Informed Consent Statement: Informed consent was obtained from all subjects involved in the study.

Data Availability Statement: The datasets used and/or analysed for the current study are available from the corresponding author on reasonable request.

Acknowledgments: We thank all the patients for their participation in the study. We would like to thank Saša Mohar, head nurse of the glaucoma unit, for contribution to patient enrolment. We would also like to thank Savica Soldat from the pharmacogenetics laboratory for help with the laboratory work.

Conflicts of Interest: The authors declare no conflict of interest.

References

1. Pinazo-Duran, M.D.; Zanon-Moreno, V.; Garcia-Medina, J.J.; Gallego-Pinazo, R. Evaluation of presumptive biomarkers of oxidative stress, immune response and apoptosis in primary open-angle glaucoma. *Curr. Opin. Pharmacol.* **2013**, *13*, 98–107. [CrossRef] [PubMed]
2. Gupta, N.; Ang, L.C.; Noel de Tilly, L.; Bidaisee, L.; Yucel, Y.H. Human glaucoma and neural degeneration in intracranial optic nerve, lateral geniculate nucleus, and visual cortex. *Br. J. Ophthalmol.* **2006**, *90*, 674–678. [CrossRef]

3. Gupta, N.; Ly, T.; Zhang, Q.; Kaufman, P.L.; Weinreb, R.N.; Yucel, Y.H. Chronic ocular hypertension induces dendrite pathology in the lateral geniculate nucleus of the brain. *Exp. Eye Res.* **2007**, *84*, 176–184. [CrossRef] [PubMed]
4. Gupta, N.; Fong, J.; Ang, L.C.; Yucel, Y.H. Retinal tau pathology in human glaucomas. *Can. J. Ophthalmol.* **2008**, *43*, 53–60. [CrossRef]
5. Gallego, B.I.; Salazar, J.J.; de Hoz, R.; Rojas, B.; Ramirez, A.I.; Salinas-Navarro, M.; Ortin-Martinez, A.; Valiente-Soriano, F.J.; Aviles-Trigueros, M.; Villegas-Perez, M.P.; et al. IOP induces upregulation of GFAP and MHC-II and microglia reactivity in mice retina contralateral to experimental glaucoma. *J. Neuroinflamm.* **2012**, *9*, 92. [CrossRef]
6. De Hoz, R.; Gallego, B.I.; Ramirez, A.I.; Rojas, B.; Salazar, J.J.; Valiente-Soriano, F.J.; Aviles-Trigueros, M.; Villegas-Perez, M.P.; Vidal-Sanz, M.; Trivino, A.; et al. Rod-like microglia are restricted to eyes with laser-induced ocular hypertension but absent from the microglial changes in the contralateral untreated eye. *PLoS ONE* **2013**, *8*, e83733. [CrossRef]
7. Rojas, B.; Gallego, B.I.; Ramirez, A.I.; Salazar, J.J.; de Hoz, R.; Valiente-Soriano, F.J.; Aviles-Trigueros, M.; Villegas-Perez, M.P.; Vidal-Sanz, M.; Trivino, A.; et al. Microglia in mouse retina contralateral to experimental glaucoma exhibit multiple signs of activation in all retinal layers. *J. Neuroinflamm.* **2014**, *11*, 133. [CrossRef] [PubMed]
8. Tezel, G. Oxidative stress in glaucomatous neurodegeneration: Mechanisms and consequences. *Prog. Retin. Eye Res.* **2006**, *25*, 490–513. [CrossRef] [PubMed]
9. Izzotti, A.; Bagnis, A.; Sacca, S.C. The role of oxidative stress in glaucoma. *Mutat. Res.* **2006**, *612*, 105–114. [CrossRef] [PubMed]
10. Ghanem, A.A.; Arafa, L.F.; El-Baz, A. Oxidative stress markers in patients with primary open-angle glaucoma. *Curr. Eye Res.* **2010**, *35*, 295–301. [CrossRef]
11. Benoist d'Azy, C.; Pereira, B.; Chiambaretta, F.; Dutheil, F. Oxidative and Anti-Oxidative Stress Markers in Chronic Glaucoma: A Systematic Review and Meta-Analysis. *PLoS ONE* **2016**, *11*, e0166915. [CrossRef]
12. Zanon-Moreno, V.; Marco-Ventura, P.; Lleo-Perez, A.; Pons-Vazquez, S.; Garcia-Medina, J.J.; Vinuesa-Silva, I.; Moreno-Nadal, M.A.; Pinazo-Duran, M.D. Oxidative stress in primary open-angle glaucoma. *J. Glaucoma* **2008**, *17*, 263–268. [CrossRef] [PubMed]
13. Li, Y.; Chen, Y.M.; Sun, M.M.; Guo, X.D.; Wang, Y.C.; Zhang, Z.Z. Inhibition on Apoptosis Induced by Elevated Hydrostatic Pressure in Retinal Ganglion Cell-5 via Laminin Upregulating beta1-integrin/Focal Adhesion Kinase/Protein Kinase B Signaling Pathway. *Chin. Med. J.* **2016**, *129*, 976–983. [CrossRef] [PubMed]
14. Nickells, R.W. Apoptosis of retinal ganglion cells in glaucoma: An update of the molecular pathways involved in cell death. *Surv. Ophthalmol.* **1999**, *43* (Suppl. 1), S151–S161. [CrossRef]
15. Ramirez, A.I.; de Hoz, R.; Salobrar-Garcia, E.; Salazar, J.J.; Rojas, B.; Ajoy, D.; Lopez-Cuenca, I.; Rojas, P.; Trivino, A.; Ramirez, J.M. The Role of Microglia in Retinal Neurodegeneration: Alzheimer's Disease, Parkinson, and Glaucoma. *Front. Aging Neurosci.* **2017**, *9*, 214. [CrossRef]
16. Halliwell, B. Free radicals, antioxidants, and human disease: Curiosity, cause, or consequence? *Lancet* **1994**, *344*, 721–724. [CrossRef]
17. Fang, Y.Z.; Yang, S.; Wu, G. Free radicals, antioxidants, and nutrition. *Nutrition* **2002**, *18*, 872–879. [CrossRef]
18. Uttara, B.; Singh, A.V.; Zamboni, P.; Mahajan, R.T. Oxidative stress and neurodegenerative diseases: A review of upstream and downstream antioxidant therapeutic options. *Curr. Neuropharmacol.* **2009**, *7*, 65–74. [CrossRef] [PubMed]
19. Ferreira, S.M.; Lerner, S.F.; Brunzini, R.; Evelson, P.A.; Llesuy, S.F. Oxidative stress markers in aqueous humor of glaucoma patients. *Am. J. Ophthalmol.* **2004**, *137*, 62–69. [CrossRef]
20. Babizhayev, M.A. Biomarkers and special features of oxidative stress in the anterior segment of the eye linked to lens cataract and the trabecular meshwork injury in primary open-angle glaucoma: Challenges of dual combination therapy with N-acetylcarnosine lubricant eye drops and oral formulation of nonhydrolyzed carnosine. *Fundam. Clin. Pharmacol.* **2012**, *26*, 86–117. [CrossRef]
21. McElnea, E.M.; Quill, B.; Docherty, N.G.; Irnaten, M.; Siah, W.F.; Clark, A.F.; O'Brien, C.J.; Wallace, D.M. Oxidative stress, mitochondrial dysfunction and calcium overload in human lamina cribrosa cells from glaucoma donors. *Mol. Vis.* **2011**, *17*, 1182–1191. [PubMed]
22. Engin, K.N.; Engin, G.; Kucuksahin, H.; Oncu, M.; Engin, G.; Guvener, B. Clinical evaluation of the neuroprotective effect of alpha-tocopherol against glaucomatous damage. *Eur. J. Ophthalmol.* **2007**, *17*, 528–533. [CrossRef] [PubMed]
23. Koliakos, G.G.; Befani, C.D.; Mikropoulos, D.; Ziakas, N.G.; Konstas, A.G. Prooxidant-antioxidant balance, peroxide and catalase activity in the aqueous humour and serum of patients with exfoliation syndrome or exfoliative glaucoma. *Graefes. Arch. Clin. Exp. Ophthalmol.* **2008**, *246*, 1477–1483. [CrossRef]
24. Abu-Amero, K.K.; Kondkar, A.A.; Mousa, A.; Osman, E.A.; Al-Obeidan, S.A. Analysis of catalase SNP rs1001179 in Saudi patients with primary open angle glaucoma. *Ophthalmic Genet.* **2013**, *34*, 223–228. [CrossRef]
25. Goth, L.; Nagy, T.; Kosa, Z.; Fejes, Z.; Bhattoa, H.P.; Paragh, G.; Kaplar, M. Effects of rs769217 and rs1001179 polymorphisms of catalase gene on blood catalase, carbohydrate and lipid biomarkers in diabetes mellitus. *Free Radic. Res.* **2012**, *46*, 1249–1257. [CrossRef]
26. Casp, C.B.; She, J.X.; McCormack, W.T. Genetic association of the catalase gene (CAT) with vitiligo susceptibility. *Pigment. Cell Res.* **2002**, *15*, 62–66. [CrossRef] [PubMed]
27. Cherry, J.D.; Olschowka, J.A.; O'Banion, M.K. Neuroinflammation and M2 microglia: The good, the bad, and the inflamed. *J. Neuroinflamm.* **2014**, *11*, 98. [CrossRef] [PubMed]
28. Cuenca, N.; Fernandez-Sanchez, L.; Campello, L.; Maneu, V.; De la Villa, P.; Lax, P.; Pinilla, I. Cellular responses following retinal injuries and therapeutic approaches for neurodegenerative diseases. *Prog. Retin. Eye Res.* **2014**, *43*, 17–75. [CrossRef] [PubMed]

29. Varnum, M.M.; Ikezu, T. The classification of microglial activation phenotypes on neurodegeneration and regeneration in Alzheimer's disease brain. *Arch. Immunol. Ther. Exp.* **2012**, *60*, 251–266. [CrossRef] [PubMed]

30. Gonzalez, H.; Elgueta, D.; Montoya, A.; Pacheco, R. Neuroimmune regulation of microglial activity involved in neuroinflammation and neurodegenerative diseases. *J. Neuroimmunol.* **2014**, *274*, 1–13. [CrossRef]

31. Jones, E.V.; Bouvier, D.S. Astrocyte-secreted matricellular proteins in CNS remodelling during development and disease. *Neural Plast.* **2014**, *2014*, 321209. [CrossRef]

32. Neufeld, A.H.; Hernandez, M.R.; Gonzalez, M. Nitric oxide synthase in the human glaucomatous optic nerve head. *Arch. Ophthalmol.* **1997**, *115*, 497–503. [CrossRef] [PubMed]

33. Shareef, S.; Sawada, A.; Neufeld, A.H. Isoforms of nitric oxide synthase in the optic nerves of rat eyes with chronic moderately elevated intraocular pressure. *Investig. Ophthalmol. Vis. Sci.* **1999**, *40*, 2884–2891.

34. Tezel, G.; Li, L.Y.; Patil, R.V.; Wax, M.B. TNF-alpha and TNF-alpha receptor-1 in the retina of normal and glaucomatous eyes. *Investig. Ophthalmol. Vis. Sci.* **2001**, *42*, 1787–1794.

35. Nakazawa, T.; Nakazawa, C.; Matsubara, A.; Noda, K.; Hisatomi, T.; She, H.; Michaud, N.; Hafezi-Moghadam, A.; Miller, J.W.; Benowitz, L.I. Tumor necrosis factor-alpha mediates oligodendrocyte death and delayed retinal ganglion cell loss in a mouse model of glaucoma. *J. Neurosci.* **2006**, *26*, 12633–12641. [CrossRef] [PubMed]

36. Vidal, L.; Diaz, F.; Villena, A.; Moreno, M.; Campos, J.G.; de Vargas, I.P. Nitric oxide synthase in retina and optic nerve head of rat with increased intraocular pressure and effect of timolol. *Brain Res. Bull.* **2006**, *70*, 406–413. [CrossRef] [PubMed]

37. Madeira, M.H.; Boia, R.; Santos, P.F.; Ambrosio, A.F.; Santiago, A.R. Contribution of microglia-mediated neuroinflammation to retinal degenerative diseases. *Mediat. Inflamm.* **2015**, *2015*, 673090. [CrossRef] [PubMed]

38. Williams, E.A.; McGuone, D.; Frosch, M.P.; Hyman, B.T.; Laver, N.; Stemmer-Rachamimov, A. Absence of Alzheimer Disease Neuropathologic Changes in Eyes of Subjects With Alzheimer Disease. *J. Neuropathol. Exp. Neurol.* **2017**, *76*, 376–383. [CrossRef] [PubMed]

39. Dinarello, C.A. A clinical perspective of IL-1beta as the gatekeeper of inflammation. *Eur. J. Immunol.* **2011**, *41*, 1203–1217. [CrossRef]

40. Dinarello, C.A. IL-1: Discoveries, controversies and future directions. *Eur. J. Immunol.* **2010**, *40*, 599–606. [CrossRef]

41. Wang, N.; Chintala, S.K.; Fini, M.E.; Schuman, J.S. Activation of a tissue-specific stress response in the aqueous outflow pathway of the eye defines the glaucoma disease phenotype. *Nat. Med.* **2001**, *7*, 304–309. [CrossRef] [PubMed]

42. Wu, C.L.; Yang, Y.T.; Wang, Y.H.; Lin, T.Y.; Lin, I.C.; Sung, C.W. Association of interleukin-6 gene polymorphisms and glaucoma: Systematic review and meta-analysis. *Eur. J. Ophthalmol.* **2020**, 1120672120940198. [CrossRef] [PubMed]

43. Abu-Amero, K.K.; Azad, T.A.; Mousa, A.; Osman, E.A.; Sultan, T.; Al-Obeidan, S.A. A catalase promoter variant rs1001179 is associated with visual acuity but not with primary angle closure glaucoma in Saudi patients. *BMC Med. Genet.* **2013**, *14*, 84. [CrossRef] [PubMed]

44. Izzotti, A.; Sacca, S.C. Glutathione S-transferase M1 and its implications in glaucoma pathogenesis: A controversial matter. *Exp. Eye Res.* **2004**, *79*, 141–142; author reply 143. [CrossRef] [PubMed]

45. Huang, W.; Wang, W.; Zhou, M.; Chen, S.; Zhang, X. Association of glutathione S-transferase polymorphisms (GSTM1 and GSTT1) with primary open-angle glaucoma: An evidence-based meta-analysis. *Gene* **2013**, *526*, 80–86. [CrossRef] [PubMed]

46. European Glaucoma Society Terminology and Guidelines for Glaucoma. Classification and terminology Supported by the EGS Foundation: Part 1: Foreword; Introduction; Glossary; Chapter 2 Classification and Terminology; 4th Edition—Chapter 2. *Br. J. Ophthalmol.* **2017**, *101*, 73–127. [CrossRef]

47. European Glaucoma Society Terminology and Guidelines for Glaucoma. Treatment principles and options Supported by the EGS Foundation: Part 1: Foreword; Introduction; Glossary; Chapter 3 Treatment principles and options; 4th Edition—Chapter 3. *Br. J. Ophthalmol.* **2017**, *101*, 130–195. [CrossRef]

48. Redensek, S.; Flisar, D.; Kojovic, M.; Kramberger, M.G.; Georgiev, D.; Pirtosek, Z.; Trost, M.; Dolzan, V. Genetic variability of inflammation and oxidative stress genes does not play a major role in the occurrence of adverse events of dopaminergic treatment in Parkinson's disease. *J. Neuroinflamm.* **2019**, *16*, 50. [CrossRef] [PubMed]

49. Chen, C.L.; Liu, Q.; Relling, M.V. Simultaneous characterization of glutathione S-transferase M1 and T1 polymorphisms by polymerase chain reaction in American whites and blacks. *Pharmacogenetics* **1996**, *6*, 187–191. [CrossRef]

50. Dupont, W.D.; Plummer, W.D., Jr. Power and sample size calculations. A review and computer program. *Control. Clin. Trials* **1990**, *11*, 116–128. [CrossRef]

51. Stamenkovic, M.; Lukic, V.; Suvakov, S.; Simic, T.; Sencanic, I.; Pljesa-Ercegovac, M.; Jaksic, V.; Babovic, S.; Matic, M.; Radosavljevic, A.; et al. GSTM1-null and GSTT1-active genotypes as risk determinants of primary open angle glaucoma among smokers. *Int. J. Ophthalmol.* **2018**, *11*, 1514–1520. [CrossRef]

52. Rocha, A.V.; Talbot, T.; Magalhaes da Silva, T.; Almeida, M.C.; Menezes, C.A.; Di Pietro, G.; Rios-Santos, F. Is the GSTM1 null polymorphism a risk factor in primary open angle glaucoma? *Mol. Vis.* **2011**, *17*, 1679–1686.

53. Safa, F.K.; Shahsavari, G.; Abyaneh, R.Z. Glutathione s-transferase M1 and T1 genetic polymorphisms in Iranian patients with glaucoma. *Iran. J. Basic Med. Sci.* **2014**, *17*, 332–336.

54. Juronen, E.; Tasa, G.; Veromann, S.; Parts, L.; Tiidla, A.; Pulges, R.; Panov, A.; Soovere, L.; Koka, K.; Mikelsaar, A.V. Polymorphic glutathione S-transferase M1 is a risk factor of primary open-angle glaucoma among Estonians. *Exp. Eye Res.* **2000**, *71*, 447–452. [CrossRef] [PubMed]

55. Unal, M.; Guven, M.; Devranoglu, K.; Ozaydin, A.; Batar, B.; Tamcelik, N.; Gorgun, E.E.; Ucar, D.; Sarici, A. Glutathione S transferase M1 and T1 genetic polymorphisms are related to the risk of primary open-angle glaucoma: A study in a Turkish population. *Br. J. Ophthalmol.* **2007**, *91*, 527–530. [CrossRef] [PubMed]
56. Jansson, M.; Rada, A.; Tomic, L.; Larsson, L.I.; Wadelius, C. Analysis of the Glutathione S-transferase M1 gene using pyrosequencing and multiplex PCR–no evidence of association to glaucoma. *Exp. Eye Res.* **2003**, *77*, 239–243. [CrossRef]
57. Malik, M.A.; Gupta, V.; Shukla, S.; Kaur, J. Glutathione S-transferase (GSTM1, GSTT1) polymorphisms and JOAG susceptibility: A case control study and meta-analysis in glaucoma. *Gene* **2017**, *628*, 246–252. [CrossRef] [PubMed]
58. Fan, B.J.; Liu, K.; Wang, D.Y.; Tham, C.C.; Tam, P.O.; Lam, D.S.; Pang, C.P. Association of polymorphisms of tumor necrosis factor and tumor protein p53 with primary open-angle glaucoma. *Investig. Ophthalmol. Vis. Sci.* **2010**, *51*, 4110–4116. [CrossRef]
59. Ravn-Haren, G.; Olsen, A.; Tjonneland, A.; Dragsted, L.O.; Nexo, B.A.; Wallin, H.; Overvad, K.; Raaschou-Nielsen, O.; Vogel, U. Associations between GPX1 Pro198Leu polymorphism, erythrocyte GPX activity, alcohol consumption and breast cancer risk in a prospective cohort study. *Carcinogenesis* **2006**, *27*, 820–825. [CrossRef]
60. Forsberg, L.; Lyrenas, L.; de Faire, U.; Morgenstern, R. A common functional C-T substitution polymorphism in the promoter region of the human catalase gene influences transcription factor binding, reporter gene transcription and is correlated to blood catalase levels. *Free Radic. Biol. Med.* **2001**, *30*, 500–505. [CrossRef]
61. Da Rocha, T.J.; Silva Alves, M.; Guisso, C.C.; de Andrade, F.M.; Camozzato, A.; de Oliveira, A.A.; Fiegenbaum, M. Association of GPX1 and GPX4 polymorphisms with episodic memory and Alzheimer's disease. *Neurosci. Lett.* **2018**, *666*, 32–37. [CrossRef] [PubMed]
62. Gong, B.; Shi, Y.; Qu, C.; Ye, Z.; Yin, Y.; Tan, C.; Shuai, P.; Li, J.; Guo, X.; Cheng, Y.; et al. Association of catalase polymorphisms with primary open-angle glaucoma in a Chinese population. *Ophthalmic Genet.* **2018**, *39*, 35–40. [CrossRef]
63. Zhou, Y.; Shuai, P.; Li, X.; Liu, X.; Wang, J.; Yang, Y.; Hao, F.; Lin, H.; Zhang, D.; Gong, B. Association of SOD2 polymorphisms with primary open angle glaucoma in a Chinese population. *Ophthalmic Genet.* **2015**, *36*, 43–49. [CrossRef]
64. Markiewicz, L.; Pytel, D.; Mucha, B.; Szymanek, K.; Szaflik, J.; Szaflik, J.P.; Majsterek, I. Altered Expression Levels of MMP1, MMP9, MMP12, TIMP1, and IL-1beta as a Risk Factor for the Elevated IOP and Optic Nerve Head Damage in the Primary Open-Angle Glaucoma Patients. *BioMed Res. Int.* **2015**, *2015*, 812503. [CrossRef]
65. Chi, W.; Li, F.; Chen, H.; Wang, Y.; Zhu, Y.; Yang, X.; Zhu, J.; Wu, F.; Ouyang, H.; Ge, J.; et al. Caspase-8 promotes NLRP1/NLRP3 inflammasome activation and IL-1beta production in acute glaucoma. *Proc. Natl. Acad. Sci. USA* **2014**, *111*, 11181–11186. [CrossRef]
66. Oliveira, M.B.; de Vasconcellos, J.P.C.; Ananina, G.; Costa, V.P.; de Melo, M.B. Association between IL1A and IL1B polymorphisms and primary open angle glaucoma in a Brazilian population. *Exp. Biol. Med.* **2018**, *243*, 1083–1091. [CrossRef] [PubMed]
67. Markiewicz, L.; Majsterek, I.; Przybylowska, K.; Dziki, L.; Waszczyk, M.; Gacek, M.; Kaminska, A.; Szaflik, J.; Szaflik, J.P. Gene polymorphisms of the MMP1, MMP9, MMP12, IL-1beta and TIMP1 and the risk of primary open-angle glaucoma. *Acta Ophthalmol.* **2013**, *91*, e516–e523. [CrossRef] [PubMed]
68. Lin, H.J.; Tsai, S.C.; Tsai, F.J.; Chen, W.C.; Tsai, J.J.; Hsu, C.D. Association of interleukin 1beta and receptor antagonist gene polymorphisms with primary open-angle glaucoma. *Ophthalmologica* **2003**, *217*, 358–364. [CrossRef]
69. Wang, C.Y.; Shen, Y.C.; Su, C.H.; Lo, F.Y.; Lee, S.H.; Tsai, H.Y.; Fan, S.S. Investigation of the association between interleukin-1beta polymorphism and normal tension glaucoma. *Mol. Vis.* **2007**, *13*, 719–723.
70. How, A.C.; Aung, T.; Chew, X.; Yong, V.H.; Lim, M.C.; Lee, K.Y.; Toh, J.Y.; Li, Y.; Liu, J.; Vithana, E.N. Lack of association between interleukin-1 gene cluster polymorphisms and glaucoma in Chinese subjects. *Investig. Ophthalmol. Vis. Sci.* **2007**, *48*, 2123–2126. [CrossRef]
71. Mookherjee, S.; Banerjee, D.; Chakraborty, S.; Mukhopadhyay, I.; Sen, A.; Ray, K. Evaluation of the IL1 Gene Cluster Single Nucleotide Polymorphisms in Primary Open-Angle Glaucoma Pathogenesis. *Genet. Test. Mol. Biomark.* **2016**, *20*, 633–636. [CrossRef] [PubMed]
72. Li, J.; Feng, Y.; Sung, M.S.; Lee, T.H.; Park, S.W. Association of Interleukin-1 gene clusters polymorphisms with primary open-angle glaucoma: A meta-analysis. *BMC Ophthalmol.* **2017**, *17*, 218. [CrossRef] [PubMed]
73. Zimmermann, C.; Weger, M.; Faschinger, C.; Renner, W.; Mossbock, G. Role of interleukin 6-174G>C polymorphism in primary open-angle glaucoma. *Eur. J. Ophthalmol.* **2013**, *23*, 183–186. [CrossRef]
74. Ye, H.; Li, X.; Wang, L.; Liao, Q.; Xu, L.; Huang, Y.; Xu, L.; Xu, X.; Chen, C.; Wu, H.; et al. Genetic associations with coronary heart disease: Meta-analyses of 12 candidate genetic variants. *Gene* **2013**, *531*, 71–77. [CrossRef]
75. Rosenberger, A.; Illig, T.; Korb, K.; Klopp, N.; Zietemann, V.; Wolke, G.; Meese, E.; Sybrecht, G.; Kronenberg, F.; Cebulla, M.; et al. Do genetic factors protect for early onset lung cancer? A case control study before the age of 50 years. *BMC Cancer* **2008**, *8*, 60. [CrossRef]
76. Malinowska, K.; Kowalski, M.; Szaflik, J.; Szaflik, J.P.; Majsterek, I. The role of Cat-262C/T, GPX1 Pro198Leu and Sod1+35A/C gene polymorphisms in a development of primary open-angle glaucoma in a Polish population. *Pol. J. Pathol.* **2016**, *67*, 404–410. [CrossRef] [PubMed]
77. Wolfs, R.C.; Klaver, C.C.; Ramrattan, R.S.; van Duijn, C.M.; Hofman, A.; de Jong, P.T. Genetic risk of primary open-angle glaucoma. Population-based familial aggregation study. *Arch. Ophthalmol.* **1998**, *116*, 1640–1645. [CrossRef] [PubMed]
78. Cheema, A.; Chang, R.T.; Shrivastava, A.; Singh, K. Update on the Medical Treatment of Primary Open-Angle Glaucoma. *Asia Pac. J. Ophthalmol.* **2016**, *5*, 51–58. [CrossRef]

79. Springelkamp, H.; Iglesias, A.I.; Mishra, A.; Hohn, R.; Wojciechowski, R.; Khawaja, A.P.; Nag, A.; Wang, Y.X.; Wang, J.J.; Cuellar-Partida, G.; et al. New insights into the genetics of primary open-angle glaucoma based on meta-analyses of intraocular pressure and optic disc characteristics. *Hum. Mol. Genet.* **2017**, *26*, 438–453. [CrossRef] [PubMed]

80. Choquet, H.; Wiggs, J.L.; Khawaja, A.P. Clinical implications of recent advances in primary open-angle glaucoma genetics. *Eye* **2020**, *34*, 29–39. [CrossRef] [PubMed]

81. Khawaja, A.P.; Cooke Bailey, J.N.; Wareham, N.J.; Scott, R.A.; Simcoe, M.; Igo, R.P., Jr.; Song, Y.E.; Wojciechowski, R.; Cheng, C.Y.; Khaw, P.T.; et al. Genome-wide analyses identify 68 new loci associated with intraocular pressure and improve risk prediction for primary open-angle glaucoma. *Nat. Genet.* **2018**, *50*, 778–782. [CrossRef]

82. Gordon, M.O.; Beiser, J.A.; Brandt, J.D.; Heuer, D.K.; Higginbotham, E.J.; Johnson, C.A.; Keltner, J.L.; Miller, J.P.; Parrish, R.K., 2nd; Wilson, M.R.; et al. The Ocular Hypertension Treatment Study: Baseline factors that predict the onset of primary open-angle glaucoma. *Arch. Ophthalmol.* **2002**, *120*, 714–720; discussion 829–830. [CrossRef] [PubMed]

83. Leske, M.C.; Heijl, A.; Hyman, L.; Bengtsson, B.; Dong, L.; Yang, Z. Predictors of long-term progression in the early manifest glaucoma trial. *Ophthalmology* **2007**, *114*, 1965–1972. [CrossRef] [PubMed]

84. Medeiros, F.A.; Meira-Freitas, D.; Lisboa, R.; Kuang, T.M.; Zangwill, L.M.; Weinreb, R.N. Corneal Hysteresis as a Risk Factor for Glaucoma Progression: A Prospective Longitudinal Study. *Ophthalmology* **2013**, *120*, 1533–1540. [CrossRef]

85. Mitchell, P.; Lee, A.J.; Rochtchina, E.; Wang, J.J. Open-angle glaucoma and systemic hypertension: The blue mountains eye study. *J. Glaucoma* **2004**, *13*, 319–326. [CrossRef] [PubMed]

86. Klein, B.E.; Klein, R.; Knudtson, M.D. Intraocular pressure and systemic blood pressure: Longitudinal perspective: The Beaver Dam Eye Study. *Br. J. Ophthalmol.* **2005**, *89*, 284–287. [CrossRef]

87. Hayreh, S.S.; Podhajsky, P.; Zimmerman, M.B. Ocular and optic nerve head ischemic disorders and hearing loss. *Am. J. Ophthalmol.* **1999**, *128*, 606–611. [CrossRef]

88. Hayreh, S.S.; Podhajsky, P.; Zimmerman, M.B. Beta-blocker eyedrops and nocturnal arterial hypotension. *Am. J. Ophthalmol.* **1999**, *128*, 301–309. [CrossRef]

89. Zhao, D.; Cho, J.; Kim, M.H.; Friedman, D.S.; Guallar, E. Diabetes, fasting glucose, and the risk of glaucoma: A meta-analysis. *Ophthalmology* **2015**, *122*, 72–78. [CrossRef]

90. Ko, F.; Boland, M.V.; Gupta, P.; Gadkaree, S.K.; Vitale, S.; Guallar, E.; Zhao, D.; Friedman, D.S. Diabetes, Triglyceride Levels, and Other Risk Factors for Glaucoma in the National Health and Nutrition Examination Survey 2005–2008. *Investig. Ophthalmol. Vis. Sci.* **2016**, *57*, 2152–2157. [CrossRef]

91. Shen, L.; Walter, S.; Melles, R.B.; Glymour, M.M.; Jorgenson, E. Diabetes Pathology and Risk of Primary Open-Angle Glaucoma: Evaluating Causal Mechanisms by Using Genetic Information. *Am. J. Epidemiol.* **2016**, *183*, 147–155. [CrossRef]

92. Song, B.J.; Aiello, L.P.; Pasquale, L.R. Presence and Risk Factors for Glaucoma in Patients with Diabetes. *Curr. Diabetes Rep.* **2016**, *16*, 124. [CrossRef]

93. Chen, Y.Y.; Hu, H.Y.; Chu, D.; Chen, H.H.; Chang, C.K.; Chou, P. Patients with Primary Open-Angle Glaucoma May Develop Ischemic Heart Disease More Often than Those without Glaucoma: An 11-Year Population-Based Cohort Study. *PLoS ONE* **2016**, *11*, e0163210. [CrossRef] [PubMed]

94. Luo, X.Y.; Dai, W.; Chee, M.L.; Tao, Y.; Chua, J.; Tan, N.Y.Q.; Tham, Y.C.; Aung, T.; Wong, T.Y.; Cheng, C.Y. Association of Diabetes With Central Corneal Thickness Among a Multiethnic Asian Population. *JAMA Netw. Open* **2019**, *2*, e186647. [CrossRef]

95. Karvonen, E.; Stoor, K.; Luodonpaa, M.; Hagg, P.; Kuoppala, J.; Lintonen, T.; Ohtonen, P.; Tuulonen, A.; Saarela, V. Prevalence of glaucoma in the Northern Finland Birth Cohort Eye Study. *Acta Ophthalmol.* **2019**, *97*, 200–207. [CrossRef]

96. Klein, B.E.; Klein, R.; Jensen, S.C. Open-angle glaucoma and older-onset diabetes. The Beaver Dam Eye Study. *Ophthalmology* **1994**, *101*, 1173–1177. [CrossRef]

97. Dielemans, I.; Vingerling, J.R.; Wolfs, R.C.; Hofman, A.; Grobbee, D.E.; de Jong, P.T. The prevalence of primary open-angle glaucoma in a population-based study in The Netherlands. The Rotterdam Study. *Ophthalmology* **1994**, *101*, 1851–1855. [CrossRef]

98. Mizzi, C.; Dalabira, E.; Kumuthini, J.; Dzimiri, N.; Balogh, I.; Basak, N.; Bohm, R.; Borg, J.; Borgiani, P.; Bozina, N.; et al. A European Spectrum of Pharmacogenomic Biomarkers: Implications for Clinical Pharmacogenomics. *PLoS ONE* **2016**, *11*, e0162866. [CrossRef] [PubMed]

99. Vidan-Jeras, B.; Jurca, B.; Dolzan, V.; Jeras, M.; Breskvar, K.; Bohinjec, M. Slovenian Caucasian Normal. In *HLA 1998*; Terasaki, P.I., Gjertson, D.W., Lenaxa, K.S., Eds.; American Society for Histocompatibility and Immunogenetics: Mount Laurel, NJ, USA, 1998; pp. 180–181.

100. Ramdas, W.D.; Schouten, J.; Webers, C.A.B. The Effect of Vitamins on Glaucoma: A Systematic Review and Meta-Analysis. *Nutrients* **2018**, *10*, 359. [CrossRef]

101. Pinazo-Duran, M.D.; Shoaie-Nia, K.; Zanon-Moreno, V.; Sanz-Gonzalez, S.M.; Del Castillo, J.B.; Garcia-Medina, J.J. Strategies to Reduce Oxidative Stress in Glaucoma Patients. *Curr. Neuropharmacol.* **2018**, *16*, 903–918. [CrossRef]

102. Hui, F.; Tang, J.; Williams, P.A.; McGuinness, M.B.; Hadoux, X.; Casson, R.J.; Coote, M.; Trounce, I.A.; Martin, K.R.; van Wijngaarden, P.; et al. Improvement in inner retinal function in glaucoma with nicotinamide (vitamin B3) supplementation: A crossover randomized clinical trial. *Clin. Exp. Ophthalmol.* **2020**, *48*, 903–914. [CrossRef]

103. Adornetto, A.; Russo, R.; Parisi, V. Neuroinflammation as a target for glaucoma therapy. *Neural Regen. Res.* **2019**, *14*, 391–394. [CrossRef]

104. Ban, N.; Siegfried, C.J.; Apte, R.S. Monitoring Neurodegeneration in Glaucoma: Therapeutic Implications. *Trends Mol. Med.* **2018**, *24*, 7–17. [CrossRef]
105. Guo, X.; Namekata, K.; Kimura, A.; Harada, C.; Harada, T. ASK1 in neurodegeneration. *Adv. Biol. Regul.* **2017**, *66*, 63–71. [CrossRef]
106. Sutton, A.; Imbert, A.; Igoudjil, A.; Descatoire, V.; Cazanave, S.; Pessayre, D.; Degoul, F. The manganese superoxide dismutase Ala16Val dimorphism modulates both mitochondrial import and mRNA stability. *Pharmacogenet. Genom.* **2005**, *15*, 311–319. [CrossRef]
107. Nebert, D.W.; Vasiliou, V. Analysis of the glutathione S-transferase (GST) gene family. *Hum Genom.* **2004**, *1*, 460–464. [CrossRef] [PubMed]
108. Kutikhin, A.G.; Yuzhalin, A.E.; Volkov, A.N.; Zhivotovskiy, A.S.; Brusina, E.B. Correlation between genetic polymorphisms within IL-1B and TLR4 genes and cancer risk in a Russian population: A case-control study. *Tumor Biol.* **2014**, *35*, 4821–4830. [CrossRef]
109. Torres-Merino, S.; Moreno-Sandoval, H.N.; Thompson-Bonilla, M.D.R.; Leon, J.A.O.; Gomez-Conde, E.; Leon-Chavez, B.A.; Martinez-Fong, D.; Gonzalez-Barrios, J.A. Association Between rs3833912/rs16944 SNPs and Risk for Cerebral Palsy in Mexican Children. *Mol. Neurobiol.* **2018**, *21*, 018–1178. [CrossRef] [PubMed]
110. Lagmay, J.P.; London, W.B.; Gross, T.G.; Termuhlen, A.; Sullivan, N.; Axel, A.; Mundy, B.; Ranalli, M.; Canner, J.; McGrady, P.; et al. Prognostic significance of interleukin-6 single nucleotide polymorphism genotypes in neuroblastoma: rs1800795 (promoter) and rs8192284 (receptor). *Clin. Cancer Res.* **2009**, *15*, 5234–5239. [CrossRef] [PubMed]
111. Szkup, M.; Chelmecka, E.; Lubkowska, A.; Owczarek, A.J.; Grochans, E. The influence of the TNFalpha rs1800629 polymorphism on some inflammatory biomarkers in 45–60-year-old women with metabolic syndrome. *Aging* **2018**, *10*, 2935–2943. [CrossRef]

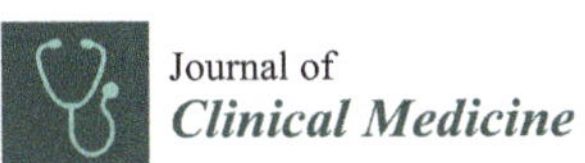

Journal of
Clinical Medicine

Article

Effects of Ripasudil on Open-Angle Glaucoma after Circumferential Suture Trabeculotomy Ab Interno

Tomoki Sato and Takahiro Kawaji *

Sato Eye and Internal Medicine Clinic, 4160-270 Arao, Arao City, Kumamoto 860-0041, Japan; zxsato@gmail.com
* Correspondence: kawag@white.plala.or.jp; Tel.: +81-968-65-5900

Abstract: We evaluated the effects of ripasudil on the distal aqueous outflow tract in patients with open-angle glaucoma (OAG) who underwent a 360° suture trabeculotomy ab interno followed by ripasudil treatment beginning 1 month postoperatively. We compared 27 of these patients, by using propensity score analysis, with 27 patients in a matched control group who had no ripasudil treatment. We assessed the changes in the mean intraocular pressure (IOP) and the relationship between the IOP changes and background factors. All eyes had a complete 360° Schlemm's canal incision and phacoemulsification. The mean IOP at 1 and 3 months after ripasudil administration were significantly reduced by -1.7 ± 1.9 mmHg ($p < 0.0001$) and -1.3 ± 2.3 mmHg ($p = 0.0081$) in the ripasudil group, respectively, but IOP in the control group was not significantly reduced. The IOP reduction was significantly associated with the IOP before ripasudil treatment ($p < 0.001$). In conclusion, the use of ripasudil for patients with OAG after circumferential incision of the Schlemm's canal produced significant IOP reductions. Ripasudil may affect the distal outflow tract, thereby leading to the IOP reduction.

Keywords: ripasudil; suture trabeculotomy ab interno; Schlemm's canal incision; aqueous outflow; open-angle glaucoma

Citation: Sato, T.; Kawaji, T. Effects of Ripasudil on Open-Angle Glaucoma after Circumferential Suture Trabeculotomy Ab Interno. *J. Clin. Med.* **2021**, *10*, 401. https://doi.org/10.3390/jcm10030401

Academic Editor: Jose Javier Garcia-Medina

Received: 26 December 2020
Accepted: 18 January 2021
Published: 21 January 2021

Publisher's Note: MDPI stays neutral with regard to jurisdictional claims in published maps and institutional affiliations.

1. Introduction

Glaucoma is an ocular condition that manifests functional and structural abnormalities of the optic nerve related to retinal ganglion cell death [1,2]. Elevated intraocular pressure (IOP) is known to be a main risk factor for the onset and progression of glaucoma, so lowering the IOP has been believed to be the main treatment strategy to prevent vision loss in patients with glaucomatous eyes [3,4]. Aqueous humor drains through the conventional outflow pathway via the trabecular meshwork and the uveoscleral pathway through the ciliary body to the suprachoroidal space. This trabecular meshwork structure is thought to be responsible for the highest resistance to aqueous outflow [5–7]. However, several experiments and surgical outcomes have suggested that one-third to one-half of the total outflow resistance is located distal to Schlemm's canal [8–10]. A number of medications, such as prostaglandin analogs, beta-blockers, carbonic anhydrase inhibitors, and α2-agonists, are used to lower IOP levels in glaucomatous eyes; however, these drugs affect the uveoscleral pathway or aqueous humor production as opposed to the conventional outflow pathway.

In addition to these IOP-lowering drugs, inhibitors of Rho-associated protein kinase (ROCK) have been developed to reduce IOP levels in animal and human eyes [11,12]. The IOP-lowering effects of ROCK inhibitors have induced alterations in cell shape, contraction, motility, attachment, and extracellular matrix production in the trabecular meshwork and Schlemm's canal endothelial cells, which have resulted in improvements in the conventional aqueous outflow [12]. Certain ROCK inhibitors, including ripasudil (Glanatec ophthalmic solution 0.4%; Kowa Company, Ltd., Nagoya, Aichi, Japan) and netarsudil (Rhopressa ophthalmic solution 0.02%; Aerie Pharmaceuticals, Bedminster, NJ, USA), are now available in the market and are used in clinical practice in a number of countries [13,14]. In animal models, enucleated human eyes and living human eyes, netarsudil increased outflow facility by expanding the juxtacanalicular trabecular meshwork and by dilating episcleral veins [15–20]. However, the effects of ripasudil, one of the ROCK inhibitors, on the distal outflow pathway in living human subjects have not yet been studied.

We have seen several reports concerning the clinical outcomes of 360° suture trabeculotomy ab interno used for open-angle glaucoma (OAG) [21,22]. This procedure can relieve the resistance to aqueous humor outflow by using an incision of the trabecular meshwork and the inner layer of Schlemm's canal. Therefore, the function of the distal outflow tract can be evaluated after the circumferential incision of Schlemm's canal via this procedure. In our previous studies, we showed that the IOP was reduced and fluctuated within 1 month after the surgery, and then, from 1 month postoperatively, the IOP stabilized in most cases [21,22]. Therefore, in the present study, we evaluated the effects of ripasudil on the distal aqueous outflow tract in patients with OAG who underwent the circumferential incision of Schlemm's canal, followed by ripasudil treatment beginning 1 month postoperatively. We then compared those patients with a matched control group, i.e., patients who had no ripasudil treatment postoperatively. We utilized a quasi-randomized propensity score analysis to minimize the influence of the confounding factors.

2. Materials and Methods

2.1. Study Design and Patients

This analysis was a retrospective, single-center, observational, comparative clinical study performed at Sato Eye and Internal Medicine Clinic (Arao City, Kumamoto, Japan) between 2014 and 2019. The study protocol adhered to the principles of the Declaration of Helsinki and was approved by the Institutional Review Board and the Ethics Committee at Sato Eye and Internal Medicine Clinic. Informed consent was obtained from all patients.

Patients were considered for admission into the study if they had OAG together with a visually significant cataract. We reviewed the medical charts of 42 consecutive patients who underwent a 360° suture trabeculotomy ab interno with phacoemulsification, and 1 month later these patients started to receive ripasudil between 2018 and 2019 (ripasudil group); alternatively, we reviewed 52 patients who underwent a 360° suture trabeculotomy ab interno with phacoemulsification without additional treatment after surgery between 2014 and 2017 (control group). Patients were followed up for at least 3 months after the start of ripasudil treatment. We did not include patients who had suture trabeculotomy ab interno alone because of the small number of these patients.

Study patients had primary open-angle glaucoma (POAG), normal-tension glaucoma, or exfoliation glaucoma. Glaucoma surgeries were performed both in medically uncontrolled eyes and in medically well-controlled eyes to reduce the medication burden. A cataract was said to be visually significant if a patient reported a glare or halos and had a best-corrected visual acuity of 20/20 or worse. If subjects had any of the following, they were excluded from this study: other types of glaucoma; a history of incisional glaucoma surgery; use of additional anti-glaucoma agents except ripasudil or surgery during a post-operative 3-month period; and being under 20 years of age at the time of the surgery. One surgeon (T.S.) performed all operations; he used the surgical procedure described here [21].

The primary outcome measure was the mean IOP change at each visit. We also assessed the relationship between the change in IOP and the background factors in the ripasudil group.

2.2. Surgical Technique

The suture trabeculotomy ab interno procedure used here was previously described in full [21]; in the present study, a modified technique for Schlemm's canal incision was used. In brief, a 1.7 mm temporal corneal incision was made, and the Schlemm's canal on the nasal side was incised at 15° by utilizing a microhook needle (HS-2167; Handaya, Tokyo, Japan) instead of the trabectome (NeoMedix, Tustin, CA, USA), as used in the original paper [21]. A standard phacoemulsification with intraocular lens implantation in the capsular bag was performed through the same or a new upper corneal incision (depending on the easier procedure in each case), with the phacoemulsification with lens implantation being performed after the suture trabeculotomy ab interno. At the end of operation, we used iCare (M.E. Technica, Tokyo, Japan) to determine that no wound leakage existed and that the IOP value in the supine position was 18 mmHg or more. Postoperative drug therapy consisted of a 2-week regimen of moxifloxacin hydrochloride, 0.1% betamethasone, and 2% pilocarpine.

2.3. Data Collection and Statistical Analysis

All potential subjects were screened for eligibility by using the following methods: slit-lamp biomicroscopy, indirect ophthalmoscopy, manifest refraction, measurement of IOP, and best-corrected visual acuity assessment (via the conventional Landolt ring chart). The surgeons or other ophthalmologists used a Goldmann tonometer to measure all IOP values. The mean of the 3 most recent measurements, acquired on separate days within 1 month before surgery, was utilized to determine the baseline IOP. An Auto Ref/Keratometer (ARK-530A; Nidek, Tokyo, Japan) was used to measure the manifest refraction; decimal visual acuity values were changed to the logarithm of the minimum angle of resolution.

All patients were evaluated on days 1, 2, and 3 after surgery, and then every 1–2 weeks for 1 month, after which ripasudil was administered. After the start of ripasudil treatment, patients were examined at 1, 2, and 3 months. The IOP was measured at every visit.

The JMP statistical package (version 14; SAS Institute Inc., Cary, NC, USA) was used to analyze all data. Cases were matched via propensity score analysis by using a genetic algorithm based on age, sex, type of glaucoma, preoperative IOP and medications, 1-month postoperative IOP, axial length, and visual field. Continuous data were expressed as means $\pm$ standard deviation, and changes in continuous variables were assessed by using the paired t-test. Multiple regression models were utilized to analyze associations between IOP changes at 3 months after ripasudil treatment and background factors. The statistical significance value was set at $p < 0.05$.

3. Results

3.1. Disposition and Characteristics of Patients

From among 40 patients in the ripasudil group and 54 patients in the control group, 54 patients were included in this study—27 patients in a ripasudil group and 27 patients in a control group. The propensity score analysis revealed no significant difference in baseline characteristics between the two groups (Table 1). Suture trabeculotomy ab interno combined with phacoemulsification was performed in all eyes, and all eyes had a complete 360° Schlemm's canal incision.

Table 1. Baseline characteristics of patients.

Characteristic	Ripasudil	Control	p-Value
No. of patients	27	27	
Age, years, mean $\pm$ SD (range)	79.7 $\pm$ 6.8 (63–88)	78.5 $\pm$ 7.6 (64–89)	0.548
Male/female, n	15/12	11/16	0.414
Right/left, n	11/16	13/14	0.352
IOP, mmHg, mean $\pm$ SD (range)			
Pre-SLOT surgery	16.4 $\pm$ 3.6 (11–26)	16.4 $\pm$ 3.4 (11–25)	0.785
Pre-ripasudil treatment	12.5 $\pm$ 3.0 (6–21)	12.1 $\pm$ 2.2 (7–16)	0.775
No. of preoperative medications, mean $\pm$ SD (range)	1.9 $\pm$ 1.3 (0–4)	1.4 $\pm$ 1.5 (0–4)	0.525
BCVA, logMAR, mean $\pm$ SD (range)	0.26 $\pm$ 0.21 (0–0.82)	0.35 $\pm$ 0.22 (0–1.10)	0.295
Visual field, MD (dB), mean $\pm$ SD (range)	-8.6 ± 5.4 (-18.4––0.2)	-9.7 ± 8.1 (-27.9––1.6)	0.106
Axial length, mm, mean $\pm$ SD (range)	23.7 $\pm$ 0.8 (22.5–25.8)	24.2 $\pm$ 1.5 (21.3–27.4)	0.569
Type of glaucoma, n (%)			0.211
POAG	10	13	
NTG	10	11	
XFG	7	3	

IOP, intraocular pressure; SLOT, suture trabeculotomy ab interno; BCVA, best-corrected visual acuity; logMAR, logarithm of minimum angle of resolution; MD, mean deviation; POAG, primary open-angle glaucoma; NTG, normal-tension glaucoma; SD, standard deviation; XFG, exfoliation glaucoma.

3.2. Efficacy

As Figure 1a shows, the mean IOP value was significantly reduced from 16.4 ± 3.6 mmHg to 12.5 ± 3.0 mmHg ($p < 0.0001$) at 1 month post-operation in the ripasudil group and from 16.4 ± 3.4 mmHg to 12.1 ± 2.2 mmHg ($p < 0.0001$) at 1 month post-operation in the control group; ripasudil treatment was then started in the ripasudil group. The mean IOP values at 1 and 3 months after the start of ripasudil treatment were significantly reduced by -1.7 ± 1.9 mmHg ($p < 0.0001$) and -1.3 ± 2.3 mmHg ($p = 0.0081$) in the ripasudil group, respectively, and there was no significant difference between at 1 and 3 months IOP ($p = 0.3013$). At these same time points, however, the IOP reductions were not significant in the control group: 0.4 ± 2.2 mmHg ($p = 0.8494$) and 0.1 ± 2.0 mmHg ($p = 0.9251$), respectively. The IOP values at 1 month ($p = 0.0003$) and 3 months ($p = 0.0317$) after ripasudil treatment were significantly different between the ripasudil group and the control group. At both 1 and 3 months after ripasudil treatment, no IOP reduction was seen in 33% of the ripasudil group; at that same time point, 60% of the control group showed no IOP reduction (Figure 1b).

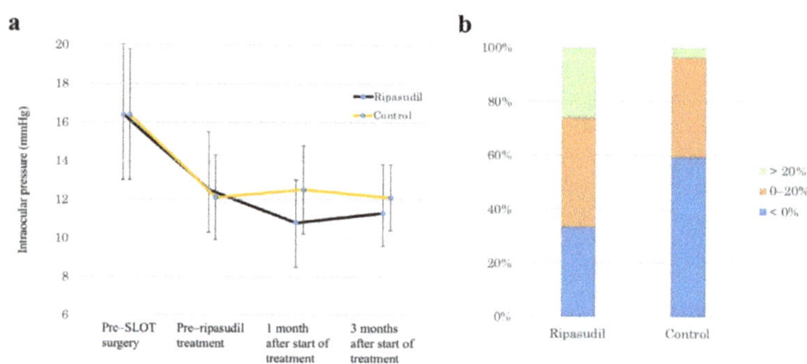

Figure 1. IOP–lowering effects of ripasudil. (**a**) Time–dependent changes in IOP at different time points: pre–SLOT surgery, pre–ripasudil treatment (i.e., 1 month post-operation), and 1 month and 3 months after the start of ripasudil treatment. (**b**) Stacked bar chart of IOP changes at 3 months after the start of ripasudil treatment. SLOT suture trabeculotomy ab interno.

Multiple regression analysis of data for the ripasudil group demonstrated that the IOP reduction at 3 months was significantly associated with the IOP value before ripasudil treatment, but not with age, visual field, preoperative medications, or IOP value before surgery (Table 2).

Table 2. Relationship between IOP changes at 3 months after the start of ripasudil treatment and background factors, as determined by multiple regression analysis.

Background Factor	T-Value	*p*-Value
IOP (mmHg) before surgery	1.67	0.097
IOP (mmHg) before ripasudil treatment	−7.28	<0.001
Medication before surgery	1.99	0.050
Age (years)	0.38	0.702
Visual field (mean deviation, dB)	−0.39	0.699

IOP intraocular pressure.

4. Discussion

In this retrospective study, we used propensity score analysis to investigate the effects of ripasudil treatment on patients with OAG after 360° suture trabeculotomy ab interno, in whom the aqueous outflow resistance caused by the trabecular meshwork should be eliminated, and we found a significant IOP reduction. This finding suggested that ripasudil may affect the distal outflow tract, with the consequence being IOP reduction.

Although IOP elevation was long thought to be caused by outflow resistance at the trabecular meshwork, which blocks the eye's drainage system, data from clinical studies of trabecular meshwork-targeted minimally invasive glaucoma surgery (MIGS) showed that the MIGS failed to lower the IOP to the pressure level in the recipient episcleral veins [23,24]. Previous studies in enucleated human eyes suggested that 25–50% of total outflow resistance is located at the conventional outflow pathway distal to Schlemm's canal [8,9]. Research utilizing multimodal two-photon-deep tissue imaging and three-dimensional analysis demonstrated that the distal aqueous drainage tract wall can contract and aid the dynamic alteration of the drainage tract, similarly to the function of blood vessel tone in blood flow regulation [25]. Another study showed that the regulation of distal vessels via the physiological vasoregulators endothelin-1 and nitric oxide dramatically affected outflow resistance in both humans and pigs [26]. Thus, distal vessels probably play an important role in regulating outflow resistance, especially after MIGS and perhaps in the pathophysiology of glaucomatous eyes.

Several reports showed the effects of netarsudil on the structure and function of the distal outflow tract; the dilation of outflow tract vessels together with a corresponding pressure reduction was observed in mouse [17], rabbit [16], porcine [19] and ennucleated human eye models [18], and living human eye [20]. However, the effects of ROCK inhibitors on the distal outflow tract in living human subjects has not been fully studied. We demonstrated here that glaucomatous eyes that had a circumferential incision of the trabecular meshwork via 360° suture trabeculotomy demonstrated a significant IOP reduction after ripasudil treatment. We started ripasudil administration 1 month post-operation, because we had found that the IOP fluctuated for 1 month after suture trabeculotomy and then, from 1 month postoperatively, the IOP stabilized in most cases [21,22]. In this study, we included a control group and used propensity score analysis to evaluate whether the IOP actually stabilized from 1 month postoperatively. Our result clearly showed that the IOP stabilized from 1 month postoperatively in the control group; therefore, a significant IOP reduction after the administration of ripasudil may be caused by the effect of ripasudil, and may not be the natural postoperative course. In addition, we excluded a patient who also required anti-glaucoma medication other than ripasudil, because such a patient may already have a non-functional distal outflow tract. Thus, our study protocol made the evaluation of the function of an almost intact distal outflow tract possible. Multiple regression analysis showed that the IOP reduction was significantly associated with only the IOP value before ripasudil treatment. As Figure 1b shows, no IOP reduction at 3 months after the start of ripasudil treatment was observed in about one-third of the eyes. The absence of IOP reduction in these eyes may be explained by a lack of efficacy of ripasudil at lower IOP values, but the reason for this finding is unknown.

Trabecular meshwork-targeted MIGS have gained popularity for lowering the IOP, so the imaging and understanding of the distal outflow tract have increased in importance. Recent publications reported intraoperative observations of fluid waves in episcleral veins, which were correlated with good postoperative IOP reduction and/or the number of medications [27,28]. Goda et al. reported that success probabilities for trabeculotomy ab externo were 100% for patients with POAG who achieved an IOP value < 21 mmHg via preoperative ripasudil administration [29]. This result suggested that whether ripasudil is effective or not before trabeculotomy may help predict to what degree the trabecular meshwork, as well as possibly the distal outflow tract, is functional, and may be used as a trabeculotomy outcome marker in patients with POAG. In this study, this hypothesis could not be evaluated because of the small number of patients who received ripasudil before surgery.

Recent MIGS procedures have been routinely performed in medically well-controlled eyes to reduce the medication burden, and as an early intervention in eyes requiring IOP reduction without medications or laser treatments at the time of cataract surgery [30,31].

Thus, such cases were included in the present study and had relatively low baseline IOP and 1-month postoperative IOP. Our data showed that the mean 1-month postoperative IOP was about 12 mmHg; no medication is usually used for eyes having such a low IOP in clinical settings. We had thought to investigate whether ripasudil could affect the distal outflow tract in living humans; on the basis of this study, however, we cannot determine whether ripasudil is clinically useful from the point of view of glaucoma management. Additional investigations of eyes with higher IOP values and/or more severe stages of glaucoma are needed to ascertain whether ripasudil should be used after circumferential incision of the Schlemm's canal, given the expected effect of ripasudil on the distal outflow tract.

The present study has certain limitations. This study is retrospective. Additionally, although we used propensity score matching to overcome the study limitations, propensity score analysis, unlike prospective randomized clinical trials, cannot randomize unknown confounding factors and loses certain samples through 1:1 matching analysis. This study also includes the possibility of selection bias because of its single institution-based nature with a small sample size. In addition, all eyes underwent suture trabeculotomy ab interno plus phacoemulsification. The eyes that underwent only suture trabeculotomy ab interno (i.e., without phacoemulsification) may have demonstrated a more dramatic result, but the number of eyes was small. Phacoemulsification may have further limited the effect of ripasudil and may have affected the IOP changes after surgery or after ripasudil administration. Therefore, eyes that underwent suture trabeculotomy ab interno with phacoemulsification, but without ripasudil treatments, were included as a control group.

In conclusion, the ripasudil treatment of patients with OAG after 360° suture trabeculotomy ab interno led to a significant reduction in IOP. Ripasudil may affect the distal outflow tract and result in an IOP reduction in living human subjects.

Author Contributions: Conceptualization, T.S. and T.K.; methodology, T.K.; software, T.S.; validation, T.S. and T.K.; formal analysis, T.S. and T.K.; investigation, T.S.; resources, T.S.; data curation, T.S. and T.K.; writing—original draft preparation, T.S.; writing—review and editing, T.K.; visualization, T.K.; supervision, T.K.; project administration, T.S.; funding acquisition, None. All authors have read and agreed to the published version of the manuscript.

Funding: This research received no external funding.

Institutional Review Board Statement: The study adhered to the tenets of the Declaration of Helsinki and was approved by the institutional Ethics Committee (CN 202001).

Informed Consent Statement: Informed consent was obtained from all subjects involved in the study.

Data Availability Statement: The data analyzed in this study are available from the corresponding author on reasonable request.

Conflicts of Interest: The authors declare no conflict of interest.

References

1. Quigley, H.A. Glaucoma. *Lancet* **2011**, *377*, 1367–1377. [CrossRef]
2. Weinreb, R.N.; Aung, T.; Medeiros, F.A. The pathophysiology and treatment of glaucoma: A review. *JAMA* **2014**, *311*, 1901–1911. [CrossRef] [PubMed]
3. Cohen, L.P.; Pasquale, L.R. Clinical characteristics and current treatment of glaucoma. *Cold Spring Harb. Perspect. Med.* **2014**, *4*, a017236. [CrossRef] [PubMed]
4. Mantravadi, A.V.; Vadhar, N. Glaucoma. *Care* **2015**, *42*, 437–449. [CrossRef]
5. Bill, A.; Phillips, C.I. Uveoscleral drainage of aqueous humour in human eyes. *Exp. Eye Res.* **1971**, *3*, 275–281. [CrossRef]
6. Tamm, E.R. The trabecular meshwork outflow pathways: Structural and functional aspects. *Exp. Eye Res.* **2009**, *88*, 648–655. [CrossRef]
7. Tektas, O.Y.; Lütjen-Drecoll, E. Structural changes of the trabecular meshwork in different kinds of glaucoma. *Exp. Eye Res.* **2009**, *88*, 769–775. [CrossRef]
8. Rosenquist, R.; Epstein, D.; Melamed, S.; Johnson, M.; Grant, W.M. Outflow resistance of enucleated human eyes at two different perfusion pressures and different extents of trabeculotomy. *Curr. Eye Res.* **1989**, *8*, 1233–1240. [CrossRef]

9. Schuman, J.S.; Chang, W.; Wang, N.; De Kater, A.W.; Allingham, R.R. Excimer laser effects on outflow facility and outflow pathway morphology. *Investig. Ophthalmol. Vis. Sci.* **1999**, *40*, 1676–1680.

10. Konopińska, J.; Kozera, M.; Kraśnicki, P.; Mariak, Z.; Rękas, M. The Effectiveness of First-Generation iStent Microbypass Implantation Depends on Initial Intraocular Pressure: 24-Month Follow-Up-Prospective Clinical Trial. *J. Ophthalmol.* **2020**, *2020*, 8164703. [CrossRef]

11. Honjo, M.; Tanihara, H.; Inatani, M.; Kido, N.; Sawamura, T.; Yue, B.Y.; Narumiya, S.; Honda, Y. Effects of rho-associated protein kinase inhibitor Y-27632 on intraocular pressure and outflow facility. *Investig. Ophthalmol. Vis. Sci.* **2001**, *42*, 137–144.

12. Inoue, T.; Tanihara, H. Rho-associated kinase inhibitors: A novel glaucoma therapy. *Prog. Retin. Eye Res.* **2013**, *37*, 1–12. [CrossRef]

13. Tanihara, H.; Inoue, T.; Yamamoto, T.; Kuwayama, Y.; Abe, H.; Fukushima, A.; Suganami, H.; Araie, M. K-115 Clinical Study Group. One-year clinical evaluation of 0.4% ripasudil (K-115) in patients with open-angle glaucoma and ocular hypertension. *Acta Ophthalmol.* **2016**, *94*, e26–e34. [CrossRef]

14. Wang, R.F.; Williamson, J.E.; Kopczynski, C.; Serle, J.B. Effect of 0.04% AR-13324, a ROCK, and norepinephrine transporter inhibitor, on aqueous humor dynamics in normotensive monkey eyes. *J. Glaucoma* **2015**, *24*, 51–54. [CrossRef]

15. Sturdivant, J.M.; Royalty, S.M.; Lin, C.W.; Moore, L.A.; Yingling, J.D.; Laethem, C.L.; Sherman, B.; Heintzelman, G.R.; Kopczynski, C.C.; DeLong, M.A. Discovery of the ROCK inhibitor netarsudil for the treatment of open-angle glaucoma. *Bioorg. Med. Chem. Lett.* **2016**, *26*, 2475–2480. [CrossRef] [PubMed]

16. Kiel, J.W.; Kopczynski, C.C. Effect of AR-13324 on episcleral venous pressure in Dutch belted rabbits. *J. Ocul. Pharmacol. Ther.* **2015**, *31*, 146–151. [CrossRef] [PubMed]

17. Li, G.; Mukherjee, D.; Navarro, I.; Ashpole, N.E.; Sherwood, J.M.; Chang, J.; Overby, D.R.; Yuan, F.; Gonzalez, P.; Kopczynski, C.C. et al. Visualization of conventional outflow tissue responses to netarsudil in living mouse eyes. *Eur. J. Pharmacol.* **2016**, *787*, 20–31. [CrossRef] [PubMed]

18. Ren, R.; Li, G.; Le, T.D.; Kopczynski, C.; Stamer, W.D.; Gong, H. Netarsudil Increases Outflow Facility in Human Eyes Through Multiple Mechanisms. *Investig. Ophthalmol. Vis. Sci.* **2016**, *57*, 6197–6209. [CrossRef] [PubMed]

19. Chen, S.; Waxman, S.; Wang, C.; Atta, S.; Loewen, R.; Loewen, N.A. Dose-dependent effects of netarsudil, a Rho-kinase inhibitor, on the distal outflow tract. *Graefes Arch. Clin. Exp. Ophthalmol.* **2020**, *258*, 1211–1216. [CrossRef]

20. Kazemi, A.; McLaren, J.W.; Kopczynski, C.C.; Heah, T.G.; Novack, G.D.; Sit, A.J. The Effects of Netarsudil Ophthalmic Solution on Aqueous Humor Dynamics in a Randomized Study in Humans. *J. Ocul. Pharmacol. Ther.* **2018**, *34*, 380–386. [CrossRef]

21. Sato, T.; Kawaji, T.; Hirata, A.; Mizoguchi, T. 360-degree suture trabeculotomy ab interno to treat open-angle glaucoma: 2-year outcomes. *Clin. Ophthalmol.* **2018**, *12*, 915–923. [CrossRef]

22. Sato, T.; Kawaji, T.; Hirata, A.; Mizoguchi, T. 360-degree suture trabeculotomy ab interno with phacoemulsification in open-angle glaucoma and coexisting cataract: A pilot study. *BMJ Open Ophthalmol.* **2018**, *3*, e000159. [CrossRef] [PubMed]

23. Parikh, H.A.; Loewen, R.T.; Roy, P.; Schuman, J.S.; Lathrop, K.L.; Loewen, N.A. Differential Canalograms Detect Outflow Changes from Trabecular Micro-Bypass Stents and Ab Interno Trabeculectomy. *Sci. Rep.* **2016**, *6*, 34705. [CrossRef] [PubMed]

24. Dang, Y.; Wang, C.; Shah, P.; Waxman, S.; Loewen, R.T.; Hong, Y.; Esfandiari, H.; Loewen, N.A. Outflow enhancement by three different ab interno trabeculectomy procedures in a porcine anterior segment model. *Graefes Arch. Clin. Exp. Ophthalmol.* **2018**, *256*, 1305–1312. [CrossRef] [PubMed]

25. Fallano, K.; Bussel, I.; Kagemann, L.; Lathrop, K.L.; Loewen, N. Training strategies and outcomes of ab interno trabeculectomy with the trabectome. *F1000Research* **2017**, *6*, 67. [CrossRef]

26. McDonnell, F.; Dismuke, W.M.; Overby, D.R.; Stamer, W.D. Pharmacological regulation of outflow resistance distal to Schlemm's canal. *Am. J. Physiol. Cell Physiol.* **2018**, *315*, C44–C51. [CrossRef]

27. Fellman, R.L.; Feuer, W.J.; Grover, D.S. Episcleral Venous Fluid Wave Correlates with Trabectome Outcomes: Intraoperative Evaluation of the Trabecular Outflow Pathway. *Ophthalmology* **2015**, *122*, 2385–2391.e1. [CrossRef]

28. Fellman, R.L.; Grover, D.S. Episcleral Venous Fluid Wave in the Living Human Eye Adjacent to Microinvasive Glaucoma Surgery (MIGS) Supports Laboratory Research: Outflow is Limited Circumferentially, Conserved Distally, and Favored Inferonasally. *J. Glaucoma* **2019**, *28*, 139–145. [CrossRef]

29. Goda, E.; Hirooka, K.; Mori, K.; Kiuchi, Y. Intraocular pressure-lowering effects of Ripasudil: A potential outcome marker for Trabeculotomy. *BMC Ophthalmol.* **2019**, *19*, 243. [CrossRef]

30. Bovee, C.E.; Pasquale, L.R. Evolving Surgical Interventions in the Treatment of Glaucoma. *Semin. Ophthalmol.* **2017**, *32*, 91–95. [CrossRef]

31. Agrawal, P.; Bradshaw, S.E. Systematic Literature Review of Clinical and Economic Outcomes of Micro-Invasive Glaucoma Surgery (MIGS) in Primary Open-Angle Glaucoma. *Ophthalmol. Ther.* **2018**, *7*, 49–73. [CrossRef] [PubMed]

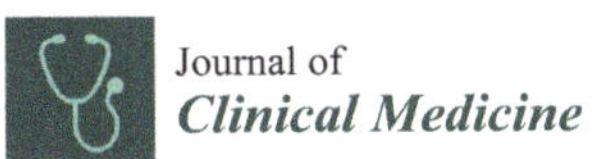
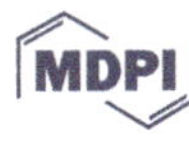

Journal of
Clinical Medicine

Review

Multifocal Visual Evoked Potentials (mfVEP) for the Detection of Visual Field Defects in Glaucoma: Systematic Review and Meta-Analysis

Haitao Liu [1], Fei Liao [1], Román Blanco [2,3] and Pedro de la Villa [1,3,*

[1] Physiology Unit, Department of Systems Biology, School of Medicine, University of Alcalá, 28005 Madrid, Spain; haitao.liu@edu.uah.es (H.L.); fei.liao@edu.uah.es (F.L.)
[2] Department of Surgery, School of Medicine, University of Alcalá, 28005 Madrid, Spain; roman.blanco@uah.es
[3] Visual Neurophysiology Group-IRYCIS, 28034 Madrid, Spain
* Correspondence: pedro.villa@uah.es

Abstract: Some discrepancies have been observed in the diagnostic efficacy of multifocal visual evoked potential (mfVEP) when evaluating visual field defects in glaucoma patients. Therefore, we evaluated the diagnostic precision of the mfVEP in glaucoma to find its best diagnostic indicator. A systematic review and meta-analysis of quantitative studies published up to 1 April 2021 was performed. The methodological quality of the included articles was assessed. Publication bias analysis and heterogeneity tests were performed. The sensitivity, specificity and diagnostic odds ratio were calculated. The area under the curve (AUC) was calculated using the summary of receiver operating characteristics curve. Six studies with a total of 241 patients were included according to the inclusion and exclusion criteria. The AUC was 0.98. There was no evidence of publication bias or threshold effect. The pooled sensitivity and pooled specificity of the mfVEP amplitude for detection of visual field defects in all studies was 0.93 and 0.89, respectively. The positive and negative likelihood ratios of mfVEP amplitude were 6.56 and 0.08, respectively. The amplitude of mfVEP showed a good diagnostic precision in the prediction of visual field defects. Interocular mfVEP amplitude analysis can be a good diagnostic indicator for visual field study.

Keywords: multifocal visual evoked potentials; mfVEP; glaucoma; perimetry

Citation: Liu, H.; Liao, F.; Blanco, R.; de la Villa, P. Multifocal Visual Evoked Potentials (mfVEP) for the Detection of Visual Field Defects in Glaucoma: Systematic Review and Meta-Analysis. *J. Clin. Med.* **2021**, *10*, 4165. https://doi.org/10.3390/jcm10184165

Academic Editors: Jose Javier Garcia-Medina and Maria Dolores Pinazo-Duran

Received: 2 September 2021
Accepted: 13 September 2021
Published: 15 September 2021

Publisher's Note: MDPI stays neutral with regard to jurisdictional claims in published maps and institutional affiliations.

1. Introduction

Background and Rationale

Glaucoma is the leading cause of irreversible visual damage in the world and incidence is expected to increase to approximately 111.8 million people by 2040 [1]. Therefore, early diagnosis of glaucoma is important to detect and treat patients in the initial stages. Early-stage treatment can prevent its progression to advanced stages and maintain healthy vision.

Glaucoma is an ocular disease characterized by the excavation of the optic nerve and defects in the visual field, constituting one of the main causes of blindness. Intraocular pressure (IOP) can be elevated or normal [2]. Although the mechanism of the pathogenesis of glaucoma is not yet clear, some researchers have proposed different theories about its pathogenesis such as: the intraocular mechanical pressure factor [3,4], the vascular factor [5], anatomical changes in the cribriform plate [6,7], autoimmune factors [8], increase of trans lamina cribrosa pressure [9] and the decrease in intracranial pressure [10].

The standard Humphrey Perimeter 24-2 (SAP) has been used as a standard criterion for measuring visual field defects and diagnosing glaucoma [11]. However, SAP has great variability between test and retest, mainly in areas with decreased visual field sensitivity [12,13]. In addition, SAP is a subjective test that detects visual field abnormalities at a late stage, when up to 25% to 35% retinal ganglion cells (RGC) are lost and statistical abnormalities of 5 dB decrease may be observed in SAP mean deviation [14,15]. Therefore, SAP is not a suitable technique for either the early diagnosis or the monitoring of the evolution of glaucoma. Patient cooperation, physical and psychological factors and the learning effect can also influence the objectivity of the SAP. Finally, the result depends ultimately on the ophthalmologist's interpretation.

Visual evoked potential (VEP) is a technique that reflects the functional integrity of the visual pathway as a whole. The light response is recorded in the visual cortex, with a flash light stimulus or pattern stimulation on the retina. Deficits in the VEP response do not provide topographical information, so it does not allow local damage to be located [16]. In 1994, Baseler applied multifocal stimuli to record from visual evoked potentials, consisting of 60 black and white checkerboard sectors and performance of VEP [17] with a pseudorandomized m-binary sequence, which allowed the topographical analysis of the response from the retina to the visual cortex. This technique is called multifocal visual evoked potential (mfVEP). It is an objective and sensitive technique to measure the visual field, which does not require manual cooperation when the patient sees the stimulus and the patient only needs to look at the fixation point in the center of the stimulus. It is not affected by physical or psychological factors and it is also observed that age and sex do not affect the objectivity of the patient mfVEP [18].

Multifocal visual evoked potential has been more effective in monitoring unilateral mild damage to ganglion cells than SAP [19,20], while other studies have shown that the amplitude of mfVEP is proportional to the loss in the perimetry of the Humphrey visual field (HVF) 24-2 [11]. The mfVEP has many more stimuli in the central and paracentral region than the traditional HVF 24-2 perimetry, making it more sensitive for detecting central and paracentral defects [21,22]. It has been also shown that mfVEP has higher repeatability reliability than HVF [23]. The mfVEP has also been useful in the diagnosis of diseases such as ischemic and compressive optic neuropathy, optic neuritis and multiple sclerosis [24,25]. Finally, it has been shown that mfVEP amplitude is proportional to glaucoma progression, but just moderately related to mfVEP latency [26–28].

To date, there is no standardized protocol for mfVEP that includes stimulation, equipment, electrode placement and the method of analyzing the result. The two types of equipment (Veris and Accumap) are the two main methods included in the literature of mfVEP. In the Veris equipment, the stimulus is a dartboard pattern consisting of 60 sectors. Each sector consists of 8 white checkerboards and 8 black checkerboards and the sizes of the different sectors and checkerboards are scaled according to the cortical magnification of the visual cortex. The patient sits in front of the screen at a viewing angle of 44.5° on the vertical and horizontal axes. Gold cup electrodes are used for recording; one electrode is located 4 cm above the inion, the other two electrodes are placed 4 cm to the left and right side from the point 1 cm above the inion, respectively. The reference electrode is placed on the inion and the ground electrode is placed on the forehead [25]. In the Accumap equipment, the stimulus consists of a cortically scaled dartboard pattern of 58 sectors, with temporal step up to 24° and nasal step up to 32° eccentrically. Each sector consists of four white checkerboards and four black checkerboards. Gold cup electrodes are used for recording; two electrodes are located 4 cm to the left and right side of the inion, one electrode is in the midline 2.5 cm above the inion, one electrode is in the midline for 4.5 cm below the inion and the ground electrode is placed in an ear lobe [29,30]. To interpret the mfVEP results, it has been proposed to calculate the amplitude root mean square (RMS) and the signal-to-noise ratio (SNR) in each sector, then compare each sector with a normative basis to determine its probability, and finally calculate its monocular and interocular cluster [25]. It has been also suggested to calculate the maximum response in each sector and compare it with a normative basis to achieve a probability graph in each sector, then calculate the monocular and interocular scotoma. Calculation of the size, depth and asymmetry of the scotomas gives an index score that is the Accumap Severity Index (ASI) [29,30]. The mfVEP response is similar to VEP, which examines the functional integrity of the visual pathway from the retina to the visual cortex. However, it is not clear which pathway (magnocellular or parvocellular) is stimulated by mfVEP [18,28]. Due to the different ways in which the mfVEP are applied and the results are interpreted, discrepancies have been observed in the diagnostic efficacy of mfVEP latency and amplitude when evaluating visual field defects in glaucoma.

A systematic review seems to be necessary to know whether or not there are significant differences between the distinct ways of applying mfVEP and interpreting its result. It seems also necessary to evaluate the diagnostic accuracy of mfVEP in glaucoma patients and seek its best diagnostic indicator through a systematic diagnostic review of the relevant literature in order to provide useful inspiration for clinical work. The main objective of the present work is to investigate the diagnostic efficacy of mfVEP latency and amplitude to assess visual field defects in glaucoma, and to seek a more precise diagnostic indicator through a systematic diagnostic review of the relevant literature.

2. Methods

2.1. Search Strategy

The search for articles in this review was performed through the available literature on mfVEP in glaucoma. We searched the online databases PubMed, Medline, Scopus, Embase, Web of Science and the Cochrane Central Register of Controlled Trials, from inception to 1 April 2021.

The search terms were ((*"mfVEP"*) OR (*"multifocal visual evoked potential"*) OR (*"multifocal VEP"*) OR (*"mfVEPs"*)) AND (*glaucoma*) AND ((*human*) OR (*individual*) OR (*patient*) OR (*people*)), later adapted for other databases, and which encompass different terms for mfVEP and glaucoma status. In addition, we examined the reference lists of included studies for potentially eligible works, as well as articles that cited the source to identify any direct/reverse citation.

2.2. Inclusion Criteria

Eligibility criteria for this review depended on the PICO framework, which corresponds to Population, Intervention, Comparison and Outcome [31]. Articles that met the inclusion criteria were included. The population included adult patients of both sexes and all ethnicities diagnosed with all types of glaucoma. With at least one eye characterized by glaucomatous optic neuropathy, defined as a cup/disc ratio >0.6, asymmetry of the cup/disc ratio between eyes >0.2, thinning of the rim, notches, excavation and defects of the nerve fiber layer of the retina. A reliable and repeatable visual field defect in SAP, defined as a standard deviation of the pattern <5% and the glaucoma hemifield test outside normal limits. The best corrected visual acuity was at least 20/40, without significant opacities of the ocular media, pupil diameter >3 mm, refractive error not greater than ±6 diopters or two cylinder diopters. No history or presence of other eye and neurological diseases.

This review focused on articles with an observational, cross-sectional and prospective study. Glaucoma patients were confirmed with reference standards such as SAP and optical coherence tomography (OCT), stereo disk photography, Heidelberg retinal tomography (HRT), fundus biomicroscopy or ophthalmoscopy, and then mfVEP with a short interval. Data were compared with a control group including healthy people without eye diseases. The reviewed results included diagnostic indicators such as mfVEP amplitude or mfVEP latency and then assay methods such as cluster or ASI, sensitivity, specificity, true positive (TP), false positive (FP), true negative (TN), false negative (FN) were estimated. TP, FN, FP, TN are defined as: in the glaucoma patient group diagnosed with the reference standard, the mfVEP analysis result is positive (TP) or negative (FN); in the control group with healthy people confirmed by the reference standard, and the mfVEP analysis result is positive (FP) or negative (TN).

2.3. Exclusion Criteria

Studies with any of the following characteristics were excluded: (a) No control group of healthy people; (b) not on human beings; (c) systematic reviews; (d) incomplete data on evaluation index; (e) reports of cases with less than 10 people.

2.4. Selection of Studies

Data selection and extraction were performed by two independent investigators based on eligibility characteristics such as population, intervention, comparison and study types. We first reviewed the titles and abstracts. If the articles matched our inclusion criteria, we read the full texts to make a final decision for the inclusion of each study. If there was any discrepancy, we requested the opinion of a third investigator. Finally, we made a selection flow diagram, the preferred items report for systematic reviews and meta-analysis (PRISMA) for the study [32].

The management of the articles was carried out in the Endnote software (Endnote X8, Clarivate Analytics, London, UK). First, we excluded duplicate items. By analyzing titles, abstracts and keywords, we eliminated articles that were not relevant to the study of mfVEP in glaucoma. We also checked the reference list of review articles so as not to miss a primary research study. Finally, we read the full text. Articles that met the strict inclusion criteria underwent data extraction.

2.5. Data Extraction

The data were extracted in a form that included the following variables:

I. Basic information on the study such as country of origin, year of publication and sample size;

II. Information on the study design, such as an observational, cross-sectional, prospective study;

III. Participant information, such as age, gender, ethnicity and severity of glaucoma;

IV. Experimental information such as reference standard, equipment, diagnostic indicator, amplitude or latency of the mfVEP and the assay method such as cluster or ASI analysis;

V. Key results such as sensitivity and specificity, TP, FP, TN, FN.

We did not have the approval of any ethical research committee, since our study was a secondary analysis of the publications, which did not directly involve any human subject.

2.6. Assessment of Risk of Bias

The assessment of the methodological quality of the included studies was carried out using the tool for assessing the Quality of Diagnostic precision Studies, version 2 (QUADAS-2) [33]. A total of 14 assessment items were established and each study was scored according to 'yes', 'no' and 'unclear'. In QUADAS-2, there are four key domains to evaluate the risk of bias: (1) the selection of patients, (2) the index test, (3) the reference standard and (4) the time between the index test and the reference standard and the flow of the patient in the study.

The first three domains above also evaluate applicability with respect to participants, equipment, performance and interpretation. Furthermore, the diagnosis of disease according to the reference standard coincides or does not coincide with our review [34]. The risk of bias section assesses the design of the included studies and their potential for bias. The applicability concerns section assesses the relationship between the included studies and our review question and whether or not the included studies matched our review question. Two investigators evaluated each article independently. If they did not reach a consensus, it was resolved with the judgment of another researcher.

2.7. Data Synthesis and Statistical Analysis

2.7.1. Heterogeneity Test

We used the chi-square (X^2) and Cochran-Q statistical tests to assess heterogeneity between the included studies; a result with a low *p* value indicated heterogeneity. The inconsistency index (I^2) was also calculated to quantify heterogeneity; an I^2 value of 0% means there is no heterogeneity and an I^2 value greater than 50% means there is heterogeneity between the included studies [35].

2.7.2. Threshold Effect

In a study for the assessment of test precision, the threshold effect may be a major cause of heterogeneity due to the lack of standardization of the definition of a positive result. To find if there is a threshold effect, we can calculate the Spearman correlation coefficient between the sensitivity logit and the 1-specificity logit; a positive correlation and a $p < 0.05$ indicate the existence of a threshold effect. Furthermore, the presence of a typical "shoulder-arm" pattern on the receiver operating characteristic (ROC) curve signifies a possible threshold effect [36,37].

2.7.3. Publication Bias

Studies with favorable and optimistic results are more likely to be accepted and published; this may be a factor that influences the conclusions [38]. We evaluated the publication biases through the funnel plot. The graph with symmetrically distributed data points means the absence of publication bias and an asymmetric graph indicates the existence of publication bias [39].

2.8. Statistical Summary

The extracted data were used to construct forest plots of sensitivity and specificity and to estimate the diagnostic accuracy of mfVEP in the diagnosis of visual field defects in glaucoma patients. The statistical summary can be calculated using the fixed effects model (FEM) or using the random effects model (REM) depending on the homogeneous characteristics of the included studies. We used the bivariate regression method to calculate sensitivity and specificity. We then summarized the corresponding positive likelihood ratio (PLR), negative likelihood ratio (NLR) and diagnostic odds ratio (DOR). Summary receiver operating characteristic curve (sROC) synthesis is based on pooled sensitivity, pooled specificity and respective variations [40,41]. The area under the curve (AUC) of sROC is used to evaluate the overall performance of the test [42]. DOR is calculated by combining sensitivity and specificity [43].

2.9. Sensitivity Analysis

We performed a sensitivity analysis by sequential elimination of the studies, in order to avoid those studies that would affect results in a statistically significant way. When there was significant heterogeneity, the source of the heterogeneity was sought and, when necessary, a subgroup analysis was performed between the included studies. Subgroup analysis was appropriate among participants of varying glaucoma severity, ethnicity, equipment, mfVEP assay method and number of populations.

The analyses of heterogeneity, sensitivity, threshold effect and calculation of the statistical estimate were performed with Meta-Disc version 1.4 (Hospital Ramón y Cajal. Madrid, Spain) [37]. The publication bias analysis was performed using Stata 15.0 (StataCorp LP, College Station, TX, USA).

3. Results

3.1. Selection of Studies

Figure 1 shows the complete flow of the selection of the studies included in the present work. Initially, 468 total articles were found by the search carried out through the different databases. Of the total articles, 303 were duplicates and 159 articles were excluded because they were not considered relevant for the systematic review proposed. The reasons for exclusion were: (i) the article did not include a control group with healthy subjects; (ii) articles written in a language other than English; (iii) systematic reviews; (iv) articles and reports of cases with a small number of participants; (v) the article provided insufficient data on the evaluation index (true positives, false positives, true negatives and false negatives). Finally, a total of six studies were included [20,44–48] which met all the inclusion criteria.

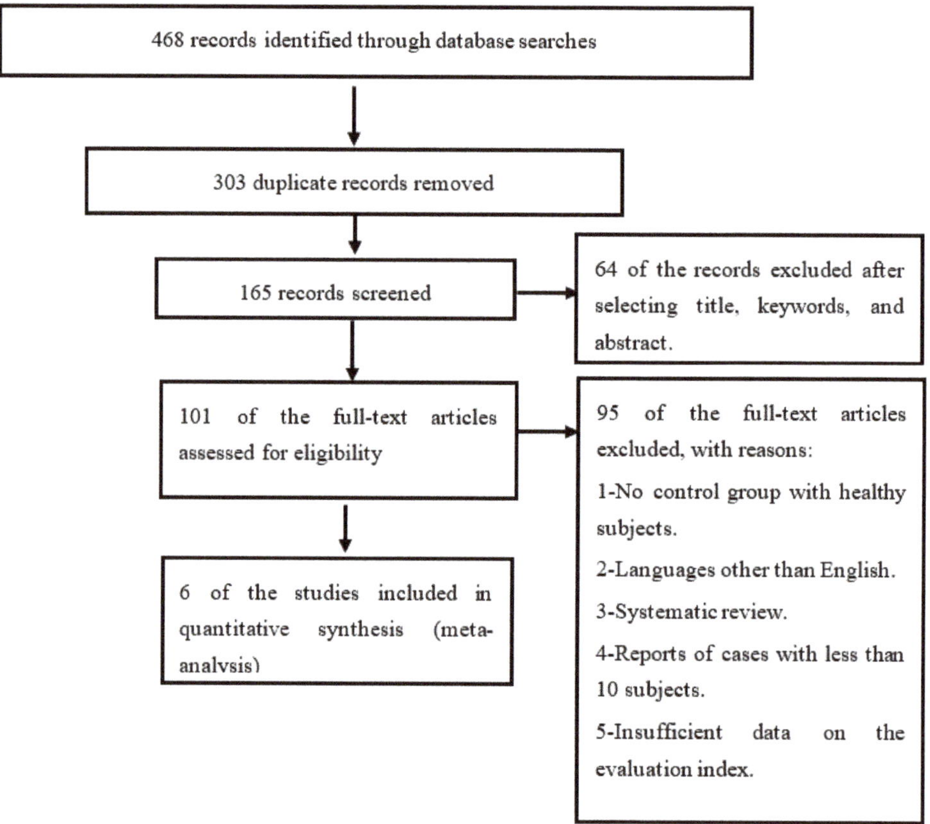

Figure 1. Flowchart of studies included through the systematic review process.

3.2. Characteristics of the Included Studies

In the six included studies, a total of 241 patients (273 eyes) diagnosed with glaucoma and 195 healthy people (202 eyes) could be counted. Of the 241 patients, 196 belonged to the mixed-type glaucoma group (different types of glaucoma), while 10 patients had normal tension glaucoma (NTG) and the other 35 patients had primary open-angle glaucoma (POAG). Table 1 shows the main characteristics of the six studies included in the meta-analysis.

Table 1. Main characteristics of the studies included in the meta-analysis.

ID Study	Type of Study	Types and No. of Glaucoma Patients	Glaucoma Severity (MD of SAP) dB	Reference Standard	Equipment for Index Test (mfVEP)	Diagnostic Indicator-Assay Method	Age (Years) Mean ± SD
Balachandran, 2006	NA	Mixed 41P 41E	-7.1 ± 6.0	SAP, stereoscopic optic nerve head photography, HRT	AccuMap version 2.0	Amplitude-ASI	65 ± 11
Goldberg, 2002	Cross	Mixed 100P 100E	-6.5 ± 4.2	SAP, stereo disk photography	AccuMap version NA	Amplitude-ASI	62.2 ± 9.8
Gutierrez-Diaz, 2012	Cross	NTG 10P 10E	-5.95 ± 11.7	SAP, OCT, ophthalmoscopy	VERIS version NA	Amplitude-Cluster	66.8 ± 6.1
Kanadani, 2014	Cross	Mixed 39P 39E	all levels	SAP, fundus biomicroscopy	VERIS version NA	Amplitude-Cluster	$66.3 \pm$ NA
Punjabi, 2008	Cross	POAG 35P 67E	-6.2 ± 0.8	SAP, indirect ophthalmoscopy, HRT	AccuMap version 2.0	Amplitude-ASI	68 ± 10
Thienprasiddhi, 2003	NA	Mixed 16P 16E	-6.8 ± 4.2	SAP, stereoscopic optic nerve head photography	VERIS version 4.3	Amplitude-Cluster	56 ± 7

NA = Not available. Cross = Cross-sectional study. P = People. E = Eyes. POAG = Primary open angle glaucoma. NTG = Normal tension glaucoma. Mixed = Different types of mixed glaucoma. SAP = Standard automated perimetry. MD = Mean deviation. OCT = Optical coherence tomography. HRT = Heidelberg Retinal Tomography. BMC = Biomicroscopy. ASI = Accumap Severity Index. The study identification (ID) numbers correspond to the study numbers in the graphs of Figures 2 and 3.

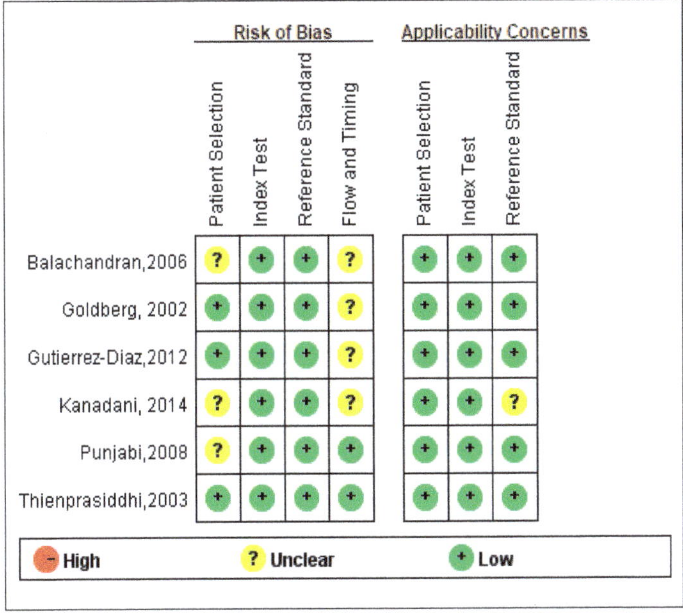

Figure 2. Quality of the included studies according to the tool for assessing the quality of diagnostic precision studies (QUADAS). The results revealed that the six studies included in this review met 9 or more of the 14 criteria of the QUADAS tool, indicating relatively good methodological quality of the included studies.

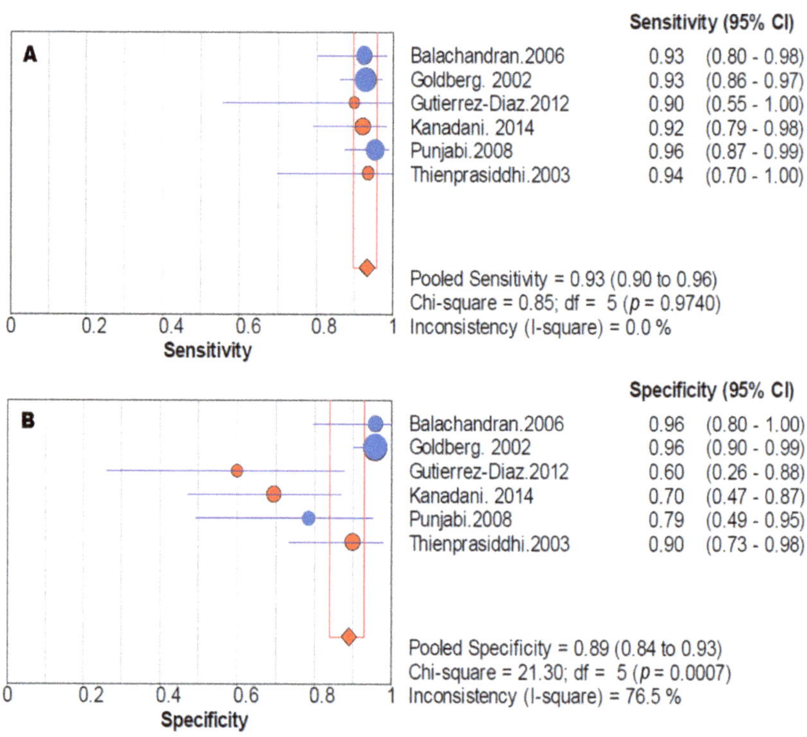

Figure 3. Sensitivity and specificity forest plots in the meta-analysis. Forest plots of sensitivity (**A**) and specificity (**B**) corresponding to the amplitude of mfVEP to diagnose visual field defects in glaucoma. Pooled sensitivity was 0.93 (95% CI: 0.90–0.96) and pooled specificity was 0.89 (95% CI: 0.84–0.93). The size of each point is proportional to the study sample size or the weight of the study in the meta-analysis. The blue points represent studies with Accumap equipment and the red points are with Veris equipment.

3.3. Methodological Quality of the Included Studies

The methodological quality of the six reviewed studies was initially assessed with the QUADAS-2 tool. Four of the six trials were cross-sectional studies; three trials enrolled patients consecutively and other enrollments were not specified. Gold standard tests included SAP to detect visual field loss, OCT, stereo disc photography, HRT, fundus biomicroscopy, or ophthalmoscopy to study the findings of the glaucomatous optic nerve. Only one of the articles mentioned the time interval between the mfVEP index test and the reference standard; the others did not mention the interval time, indicating a high risk of bias in the flow and time domain. The result of the evaluation of the methodological quality of the included studies is shown in Figure 2.

3.4. Synthesis of Diagnostic Data

The summary estimates of the mfVEP amplitude for the diagnosis of visual field defects in the six studies corresponded to a sensitivity of 0.93 (95% confidence interval, CI: 0.90–0.96) and a specificity of 0.89 (95% CI: 0.84–0.93). The positive likelihood ratio was 6.56 (95% CI: 2.67–16.10), the negative likelihood ratio was 0.08 (95% CI: 0.05–0.12) and the diagnostic odds ratio was 90.00 (95% CI: 31.51–257.11) (Table 2). Figure 3 shows the forest plots of sensitivity and specificity.

Table 2. Statistical summary of the diagnostic precision parameters in the meta-analysis.

Parameter	Estimates
Total eyes (n)	475
True positive (n)	255
False negative (n)	18
False positive (n)	22
True negative (n)	180
Accuracy (n)	0.92 (95% CI: 0.89 to 0.94)
Sensitivity	0.93 (95% CI: 0.90 to 0.96)
Specificity	0.89 (95% CI: 0.84 to 0.93)
PLR	6.56 (95% CI: 2.67 to 16.10)
NLR	0.08 (95% CI: 0.05 to 0.12)
DOR	90.00 (95% CI: 31.51 to 257.11)

Statistical summary of diagnostic accuracy parameters for mfVEP amplitude in diagnosing visual field defects in glaucoma patients included accuracy, pooled sensitivity, pooled specificity, positive likelihood ratio (PLR), negative likelihood ratio (NLR), the diagnostic odds ratio (DOR) and their 95% confidence interval (CI), respectively.

3.5. Heterogeneity and Threshold Effect

In our meta-analysis, no signs of heterogeneity were observed for sensitivity results ($I^2 = 0\%$), but substantial heterogeneity was observed for specificity ($I^2 = 73.4\%$).

To find the source of heterogeneity, we performed a subgroup analysis based on the mfVEP registry team (Veris and Accumap), assay methods (ASI and Cluster) and glaucoma severity depending on SAP mean deviation (MD). However, heterogeneity for specificity remained high, with an inconsistency rate (I^2) greater than 50%, while heterogeneity for sensitivity in all subgroups was $I^2 = 0\%$. Our review includes just 241 glaucoma patients and six articles in the meta-analysis, and we are aware that when a meta-analysis includes fewer than 500 patients and fewer than 15 trials, there may be fluctuations in I^2 estimates [49].

After excluding articles one by one through sensitivity analysis, the inconsistency rate for sensitivity heterogeneity was found to be 0%. However, the inconsistency rate for specificity was greater than 50%. Sensitivity, specificity, area under the curve (AUC) and 95% confidence interval (CI) were similar and overlapped with each other. The heterogeneity remained the same. Sensitivity analysis showed that the pooled estimates were stable and reliable.

A Spearman rank correlation was performed, which provided a value of -0.464 ($p = 0.354$); in addition to the sROC, a "shoulder-arm" pattern was not appreciated, which means that there was no threshold effect between the included studies.

We calculated the AUC of the sROC to evaluate the overall performance of the mfVEP amplitude for the diagnosis of visual field defects in glaucoma (Figure 4) and the value was 0.97. Due to the heterogeneity that existed in specificity, we did the statistical summary using the random effects model.

A funnel plot was also constructed to assess publication bias in the meta-analysis. The data points had a symmetric funnel shape, meaning the absence of publication bias. However, we must point out that in our study we only included six articles, which is a relatively small study group to do a publication bias analysis, since it is recommended that there be a minimum of 10 studies [50,51].

From the obtained results, we can confirm that the quality of the six included studies was relatively good. Diagnostic data, including sensitivity, specificity, likelihood ratio and area under the sROC curve, demonstrated that mfVEP amplitude had good diagnostic accuracy in predicting visual field defects in glaucoma patients and in the analysis of the interocular mfVEP amplitude. Therefore, it can be a good diagnostic indicator for the visual field study.

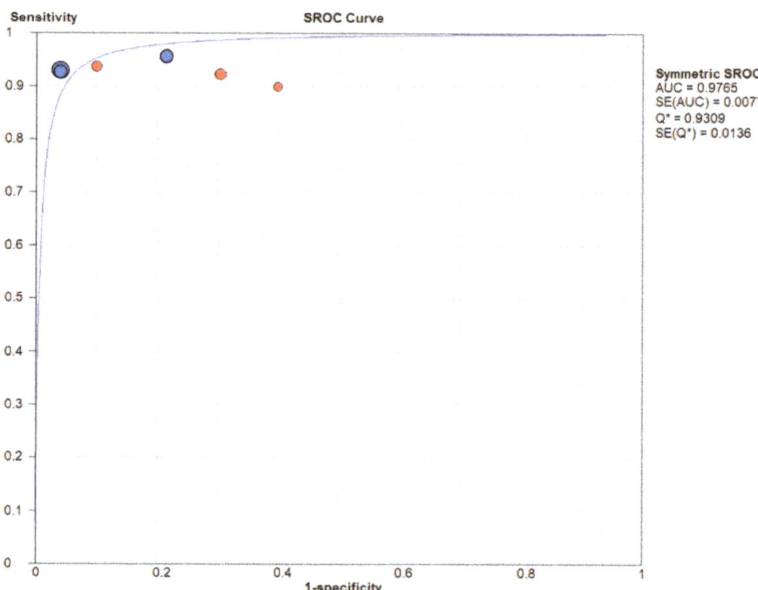

Figure 4. Summary receiver operating characteristic (sROC) curve for the six included studies. The area under the ROC summary curve was observed to be approximately 1.0. The sROC synthesis was based on pooled sensitivity, pooled specificity and respective variances. The size of each point is proportional to the study sample size or the weight of the study in the meta-analysis. The blue points represent studies with Accumap equipment and the red points are with Veris equipment. AUC = Area Under the Curve. Q = Index Q. SE = Standard Error.

4. Discussion

In this systematic review, the diagnostic efficacy of mfVEP in evaluating visual field defects in glaucoma patients was reviewed, using the amplitude and latency of its responses as diagnostic indicators. Regarding the amplitude, the results show a pooled sensitivity of 0.93 (95% CI: 0.90–0.96) and a pooled specificity of 0.89 (95% CI: 0.84–0.93). The positive likelihood ratio was 6.56 (95% CI: 2.67–16.10), the negative likelihood ratio was 0.08 (95% CI: 0.05–0.12) and the diagnostic odds ratio was 90.00 (95% CI: 31.51–257.11). The area under the curve of the summary receiver operating characteristic was 0.97, indicating a good performance of the amplitude recorded by the mfVEP in the prediction of visual field defects in glaucoma. The results of the sensitivity analysis demonstrated that the pooled estimates are stable and reliable.

In our meta-analysis, the heterogeneity for pooled specificity was somewhat high (I^2 = 73.4%) and no heterogeneity was observed for pooled sensitivity (I^2 = 0%). However, it is important to note that our study does not include a high number of patients, which may have been the cause of fluctuations in the estimate of I^2 [49]. The existence of heterogeneity in the pooled specificity indicates that the low number of people in the control group may be the cause of variation in specificity between the different studies. In our study, both pooled specificity and heterogeneity are high, in contrast to those observed in some studies when very low specificity was found [21,52]. We also found a wide variety of specificity between different studies [52]. In fact, it was suggested that the low number of people evaluated may be a possible cause of the variability observed in the specificity. Another possible cause is the lack of operator training or the erroneous or too narrow normal limits in the amplitudes recorded by the mfVEP [52].

The analysis of the subgroups evaluated with different equipment (Veris and Accumap) and test methods (ASI and Cluster) are the two main methods included in the literature on mfVEP, which show certain differences such as the number of stimulus sectors, the placement of the electrodes or how to interpret the results [25,29,30]. However, no significant differences were observed in their visual field diagnostic accuracy.

Regarding the latency of mfVEP in the diagnosis of visual field defects, some articles found a low correlation with the result of SAP [26–28]. In our review, we did not find enough articles with diagnostic data to perform a meta-analysis of the latency recorded by mfVEP.

In all the studies included in our review, both mono and interocular amplitude analysis are included. However, according to the data obtained in the study, diagnostic precision could not be assessed with the monocular amplitude analysis alone. The results showed significant variability among the patients, mainly due to the existing anatomical differences in the visual cortex and the position of the calcarine cortex in relation to the location of the external electrodes, as well as differences in the cortical folds [53]. The interocular analysis of the same individual makes it possible to reduce the variability between participants. In fact, this can be a disadvantage of mfVEP compared to SAP. On the other hand, mfVEP is more sensitive in patients with glaucoma and asymmetric visual field loss [19,54]. Furthermore, the mfVEP has more stimulus sectors at a center of 10 degrees. Therefore, it is more sensitive to the detection of central damage [55]. However, the detection of damage in the superior and peripheral campimetries is more complex, since it corresponds to the deep cortical area, located behind the calcarine fissure.

Our systematic review has confirmed that mfVEP amplitude may be a diagnostic or prognostic biomarker of visual defects in glaucoma. Doubtful clinical cases due to unconfirmed visual field defects based on dissociation between OCT-SAP, cases of unreliable SAP, concentration or motor problem of the patient to perform SAP, should use mfVEP amplitude as a complementary, reliable and objective tool. In this sense, the mfVEP technique is non-invasive, does not require subjective patient cooperation and each test is inexpensive. Its main disadvantage is that its application requires a well-trained expert.

We cannot discard some limitations in our systematic review. The meta-analysis only included 241 patients and six articles, which in our opinion is few cases if we want to evaluate the diagnostic efficacy of mfVEP in predicting visual field defects in glaucoma. Moreover, several studies used different techniques to study glaucomatous findings of the optic nerve, such as OCT, optic disc photography, HRT, fundus biomicroscopy or ophthalmoscopy. Just one article mentions the time interval between the index test and the reference standard, while the others do not indicate the time of the interval, which means a high risk of bias in the domain flow and timing. Furthermore, several articles did not mention whether they interpreted the results of the index test and the reference standard without knowing the results of the others, which is a factor that can cause inflamed measures in the diagnostic test. Finally, there are also different mfVEP parameters, such as being divided into four quadrants, six sectors, several rings, percentage of abnormal points, hemifields, etc., but we could not analyze them because few publications met our criteria.

5. Conclusions

The amplitude of mfVEP has shown good diagnostic accuracy in predicting visual field defects in glaucoma patients. Interocular mfVEP amplitude analysis can be a diagnostic indicator for visual field study in doubtful or unreliable cases of automated standard perimetry.

Author Contributions: Conceptualization, P.d.l.V. and H.L.; methodology, H.L. and F.L.; formal analysis, P.d.l.V., H.L. and F.L.; data curation, H.L. and F.L.; writing—original draft preparation, P.d.l.V. and H.L.; writing—review and editing, P.d.l.V., R.B. and H.L.; supervision, P.d.l.V. and R.B.; project administration, P.d.l.V.; funding acquisition, P.d.l.V. All authors have read and agreed to the published version of the manuscript.

Funding: This study was funded by the Instituto de Salud Carlos III and cofounded with the European Regional Development Fund "A way to make Europe", within the "Plan Estatal de Investigación Científica y Técnica y de Innovación 2017–2020" (RD16/0008/0020; FIS/PI18-00754).

Institutional Review Board Statement: Not applicable.

Informed Consent Statement: Not applicable.

Data Availability Statement: Not applicable.

Conflicts of Interest: The authors declare no conflict of interest.

References

1. Tham, Y.-C.; Li, X.; Wong, T.Y.; Quigley, H.A.; Aung, T.; Cheng, C.-Y. Global Prevalence of Glaucoma and Projections of Glaucoma Burden through 2040. *Ophthalmology* **2014**, *121*, 2081–2090. [CrossRef]
2. Von Graefe, A. Ueber die Iridectomie bei Glaucom und über den glaucomatosen Process. *Arch. Ophthalmol.* **1857**, *3*, 456–555.
3. Quigley, H.A.; Addicks, E.M. Chronic experimental glaucoma in primates. II. Effect of extended intraocular pressure elevation on optic nerve head and axonal transport. *Investig. Ophthalmol. Vis. Sci.* **1980**, *19*, 137–152.
4. Drance, S.M.; Douglas, G.R.; Wijsman, K.; Schulzer, M.; Britton, R.J. Response of Blood Flow to Warm and Cold in Normal and Low-Tension Glaucoma Patients. *Am. J. Ophthalmol.* **1988**, *105*, 35–39. [CrossRef]
5. Flammer, J.; Orgül, S.; Costa, V.P.; Orzalesi, N.; Krieglstein, G.K.; Serra, L.M.; Renard, J.-P.; Stefánsson, E. The impact of ocular blood flow in glaucoma. *Prog. Retin. Eye Res.* **2002**, *21*, 359–393. [CrossRef]
6. Miller, K.M.; Quigley, H.A. Comparison of optic disc features in low-tension and typical open-angle glaucoma. *Ophthalmic Surg.* **1987**, *18*, 882–889. [PubMed]
7. Park, H.-Y.L.; Park, C.K. Diagnostic Capability of Lamina Cribrosa Thickness by Enhanced Depth Imaging and Factors Affecting Thickness in Patients with Glaucoma. *Ophthalmology* **2013**, *120*, 745–752. [CrossRef] [PubMed]
8. Yang, J.; Patil, R.V.; Yu, H.; Gordon, M.; Wax, M.B. T cell subsets and sIL-2R/IL-2 levels in patients with glaucoma. *Am. J. Ophthalmol.* **2001**, *131*, 421–426. [CrossRef]
9. Morgan, W.H.; Yu, D.Y.; Balaratnasingam, C. The Role of Cerebrospinal Fluid Pressure in Glaucoma Pathophysiology: The Dark Side of the Optic Disc. *J. Glaucoma* **2008**, *17*, 408–413. [CrossRef] [PubMed]
10. Ren, R.; Jonas, J.B.; Tian, G.; Zhen, Y.; Ma, K.; Li, S.; Wang, H.; Li, B.; Zhang, X.; Wang, N. Cerebrospinal Fluid Pressure in Glaucoma: A Prospective Study. *Ophthalmology* **2010**, *117*, 259–266. [CrossRef] [PubMed]
11. Hood, D.C.; Greenstein, V.C.; Odel, J.G.; Zhang, X.; Ritch, R.; Liebmann, J.M.; Hong, J.E.; Chen, C.S.; Thienprasiddhi, P. Visual Field Defects and Multifocal Visual Evoked Potentials: Evidence of a linear relationship. *Arch. Ophthalmol.* **2002**, *120*, 1672–1681. [CrossRef] [PubMed]
12. Chauhan, B.C.; Johnson, C.A. Test-retest variability of frequency-doubling perimetry and conventional perimetry in glaucoma patients and normal subjects. *Investig. Ophthalmol. Vis. Sci.* **1999**, *40*, 648–656.
13. Spry, P.G.D.; Johnson, C.A.; McKendrick, A.; Turpin, A. Measurement error of visual field tests in glaucoma. *Br. J. Ophthalmol.* **2003**, *87*, 107–112. [CrossRef] [PubMed]
14. Quigley, H.A.; Dunkelberger, G.R.; Green, W.R. Retinal Ganglion Cell Atrophy Correlated With Automated Perimetry in Human Eyes with Glaucoma. *Am. J. Ophthalmol.* **1989**, *107*, 453–464. [CrossRef]
15. Kerrigan-Baumrind, L.A.; Quigley, H.A.; Pease, M.; Kerrigan, D.F.; Mitchell, R.S. Number of ganglion cells in glaucoma eyes compared with threshold visual field tests in the same persons. *Investig. Ophthalmol. Vis. Sci.* **2000**, *41*, 741–748.
16. Odom, J.V.; Bach, M.; Brigell, M.; Holder, G.E.; McCulloch, D.L.; Mizota, A.; Tormene, A.P.; International Society for Clinical Electrophysiology of Vision. ISCEV standard for clinical visual evoked potentials: (2016 update). *Doc. Ophthalmol.* **2016**, *133*, 1–9. [CrossRef] [PubMed]
17. Baseler, H.A.; Sutter, E.E.; Klein, S.A.; Carney, T. The topography of visual evoked response properties across the visual field. *Electroencephalogr. Clin. Neurophysiol.* **1994**, *90*, 65–81. [CrossRef]
18. Klistorner, A.; Graham, S.L. Objective perimetry in glaucoma. *Ophthalmology* **2000**, *107*, 2283–2299. [CrossRef]
19. Graham, S.L.; Klistorner, A.I.; Grigg, J.R.; Billson, F.A. Objective VEP Perimetry in Glaucoma: Asymmetry Analysis to Identify Early Deficits. *J. Glaucoma* **2000**, *9*, 10–19. [CrossRef]
20. Goldberg, I.; Graham, S.L.; Klistorner, A.I. Multifocal objective perimetry in the detection of glaucomatous field loss. *Am. J. Ophthalmol.* **2002**, *133*, 29–39. [CrossRef]
21. Hood, D.C.; Thienprasiddhi, P.; Greenstein, V.C.; Winn, B.J.; Ohri, N.; Liebmann, J.M.; Ritch, R. Detecting Early to Mild Glaucomatous Damage: A Comparison of the Multifocal VEP and Automated Perimetry. *Investig. Opthalmol. Vis. Sci.* **2004**, *45*, 492–498. [CrossRef]
22. Thonginnetra, O.; Greenstein, V.C.; Chu, D.; Liebmann, J.M.; Ritch, R.; Hood, D.C. Normal Versus High Tension Glaucoma: A comparison of functional and structural defects. *J. Glaucoma* **2010**, *19*, 151–157. [CrossRef]
23. Chen, C.S.; Hood, D.C.; Zhang, X.; Karam, E.Z.; Liebmann, J.M.; Ritch, R.; Thienprasiddhi, P.; Greenstein, V.C. Repeat Reliability of the Multifocal Visual Evoked Potential in Normal and Glaucomatous Eyes. *J. Glaucoma* **2003**, *12*, 399–408. [CrossRef] [PubMed]
24. Frederiksen, J.L.; Petrera, J. Serial Visual Evoked Potentials in 90 Untreated Patients with Acute Optic Neuritis. *Surv. Ophthalmol.* **1999**, *44*, S54–S62. [CrossRef]
25. Hood, D.C.; Greenstein, V.C. Multifocal VEP and ganglion cell damage: Applications and limitations for the study of glaucoma. *Prog. Retin. Eye Res.* **2003**, *22*, 201–251. [CrossRef]

26. Grippo, T.M.; Hood, D.C.; Kanadani, F.N.; Ezon, I.; Greenstein, V.C.; Liebmann, J.M.; Ritch, R. A Comparison between Multifocal and Conventional VEP Latency Changes Secondary to Glaucomatous Damage. *Investig. Opthalmol. Vis. Sci.* **2006**, *47*, 5331–5336. [CrossRef]

27. Hood, D.C.; Chen, J.Y.; Yang, E.B.; Rodarte, C.; Wenick, A.S.; Grippo, T.M.; Odel, J.G.; Ritch, R. The role of the multifocal visual evoked potential (mfVEP) latency in understanding optic nerve and retinal diseases. *Trans. Am. Ophthalmol. Soc.* **2006**, *104*, 71–77. [PubMed]

28. Rodarte, C.; Hood, D.C.; Yang, E.B.; Grippo, T.; Greenstein, V.C.; Liebmann, J.M.; Ritch, R. The effects of glaucoma on the latency of the multifocal visual evoked potential. *Br. J. Ophthalmol.* **2006**, *90*, 1132–1136. [CrossRef]

29. Klistorner, A.; Graham, S.; Grigg, J.; Billson, F.A. Multifocal topographic visual evoked potential: Improving objective detection of local visual field defects. *Investig. Ophthalmol. Vis. Sci.* **1998**, *39*, 937–950.

30. Graham, S.L.; Klistorner, A.I.; Goldberg, I. Clinical Application of Objective Perimetry Using Multifocal Visual Evoked Potentials in Glaucoma Practice. *Arch. Ophthalmol.* **2005**, *123*, 729. [CrossRef]

31. Richardson, W.S.; Wilson, M.C.; Nishikawa, J.; Hayward, R.S. The well-built clinical question: A key to evidence-based decisions. *ACP J. Club* **1995**, *123*, A12–A13. [CrossRef] [PubMed]

32. Moher, D.; Shamseer, L.; Clarke, M.; Ghersi, D.; Liberati, A.; Petticrew, M.; Shekelle, P.; Stewart, L.A.; PRISMA-P Group. Preferred reporting items for systematic review and meta-analysis protocols (PRISMA-P) 2015 statement. *Syst. Rev.* **2015**, *4*, 1. [CrossRef] [PubMed]

33. Whiting, P.F.; Rutjes, A.W.S.; Westwood, M.E.; Mallett, S.; Deeks, J.J.; Reitsma, J.B.; Leeflang, M.M.G.; Sterne, J.A.C.; Bossuyt, P.M.M. QUADAS-2: A Revised Tool for the Quality Assessment of Diagnostic Accuracy Studies. *Ann. Intern. Med.* **2011**, *155*, 529–536. [CrossRef] [PubMed]

34. Fallon, M.; Valero, O.; Pazos, M.; Antón, A. Diagnostic accuracy of imaging devices in glaucoma: A meta-analysis. *Surv. Ophthalmol.* **2017**, *62*, 446–461. [CrossRef] [PubMed]

35. Higgins, J.P.T.; Thompson, S.G.; Deeks, J.; Altman, D.G. Measuring inconsistency in meta-analyses. *BMJ* **2003**, *327*, 557–560. [CrossRef]

36. Moses, L.E.; Shapiro, D.; Littenberg, B. Combining independent studies of a diagnostic test into a summary roc curve: Data-analytic approaches and some additional considerations. *Stat. Med.* **1993**, *12*, 1293–1316. [CrossRef]

37. Zamora, J.; Abraira, V.; Muriel, A.; Khan, K.; Coomarasamy, A. Meta-DiSc: A software for meta-analysis of test accuracy data. *BMC Med. Res. Methodol.* **2006**, *6*, 31. [CrossRef]

38. Song, F.; Khan, K.S.; Dinnes, J.; Sutton, A.J. Asymmetric funnel plots and publication bias in meta-analyses of diagnostic accuracy. *Int. J. Epidemiol.* **2002**, *31*, 88–95. [CrossRef] [PubMed]

39. Song, F.; Eastwood, A.J.; Gilbody, S.; Duley, L.; Sutton, A.J. Publication and related biases. *Health Technol. Assess.* **2000**, *4*, 1–115. [CrossRef]

40. Rutter, C.M.; Gatsonis, C.A. A hierarchical regression approach to meta-analysis of diagnostic test accuracy evaluations. *Stat. Med.* **2001**, *20*, 2865–2884. [CrossRef]

41. Harbord, R.M.; Deeks, J.J.; Egger, M.; Whiting, P.; Sterne, J.A.C. A unification of models for meta-analysis of diagnostic accuracy studies. *Biostatistics* **2006**, *8*, 239–251. [CrossRef] [PubMed]

42. Swets, J.A. Measuring the accuracy of diagnostic systems. *Science* **1988**, *240*, 1285–1293. [CrossRef] [PubMed]

43. Glas, A.S.; Lijmer, J.G.; Prins, M.H.; Bonsel, G.J.; Bossuyt, P.M. The diagnostic odds ratio: A single indicator of test performance. *J. Clin. Epidemiol.* **2003**, *56*, 1129–1135. [CrossRef]

44. Thienprasiddhi, P.; Greenstein, V.C.; Chen, C.S.; Liebmann, J.M.; Ritch, R.; Hood, N.C. Multifocal visual evoked potential responses in glaucoma patients with unilateral hemifield defects. *Am. J. Ophthalmol.* **2003**, *136*, 34–40. [CrossRef]

45. Balachandran, C.; Graham, S.; Klistorner, A.; Goldberg, I. Comparison of Objective Diagnostic Tests in Glaucoma: Heidelberg retinal tomography and multifocal visual evoked potentials. *J. Glaucoma* **2006**, *15*, 110–116. [CrossRef]

46. Punjabi, O.S.; Stamper, R.L.; Bostrom, A.G.; Han, Y.; Lin, S.C. Topographic Comparison of the Visual Function on Multifocal Visual Evoked Potentials with Optic Nerve Structure on Heidelberg Retinal Tomography. *Ophthalmology* **2008**, *115*, 440–446. [CrossRef]

47. Gutiérrez-Díaz, E.; Pérez-Rico, C.; de Atauri, M.J.D.; Mencía-Gutiérrez, E.; Blanco, R. Evaluation of the visual function in obstructive sleep apnea syndrome patients and normal-tension glaucoma by means of the multifocal visual evoked potentials. *Graefe's Arch. Clin. Exp. Ophthalmol.* **2012**, *251*, 1459–1460. [CrossRef] [PubMed]

48. Kanadani, F.N.; Mello, P.A.; Dorairaj, S.K.; Kanadani, T.C. Frequency-doubling technology perimetry and multifocal visual evoked potential in glaucoma, suspected glaucoma, and control patients. *Clin. Ophthalmol.* **2014**, *8*, 1323–1330. [CrossRef] [PubMed]

49. Thorlund, K.; Imberger, G.; Johnston, B.C.; Walsh, M.; Awad, T.; Thabane, L.; Gluud, C.; Devereaux, P.; Wetterslev, J. Evolution of Heterogeneity (I2) Estimates and Their 95% Confidence Intervals in Large Meta-Analyses. *PLoS ONE* **2012**, *7*, e39471. [CrossRef]

50. Macaskill, P.; Walter, S.D.; Irwig, L. A comparison of methods to detect publication bias in meta-analysis. *Stat. Med.* **2001**, *20*, 641–654. [CrossRef]

51. Lau, J.; Ioannidis, J.P.A.; Terrin, N.; Schmid, C.; Olkin, I. The case of the misleading funnel plot. *BMJ* **2006**, *333*, 597–600. [CrossRef]

52. Bengtsson, B. Evaluation of VEP perimetry in normal subjects and glaucoma patients. *Acta Ophthalmol. Scand.* **2002**, *80*, 620–626. [CrossRef]

53. Hood, D.C.; Zhang, X.; Greenstein, V.C.; Kangovi, S.; Odel, J.G.; Liebmann, J.M.; Ritch, R. An interocular comparison of the multifocal VEP: A possible technique for detecting local damage to the optic nerve. *Investig. Ophthalmol. Vis. Sci.* **2000**, *41*, 1580–1587.
54. Hood, D.C.; Zhang, X. Multifocal ERG and VEP responses and visual fields: Comparing disease-related changes. *Doc. Ophthalmol.* **2000**, *100*, 115–137. [CrossRef] [PubMed]
55. Yu, M.; Brown, B.; Edwards, M.H. Investigation of multifocal visual evoked potential in anisometropic and esotropic amblyopes. *Investig. Ophthalmol. Vis. Sci.* **1998**, *39*, 2033–2040.

MDPI
St. Alban-Anlage 66
4052 Basel
Switzerland
Tel. +41 61 683 77 34
Fax +41 61 302 89 18
www.mdpi.com

Journal of Clinical Medicine Editorial Office
E-mail: jcm@mdpi.com
www.mdpi.com/journal/jcm

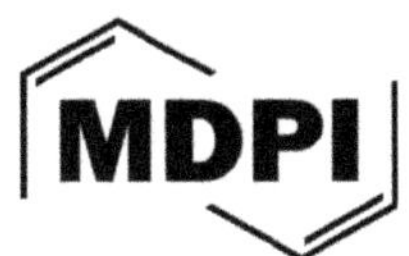